OXFORD MEDICAL PUBLICATIONS
Surgery for ischaemic heart disease

Surgery for ischaemic heart disease

Edited by

Ravi Pillai

Consultant Cardiothoracic Surgeon
John Radcliffe Hospital, Oxford

and

John E.C. Wright

Consultant Cardiothoracic Surgeon
The London Chest Hospital (Royal Hospital NHS Trust), London

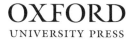

OXFORD
UNIVERSITY PRESS

OXFORD
UNIVERSITY PRESS

Great Clarendon Street, Oxford OX2 6DP

Oxford New York

Athens Auckland Bangkok Bogota Bombay Buenos Aires Calcutta
Cape Town Chennai Dar es Salaam Delhi Florence Hong Kong Istanbul
Karachi Kuala Lumpur Madrid Melbourne Mexico City Mumbai
Nairobi Paris São Paulo Singapore Taipei Tokyo Toronto Warsaw

and associated companies in Berlin Ibadan

Oxford is a trade mark of Oxford University Press

Published in the United States
by Oxford University Press, Inc., New York

A catalogue record for this book is available from the British Library

Library of Congress Cataloging in Publication Data
(Data applied for)

ISBN 0 19 262466 0 (Hbk)

Typeset by EXPO Holdings, Malaysia

Printed in Great Britain by
Bookcraft Ltd., Midsomer Norton, Avon

Preface

Ischaemic heart disease remains the most important cause of death in Britain and in most developed countries. Alongside preventive measures, the advent of coronary artery surgery has sought to improve the symptomatic status and long-term survival in patients suffering from coronary artery disease and those that suffer from myocardial infarction. The long-term results published following the Coronary Artery Surgery Study, the Veterans Administration Study, and the European Coronary Artery Study support the central position of surgery in the management of patients with triple-vessel disease, left main stem disease, and impaired ventricular function.

Attempts at surgical revascularization of the ischaemic myocardium extend back over 30 years. Early attempts included epicardial and pericardial abrasion, omental wrapping, and attempts by Vineberg to bury the internal mammary artery into a myocardial tunnel. The use of the long saphenous vein directly anastomosed to the coronary artery by Favoloro in 1967 heralded the present era of coronary artery surgery. The last 20 years have also seen improvement in cardiac surgical techniques in general and more specifically a greater understanding of cardiopulmonary bypass and cardiac anaesthesia. These developments have led to a less than 5% operative mortality in patients undergoing routine and elective surgery.

With the procedure established, attention more recently has been focused on long-term graft patency and the conduits used. Such evaluations have included not only clinical studies but also laboratory investigation of the endothelium and its role in graft occlusion. Global and regional myocardial ischaemia as well as injury caused by reperfusion have more recently been addressed at the molecular level.

Advances in anaesthetic techniques have altered the requirements of postoperative care. Since coronary artery surgery remains the 'bread and butter' of any adult cardiac surgical practice, the number of patients passing through a surgical service is significant. Current estimates of the actual demand for surgery in Britain vary between 450 and 600 cases per million of the population per year. These figures have important resource implications for the community and governments.

The developments in this field therefore are wide and varied. This book sets out to bring together more recent advances in surgical techniques, protection of the heart, and post-operative care and also introduces links with molecular biology.

The editors of this book are both involved in the teaching and training of junior cardiothoracic surgeons. At the same time we also have a large clinical practice with a major interest in operative surgery. We have felt for some time that there is a need for a book aimed at trainees both for the purpose of day-to-day reference and to assist with postgraduate examinations.

Single authors or even small groups cannot hope to cover all the aspects of such a book. We have therefore turned to our colleagues to prepare the sections on which they are recognized experts. We do not pretend to provide a comprehensive and exhaustive coverage of our subject. Rather we hope to give our readers a broad overview of coronary artery surgery as it is practised today. The contents may sometimes prove to be accepted general practice and sometimes may seem controversial. If the book helps trainees through their development stages and at the same time can stimulate diversity of thought, then we will have succeeded.

We give our sincere thanks to all our contributors who have so readily given of their time and expertise. Without them a book such as this could not be prepared.

Oxford   R.P.
London   J.E.C.W.
February 1999

Contents

Contributors

S.M. Allen Cardiothoracic Surgical Unit, Queen Elizabeth Hospital, Edgbaston, Birmingham B15 2TH, UK

Gianni D. Angelini Department of Cardiac Surgery, Bristol Royal Infirmary, Bristol BS2 8HW, UK

Adrian P. Banning Department of Cardiology, John Radcliffe Hospital, Headington, Oxford OX3 9DU, UK

Nicola Batrick South West Thames Regional Cardiothoracic Unit, St Georges Hospital, Tooting, London, UK

R.S. Bonser Cardiothoracic Surgical Unit, Queen Elizabeth Hospital, Edgbaston, Birmkngham B15 2TH, UK

Alan J. Bryan Department of Cardiac Surgery, Bristol Royal Infirmary, Bristol BS2 8HW, UK

F. Duncan The London Chest Hospital (Royal Hospital NHS Trust), Bonner Road, London E2 9JX, UK

John J. Dunning Department of Cardiothoracic Surgery, Papworth Hospital, Papworth Everard, Cambridge CB3 8RE, UK

R.O. Feneck The London Chest Hospital (Royal Hospital NHS Trust), Bonner Road, London E2 9JX, UK

Timothy J. Gardner Cardiac Surgery Unit, University of Pennsylvania Medical Center, Philadelphia, USA

Robert C. Gorman Cardiac Surgery Unit, University of Pennysylvania Medical Center, Philadelphia, USA

Catherine R. Grebenik Oxford Heart Centre, John Radcliffe Hospital, Headington, Oxford OX3 9DU, UK

Andrew Murday South West Thames Regional Cardiothoracic Unit, St Georges Hospital, Tooting, London, UK

John N. Newton Unit of Health-Care Epidemiology, Department of Public Health, University of Oxford

Oliver Ormerod Department of Cardiology, John Radcliffe Hospital, Headington, Oxford OX3 9DU, UK

John Pepper Cardiothoracic Surgery Unit, Royal Brompton Hospital, London SW3 6NP, UK

Ravi Pillai Oxford Heart Centre, The John Radcliffe Hospital, Headington, Oxford OX3 9DU, UK

Tom Treasure South West Thames Regional Cardiothoracic Unit, St George's Hospital, Tooting, London, UK

G.M.K. Tsang Queen Elizabeth Hospital, Birmingham

Steven S.L. Tsui Department of Cardiothoracic Surgery, John Radcliffe Hospital, Headington, Oxford OX3 9DU, UK and Papworth Hospital, Cambridge

J.E.C. Wright The London Chest Hospital (Royal Hospital NHS Trust), Bonner Road, London E2 9JX, UK

1 Investigating ischaemic heart disease

Oliver Ormerod

Cardiovascular disease is one of the major causes of death in western societies. In recent years there has been immense progress in diagnosis and pharmacological and surgical treatment of ischaemic heart disease. Vascular events are unpredictable and an acute coronary occlusion carries a high risk of mortality and possible subsequent morbidity for the individual, their family, and society should the patient survive. The proven benefit of therapeutic interventions in controlling symptoms and also improving prognosis in certain patient groups has encouraged physicians to seek out the symptoms of ischaemic heart disease and consider intervention earlier in the natural history of this disease.

Although the diagnosis of ischaemic heart disease may be secure on clinical grounds, the cardiologist has a large range of special investigations to help more accurately define the differential diagnosis, assess severity, prognosis and plan further treatment. Although there is some overlap between different investigations, they all have their particular advantages. The complete cardiologist needs to understand and be familiar with all these investigative techniques so that the investigation best able to answer the question posed is selected. Much of this chapter will address the merits and indications of special investigations in cardiology and in which instances they may be applied.

Principles of investigating ischaemic heart disease

All investigations can produce misleading results: false positives and negatives. The more invasive the technique the less prone it is to non-specific results, but this must be balanced against the greater likelihood of serious complications. The reliability of the results of an investigation depends upon the likelihood of the patient's having the disease being looked for, that is the prevalence of the disease in a population representative of the individual (1) (Bayes' theorem). For instance, if a non-smoking 25 year old female with atypical chest pain is subjected to an ECG stress test, any ECG changes that occur will increase the probability of the woman having coronary artery disease only marginally because the symptom is unlikely to be angina and the ECG changes are probably falsely positive. On the other hand, if the exercise ECG of a 60 year old male, who has smoked for 40 years and has typical angina, is positive, the ECG changes are highly likely to reflect myocardial ischaemia; a true positive. The presence of typical symptoms plus a positive stress test makes the probability of coronary artery disease very high. Estimating pre-test probability of the diagnosis is an important principle in investigation, and particularly so in ischaemic heart disease. It also emphasizes the central importance of thorough clinical assessment of the patient before investigations are planned.

The history in a patient with chronic stable ischaemic heart disease is nearly always typical. Patients complain of chest pain and often breathlessness. The pain may be anywhere between the costal margins and the lower jaw; in the back, neck, or arms. However, the pain is reliably related to physical or emotional stress. Patients with stable angina, particularly those with severe disease, may suffer from postural pain, for example decubitus pain on going to bed, but this is usually in the context of typical effort angina. A long history of pain poorly related to effort is unlikely to be due to myocardial ischaemia.

Patients may find it difficult to describe the quality of the pain and may prefer the term 'discomfort', but they usually recognize it as being a most unpleasant sensation which rapidly stops them from exercising. In more advanced disease, particularly with significant left ventricular damage, the symptoms move more towards those of heart failure.

Patients with a recent increase in the severity of a coronary artery stenosis may present with unpredictable pain, possibly at rest. Unstable angina reflects a sudden change in the nature of the culprit stenosis, often with plaque rupture with thrombus on the exposed atheromatous material which may wax and wane or fragment and embolize the distal vascular bed (2–3). In this case the character of the pain may be all-important in the diagnosis being considered. Indeed, the patient may put the pain down to 'indigestion' and unfortunately many do not consult their doctor until the thrombus becomes occlusive causing a myocardial infarction.

A full history of risk factors is essential to support the probability of the clinical diagnosis, although some patients may not display any conventional risk factors.

Although physical examination may be normal in patients with early ischaemic heart disease, there may be signs of cardiac damage or signs suggesting other pathologies that share the same symptoms as ischaemic heart disease. It should be remembered that angina is a symptom not a diagnosis and may be caused by, for example, aortic stenosis or hypertrophic cardiomyopathy. Physical examination may detect evidence of an incidental process causing a high cardiac output. A classic example is of a carcinoma of the caecum causing an iron-deficiency anaemia exposing mild coronary artery disease. Other examples include thyrotoxicosis and intercurrent infection.

After taking a careful history and having examined the patient, the cardiologist is likely to come to one of four possible conclusions:

- The symptom is not due to ischaemic heart disease.
- The symptom is due to ischaemic disease and either medical management or surgical assessment with coronary arteriography is clearly indicated in this individual.
- Ischaemic heart disease is possible but the diagnosis needs more support.
- The diagnosis is secure but it not yet clear whether the patient has a good prognosis and can be managed medically or whether the prognosis could be improved by revascularization.

The first two cases are straightforward. If the symptom is believed not to be due to ischaemic heart disease, the patient can be reassured that the symptom is unlikely to be a threat but other investigations may be necessary to establish the cause. However, it is important that the patient is not left feeling that their symptom will be ignored and that other investigations are instituted or the general practitioner is asked to make the necessary arrangements.

In the second case, the decision to recommend medical or surgical treatment may be influenced by a number of factors such as the patient's age and general health, but is mainly based on the degree of limitation that the patient is experiencing. Surgical revascularization is very successful at controlling angina, and symptomatic control is one of the main indications for coronary artery surgery. No further investigation other than coronary arteriography is strictly necessary, although many cardiologists like to have the support of a positive exercise test before embarking upon invasive investigation.

Clearly, further investigation is called for in the other two cases. Ultimately, coronary arteriography may be required to establish or exclude a diagnosis of ischaemic heart disease. This is sometimes justified and in most cardiac catheter laboratories a small proportion of cases are undertaken to make a definite diagnosis. However, in view of the cost of the procedure, the risk of vascular complications, and the radiation dose to the patient, invasive investigation should be kept in reserve until non-invasive methods have been tried.

Non-invasive investigations attempting to make a diagnosis of ischaemic heart disease centre around some form of stress test whilst the patient is observed for symptoms, haemodynamic changes, and workload achieved. A 12-lead-electrocardiogram (ECG) is also monitored to detect repolarization changes and rhythm disturbances. Sometimes a stress test will be supplemented by myocardial perfusion scintigraphy to improve the specificity of the result and to add additional information regarding the extent of reversible myocardial ischaemia. A more detailed discussion of stress testing will follow.

The final case hangs on the assessment of the patient's prognosis. It is perhaps not surprising that patients who have already suffered left ventricular damage and who have further territory at risk from disease in other vessel, or who have symptoms from proximal disease of the left main or anterior descending coronary arteries, have a poor prognosis (4). It has been demonstrated that the prognosis can be improved by coronary artery surgery (5). If the prognosis is a consideration in the patient's management, as it usually is, the cardiologist will want objective information regarding the state of left ventricular function and the extent of myocardium at risk. There are a number of methods of assessing left ventricular function, including echocardiography, radionuclide, and angiographic techniques, which will be compared later.

Establishing the amount of myocardium at risk is more difficult. The patient tends to be limited by the most severe coronary stenosis, which may mask less severe lesions elsewhere in the coronary tree that could be equally or more important to the prognosis should they rupture and occlude the coronary artery. A best attempt at this can be made using the workload achieved during an exercise test (6), reversible left ventricular dysfunction during exercise using either radionuclide or echocardiographic imaging, or coronary arteriography. The relative merits will be discussed in more detail later.

Special investigations

Chest radiograph

For many years the plain radiograph of the chest was one of the few investigations available to the clinician. Certainly the chest radiograph can detect dilatation of the heart as a whole and to some extent dilatation of individual chambers including the aorta as well as calcification of valves. However, this investigation is substantially less sensitive than echocardiography which has largely superseded it. Nevertheless, the chest radiograph remains the best method of documenting venous congestion and pulmonary interstitial oedema, a point which may be important in distinguishing between cardiac and pulmonary causes of breathlessness.

Of course the chest radiograph is of value in detecting other incidental pathologies. In particular, carcinoma of the bronchus and coronary artery disease share the same aetiological risk factor, cigarette smoking, and a carcinoma is detected from time to time. However, the frequency of such incidental findings is low and there is debate about whether it is justified to routinely include a chest radiograph in the work-up of patients with coronary artery disease (7).

The electrocardiogram

The standard 12-lead ECG seems very 'low tech' compared to other investigative techniques in cardiology, but it remains of use and because it is effectively harmless it is almost part of clinical examination. The problem with the ECG is that it is the most distant reflection of the state of the coronary arteries and the myocardium and is very sensitive to non-ischaemic pathologies and systemic influences such as hypertension, drugs such as digitalis, and changes in sympathetic tone, and so can pick up 'extraneous changes' along the way. Furthermore, the pattern of the normal ECG depends upon the physiognomy of the individual. For these reasons the ECG has a reputation for being difficult to interpret. Nevertheless, because of its ease of recording, harmlessness, repeatability, and economy, variations of the ECG are ubiquitous in cardiology. Recording the ECG is essential in establishing the patient's rhythm, and it is the first investigation to show abnormalities in acute ischaemia or infarction. It remains central to the assessment of the patient with acute chest pain. There may also be evidence of previous myocardial infarction, recent severe ischaemia, or hypertension which will reinforce a clinical impression of coronary artery disease.

The principles of stress testing

As the ECG is completely non-invasive it is used for the simplest form of stress testing and is recorded alongside many of the more sophisticated investigations. The stress ECG is a good template for the more general discussion of stress testing. The main problem with the ECG is that it is so sensitive to physiological changes with stress as well as those due to pathology. As a result there is a very high incidence of non-specific changes which may mimic changes due to myocardial ischaemia, resulting in false positives. Interpreting an exercise ECG in the light of the pre-test probability is particularly important (8). The incidence of false positive ECG changes is so high that this investigation is valueless as a screening tool and of limited value in diagnosis (8). Cardiologists often perform an exercise test in patients with undiagnosed chest pain, hoping that the patient will exercise to a high workload without ECG changes so that, at least, the patient can be reassured the prognosis is excellent (6). If an unequivocal diagnosis is really necessary, the ECG stress test is not reliable enough, so other techniques will be necessary.

Stress testing is much more effective as a means of assessing the impact of coronary artery disease in an individual in whom the diagnosis is secure.

The purpose of a stress test is to bring out deficiencies in cardiac function that may not be apparent at rest. The chief aim of a stress test is to quantify the extent of myocardial ischaemia and thus the risk to the patient from their coronary artery disease. In practice a patient's exercise capacity will reflect a number of factors including general ability to exercise, cardiovascular fitness, and myocardial reserve as well as myocardial ischaemia. In addition, as mentioned before, the patient is likely to be limited by ischaemia due to the most severe stenosis in the coronary tree, which may not be the most important prognostically. As a result, a stress test is better at identifying those at low risk than separating those with a poor prognosis.

Whether or not to exercise the patient on medical treatment remains debatable. Medical treatment, particularly β-adrenergic blocking drugs, will blunt the sympathetic response to exercise, so might reduce the diagnostic sensitivity of the test and possibly limit the patient's exercise capacity. On the other hand, medical treatment may reduce the tendency for patients to be limited by ischaemia of a small, and thus prognostically less important, volume of myocardium improving the specificity. If, as is usually the case, the stress test is being undertaken to contribute to assessing the prognostic significance of the disease, it seems logical to perform the stress test on medical treatment (9).

Most stress tests are performed with the patient exercising on a treadmill with gradually increasing gradient and belt speed. The Bruce protocol is almost standard for patients with angina although others exist and may be used in other circumstances.

Performing an exercise test

In recent years exercise testing has become largely standardized. The commonest means of stressing is on a moving belt treadmill which is controlled by a computer. Sometimes the patient may cope better on an upright bicycle and sometimes it may be necessary to stress the patient in the supine position if imaging is to take place during exercise. Upright exercise on a treadmill is considered to be the most physiological. The ECG trace is often signal-averaged to improve the quality of the recording. This helps to detect ST segment changes during exercise which might otherwise be concealed by movement artefact, but the signal averaging can be confusing if the rhythm changes. Some machines record a raw rhythm strip along the bottom of the 12-lead tracing to help get around this problem.

Although stress testing is safe in patients with stable angina, it can be hazardous in patients with very poor cardiac reserve or unstable angina particularly when not stabilized on medical treatment. It is good practice to take a brief history to establish the stability of the angina and to see if there are symptoms suggesting heart failure. The patient's current drug treatment should be noted. The blood pressure should be recorded at rest and a brief physical examination undertaken if there is a suspicion of significant heart failure or the possibility of an alternative diagnosis such as aortic stenosis. The ECG is recorded with the patient sitting and standing. At this point a final decision should be made as to whether to go ahead with the stress test. The test should be aborted if there is evidence of overt heart failure or aortic stenosis and performed with extreme caution, if at all, if the patients has severe or unstable symptoms.

The Bruce protocol is the most widely used treadmill stress test. This protocol consists of how many 3 minute stages although even very fit people rarely get beyond stage 5 and the point is usually made by the end of stage 4. The ECG is recorded every minute and the blood pressure every 3 minutes, usually towards the end of each stage. The clinical indication for the test may influence the individual end-point but in the majority of cases the purpose of the test is to deter-

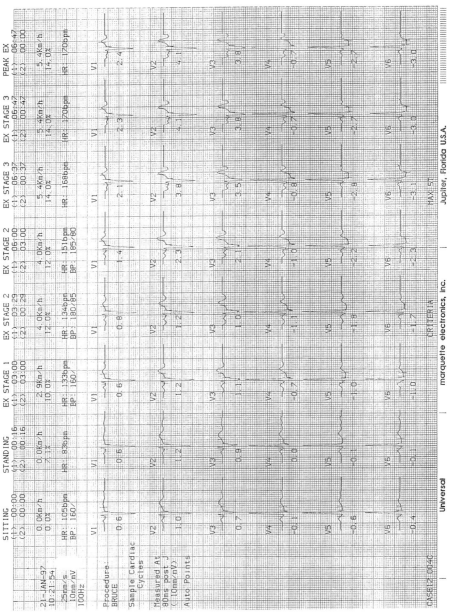

Fig. 1.1 A technically positive exercise electrocardiographic trace. Representative signal averaged QRS complexes from six ECG leads are displayed from the resting trace and at the end of each stage. Progressive inferolateral horizontal ST depression is demonstrated.

mine the patient's exercise capacity. The patient should be encouraged to exercise for as long as possible, provided no other definite reason to terminate the test intervenes. The test may need to be terminated either because of a rhythm disturbance, particularly sustained ventricular arrhythmias or evidence of haemodynamic decompensation, often detected as a fall in systolic blood pressure. Neither the onset of angina nor ST segment changes *pe se* are a sufficient indication to stop the patient if they feel they can carry on and are haemodynamically stable. There may be a reflex increase in vagal tone at peak exercise or immediately after exercise, causing a fall in blood pressure. This does not carry the prognostic significance of a fall in blood pressure early in the test but the patient may need to sit or lie down abruptly! The patient should be monitored clinically and with ECG recordings every minute at least until the values return to base line and ideally for 10 minutes. Severe arrhythmias are more likely to occur during recovery, up to 10 minutes after exercise, and definite ECG changes may appear in recovery rather than during exercise. In addition the length of time that ECG changes persist into recovery is important in deciding if they are truly positive. ST depression that disappears very quickly is often not due to myocardial ischaemia.

Reporting a stress test

The stress test provides the physician with the opportunity to observe the patient during a period of potential myocardial ischaemia. A careful record should be made of the amount of exercise achieved as well as the timing of the onset of symptoms and ECG changes. The patient's haemodynamic state during exercise should be noted. This includes their general state, whether breathless or distressed, as well as the blood pressure response. Finally, the ECG should be examined for ST segment changes.

A technically positive exercise test is one which elicits significant ECG changes (*Fig. 1.1*). Horizontal or downward sloping ST depression is more specific than upward sloping changes or J-point depression (10). The deeper the ST segment depression the more reliably positive the test becomes (11). A clinically positive test should also elicit the patient's symptoms. Significant ECG changes are regarded as horizontal or down-sloping ST segment depression of at least 1 mm, 80 ms after the J point (junction between the QRS complex and the ST segment). Of course, if the stress test is being performed on a patient in whom the diagnosis of angina seems likely, the important observation is not just that the test is positive but what is the patient's exercise capacity.

Follow-up studies of patients with angina have shown that there is a useful correlation between the stage of exercise achieved and the prognosis (12). The following is a useful rule of thumb. If the patient is limited by myocardial ischaemia, haemodynamic decompensation or arrhythmia in stage 1, they are highly likely to have severe coronary artery disease and should be considered for urgent invasive investigation. Those limited to stage 2 may have prognostically important disease and should be considered for investigation leading to revascularization even if their symptoms do not seem that limiting. Of course these patients will probably benefit from revascularization for symptoms as they are unlikely to be comfortable on medical treatment. Patients who can complete stage 4 of the Bruce protocol fall into a low risk group with an excellent prognosis and may well be suitable for medical management. Patients who stop in stage 3 or the early part of stage 4 fall into an intermediate risk group. Further investigation with radionuclide imaging may be helpful in deciding on the management of this group of patients.

Ambulatory ECG monitoring (Holter monitoring or 24 hour tape)

Ambulatory monitoring is another manifestation of the use of the ECG. The purpose of the 24 hour tape is to maximize the chances of detecting an unpredictable and intermittent problem. Of course the main indication is to detect rhythm abnormalities which may cause symptoms of their own. Occasionally a rhythm disturbance can cause unpredictable angina because of the high oxygen demand of a tachycardia.

Frequency modulated equipment can reliably record ST segment changes. Assuming that these ST segment changes correlate with myocardial ischaemia, which is subject to the same limitations as stress testing, ambulatory monitoring may provide information about the proportion of the time that the myocardium is ischaemic (ischaemic burden) which may be helpful, particularly in patients who either have symptomless ischaemia (silent ischaemia) or experience their ischaemia as symptoms other that chest pain, usually breathlessness (angina equivalent symptoms). Although a large ischaemic burden may correlate with more severe disease and thus a worse prognosis, ambulatory ST segment monitoring seems to have found itself a more useful role in research than in clinical practice.

Non-invasive cardiac imaging

Although non-invasive imaging techniques do not carry the diagnostic accuracy of arteriography, they are particularly helpful in directing the management of a patient who falls into a grey area regarding the indication for arteriography. They have a useful place in supporting a diagnosis of coronary artery disease, perhaps after an intermediate result from a treadmill stress test, providing information about left ventricular function which might well influence a decision about the use of arteriography or the functional significance of known coronary artery disease either in terms of the response of left ventricular function to stress (exercise radionuclide ventriculography) or the extent of myocardium that becomes ischaemic during stress (myocardial perfusion scintigraphy).

Echocardiography

Although echocardiography has been available for more than two decades and has revolutionized cardiac imaging in general, its place in the assessment of patients with coronary artery disease was severely restricted until the advent of two-dimensional technology; even now in routine practice its place is limited to assessing resting left ventricular function.

The great strength of echocardiography is its safety and convenience. Ultrasound is to all intents and purposes harmless, giving it a large safety advantage over techniques involving the use of ionizing radiation. In addition it is very quick and repeatable. An estimate of left ventricular function can be achieved in a matter of minutes. Beyond this, its place is limited to detecting incidental valvular lesions. With the addition of Doppler some functional data can be collected which may have relevance, for instance estimating pulmonary artery pressure. Multigated (colour flow) Doppler may detect the presence of ischaemic mitral reflux but can be rather over-sensitive to mild degrees of valvular regurgitation and is qualitative rather than reliably quantitative.

The disadvantages of echocardiography are that it is significantly operator dependent and lacks the reproducibility of other, particularly nuclear techniques. One reason for both of these is that the endocardium is more difficult to see on ultrasound than the epicardium. During systole, most of the reduction in the volume of the left ventricle is achieved by thickening of the myocardium rather than movement of the epicardium. If the true degree of thickening is underestimated then left ventricular impairment will be overestimated. Echocardiography, as a technique, tends to underestimate the ejection fraction.

M-mode echocardiography is still used to make measurements of left ventricular dimensions (as well as those of other cardiac structures). The endocardium is better appreciated by this form of recording but as left ventricular damage in coronary artery disease is typically regional and M-mode echocardiography measures left ventricular dimensions at essentially one place, just below the mitral valve, these measurements often do not truly reflect left ventricular function.

The myocardium is much better seen using transoesophageal echocardiography, but this approach lacks many of the advantages of transthoracic echocardiography as it is much more invasive and requires the patient to be sedated, prolonging the total procedure. Furthermore it is not usually possible to obtain standard views of the left ventricle to assess function with the current technology, although this may improve with the use of multiplane probes.

Over the years there has been a steady effort to bring echocardiography into the field of stress testing. The chief problem with echocardiography is getting adequate images during exercise. In many patients, it is necessary to image the patient rolled to their left; it is not easy to exercise in this position. In addition, dynamic exercise will make the patient breathless, severely interfering with the acoustic windows. One solution to this problem is to stress the patient pharmacologically using vasodilators such as adenosine or dipyridamole or a β-adrenergic agonist such as dobutamine which gets around many of the problems of dynamic exercise. The resting and stress images can be played side by side to detect reversible regional abnormalities (13). Improving technology may make this a more attractive option but, as a technique, it is likely to continue to suffer from the usual problems of echocardiography used to assess left ventricular function, those of inaccuracy and poor reproducibility.

Radionuclide imaging

For routine purposes there are two main forms of cardiac scintigraphy — radionuclide ventriculography and myocardial perfusion scintigraphy, and one minor form — ^{99m}Tc pyrophosphate myocardial scintigraphy. The latter is occasionally used to detect myocardial infarction if the ECG is unavailable (e.g. left bundle branch block) or the enzyme release has been missed as pyrophosphate imaging is most sensitive 72 hours after a myocardial infarction and remains positive for up to 10 days.

Radionuclide imaging techniques look directly at the consequences of coronary artery disease on either left ventricular function or myocardial perfusion. For this reason they are much more reliable than ECG stress testing. As the practical difficulties of imaging during stress are considerably less than with echocardiography, they are intrinsically better suited to stress testing. Of course they cannot be regarded as an alternative to coronary arteriography but they carry a smaller radiation dose, do not risk vascular injury, and do not require hospital admission.

Furthermore, as these techniques look at the functional consequences of coronary artery disease rather than just anatomy, they are a useful complement to angiography.

In the patient with ischaemic symptoms, radionuclide imaging has two main uses. The first could be considered, broadly speaking, as clarifying the results of an equivocal ECG stress test and the indications of coronary arteriography. The second is to clarify the indications for an intervention after coronary arteriography if doubt remains about the patient's management. These considerations will be followed up after a discussion of the individual techniques.

Radionuclide ventriculography

There are two techniques in radionuclide ventriculography, which are performed in different ways and may require different equipment although the results are similar. Both assess left ventricular function at rest and during stress, allowing any degree of resting left ventricular damage and the effect of inducible ischaemic left ventricular dysfunction to be quantified. As left ventricular function has a major impact on prognosis, both of these values may be central to deciding on management.

The more widely used technique is equilibrium radionuclide ventriculography, otherwise known as multiple gated cardiac scintigraphy (MUGA scan). As the gamma camera is unable to collect sufficient counts (scintillations) to image the heart beat by beat, a representative image is built up over several hundred cardiac cycles. The patient's blood (usually red blood cells) is labelled with ^{99m}technetium (Tc). After a few minutes the labelled blood reaches equilibrium within the circulation so that counts density is proportion to volume. The image is built up in the memory of a computer. The computer image is gated using the ECG. The computer measures the time between R waves of the ECG and divides the cardiac cycle into a number of frames, usually around 20 which is a similar frame rate to contrast ventriculography. With each cardiac cycle the computer collects the scintillations detected by the gamma camera within each frame until the next R wave when the process starts again. The process is repeated until a predetermined number of counts has been collected. The more counts that are collected the less noisy the image becomes. If only measures of global function are needed, such as an ejection fraction, then fewer counts are needed to obtain statistically reliable data than if more detailed analysis of wall movement is to be undertaken. The total number of counts is usually a compromise between maximum accuracy and collection time particularly during stress studies.

As the computer is collecting a representative cardiac cycle the heart rate must be reasonably constant. It may be impossible to collect an image if the patient is in atrial fibrillation and even if it is technically achievable, it is doubtful if the image is a true representation of left ventricular function. Atrial fibrillation is regarded as a contraindication to MUGA scanning. Isolated extrasystoles are catered for by allowing a window of about 10% either side of the regular R–R interval. If a particular beat falls outside this window it is rejected. The system can manage a few extrasystoles but if these are frequent enough to make the heart rate sufficiently variable, it may be impossible to acquire an image. ^{99m}Tc has a half life of 6 hours, so there is ample time to collect resting and exercise images with a single isotope dose to the patient.

As the whole blood pool is active, overlapping structures cannot be separated. Calculations of left ventricular function must be made from a 30° left anterior oblique (LAO) view. This separates the right and left ventricles. Some degree of cranial angulation is included to improve separation of the left atrium and ventricle. It is from the LAO projection that the left ventricular

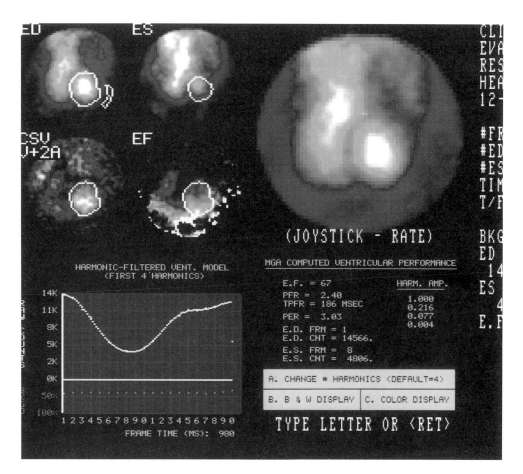

Fig. 1.2 An example of a LAO image from an equilibrium radionuclide ventriculogram is shown. On the top left are the end diastolic (ED) and the end systolic (ES) frames. Below this is the activity–time curve from which the ejection fraction (bottom right) is calculated. On the computer screen, the image on the top right is a moving closed loop cine of the heart contracting. See also colour plate section (Plate 1).

region of interest is drawn and the ejection fraction calculated. The ejection fraction is the proportion of the end diastolic volume that is ejected during systole (*Fig. 1.2*). As count rate is proportional to volume and the ejection fraction involves dividing one volume by another, it is not necessary to calculate actual volumes. The ejection fraction is calculated as the ratio of the stroke counts (end diastolic counts – end systolic counts) and the end diastolic counts, all with suitable correction for background activity outside the heart. A typical normal range for the ejection fraction is 0.50–0.70 (sometimes expressed as a percentage). Resting right anterior oblique and left lateral views are also usually collected to reveal the movement of the left ventricular anterior wall. As the right ventricle always overlaps the inferior wall it may not be possible to diagnose inferior wall movement abnormalities with any degree of certainty.

Stress images are collected during sub-maximal exercise in the left anterior oblique projection. As imaging takes 2–4 minutes, during which time exercise must continue at a steady heart rate, it is not possible to stress the patient maximally.

The ejection fraction is the simplest calculation of ventricular function. Wall movement can also be analysed, either from a closed-loop cine of the frames of the image (usually mathematically smoothed) or from static images in which some attribute of regional movement has been coded, usually in colour. Various attributes are available but perhaps the most popular is single harmonic Fourier analysis or phase analysis (14). In phase analysis it is assumed that the activity curve recorded in each pixel of the image can be represented by a cosine value. The computer calculates both the phase angle and the amplitude of each cosine and displays each value as a colour coded image. The phase image represents the timing of movement, with the atria having a different phase angle and thus colour from the ventricles and the amplitude image the degree of movement in that region. Damaged myocardium will have an abnormal phase angle with a different colour on the phase image and a reduced amplitude on the amplitude image.

Closed-loop cines and phase analysis images are calculated for all resting images and left anterior oblique stress image. The study report includes analysis of ejection fraction and regional wall movement. If the study included exercise the workload achieved, symptoms experienced, haemodynamic changes and ECG changes are reported.

The alternative method of radionuclide ventriculography is the first pass technique. In this technique a bolus of isotope is injected into a peripheral vein and imaging takes place as the bolus passes through the right heart, pulmonary circulation and left heart. As the bolus is within the right and left heart cavities at different times, overlap of structures is not a problem and imaging can take place in the anteroposterior plane. Of course repeat studies, for instance during stress, need a further dose of isotope and the subsequent data needs to be corrected for background activity from previous injections.

The advantage of first pass imaging is that the data reflects cardiac function over a much shorter time frame than the equilibrium technique which smoothes complex changes in ejection fraction taking place during stress. On the other hand, single crystal gamma cameras, i.e. the vast majority of cameras in clinical use, have a count rate capability that restricts them to calculations of the ejection fraction only during first pass studies.

Myocardial perfusion scintigraphy

Myocardial perfusion scintigraphy relies on the principle that the isotope or radiopharmaceutical is extracted by the myocardium in proportion to blood flow. Ischaemic myocardium will extract less isotope than normally perfused myocardium, and severely ischaemic or infarcted myocardium will extract negligible amounts. As the difference in blood flow between normal and abnormal coronary arteries is maximal during stress, evidence of ischaemia is detected by administering the isotope at peak exercise during a stress test, usually on a treadmill. Stress images are compared with images obtained at restwhen the difference in blood flow between normal and stenosed coronary arteries will be minimal. At rest, reversibly ischaemic myocardium will be 'filled in' distinguishing it from infarcted myocardium which will remain photon deficient. Exactly how the resting images are obtained depends upon the isotope or radiopharmaceutical used.

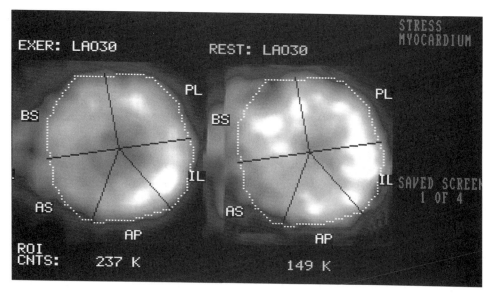

Fig. 1.3 The figure shows an example of a thallium scan. There is a reversible defect of the distal septum due to disease of the left anterior descending coronary artery. See also colour plate section (Plate 2).

Thallium myocardial perfusion scintigraphy

Thallium (^{201}Tl) behaves as an intracellular cation like potassium. Thallium has a high first pass extraction into the myocardium from the blood (around 80%) but does not remain fixed in the myocytes and will redistribute itself to all viable myocardium in time. Advantage is taken of this in thallium scanning with the stress images, identifying ischaemic myocardium, collected immediately after administering the isotope at peak effort on a stress test. After 4 hours the isotope has redistributed to previously ischaemic myocardium, distinguishing ischaemic from infarcted tissue. The long half-life of thallium (72 hours) means that very late images (as late as 24 hours) can be used to identify viable, although non-contractile, myocardium that is ischaemic at rest; so-called hibernating myocardium. The importance of hibernating myocardium will be discussed in detail under a separate heading. Thallium is also extracted by congested lung tissue. A high lung uptake may indicate pulmonary congestion during stress implying particularly severe stress-induced left ventricular dysfunction, which may have prognostic significance (15).

Stress and redistribution images are collected in three or four planes (e.g. 30° LAO, 60° LAO, left lateral and RAO) in order to interrogate different myocardial segments. Once stress and redistribution images have been collected the images are analysed. The stress and redistribution images can be compared side by side, both as raw data and smoothed images (*Fig. 1.3*). The relative counts density per segment is usually calculated and compared to normal values to make interpretation more objective.

The heart can also be imaged by tomography with a rotating head gamma camera. In recent years the value of tomography has been increasingly recognized (16) and many units have the necessary equipment and routinely use this approach to imaging.

Although thallium scanning remains a widely used isotope for myocardial perfusion imaging, it has a number of drawbacks. The energy level of the emitted gamma ray is lower than ^{99m}Tc and not well suited for gamma cameras. Furthermore, the long half-life and very long biological half-life (time that it remains in the body) means that it has far from ideal dosimetry characteristics, resulting in a substantial radiation dose to the patient approaching that of angiography. Recently, alternative radiopharmaceuticals that use ^{99m}Tc, a much cheaper isotope that is usually available from an inhouse generator, with better dosimetry and energy level, have become available. These radiopharmaceuticals have significantly different characteristics from ^{201}Tl. They have a lower first pass extraction with more visceral uptake and to all intents and purposes do not redistribute: they remain fixed within the myocyte. As a result a second injection is necessary for resting or stress images, depending upon which is done first, and it remains to be seen if they are suitable agents for the detection of hibernating myocardium. Nevertheless, the lower radiation dose to the patient is advantageous. Extraction by tissues other than the heart, particularly the liver, may cause problems in some patients due to overlap with the heart.

The practical value of nuclear imaging

Despite the theoretical advantages of direct imaging of the heart over ECG based techniques, all forms of non-invasive imaging are capable of producing unexpected results. This is particularly likely to occur if an inappropriate investigation is requested, although some may be frank false positives or negatives. Clearly it is important to request the right test.

Although there must be a sufficiently large volume of myocardium subject to reduce blood flow to be detected by perfusion scintigraphy, because this technique directly detects reduced flow it is most suitable for diagnosing the presence of flow-limiting coronary artery disease. Ventriculography demonstrates the consequences of ischaemia on myocardial function. As this is one step removed from ischaemia, these techniques are likely to be less sensitive as a diagnostic test than perfusion scintigraphy and are better suited to detecting the functional consequences of stress-induced ischaemia on left ventricular function and as such may be more valuable in assessing the prognostic significance of the disease in the individual patient. Of course, perfusion scintigraphy may show markers of prognostic significance; the size of the defect, multiple defects and lung uptake are valuable observations (15). Nevertheless, these markers are difficult to quantify and are less reliable than a significant fall in ejection fraction demonstrated by ventriculography. Furthermore, perfusion scintigraphy measures relative rather than absolute blood flow. Interpretation is based on regional differences in isotope uptake. Should the entire myocardium become ischaemic, because of either diffuse multivessel disease or severe proximal disease involving the left main or proximal left anterior descending coronary artery, the perfusion image may lack regional differences and appear normal. This possibility should be born in mind if the interpretation of the image appears out of step with the history, likelihood of the disease, and the results of the exercise ECG.

As a rule, perfusion scintigraphy is better at diagnosis and ventriculography is better at assessing prognosis.

Stunned and hibernating myocardium

In recent years there has been increasing interest in the realization that not all akinetic myocardium is irreversibly damaged. Viable myocardium may become non-contractile either because of an acute but transient loss of perfusion, so-called 'stunned' myocardium, which is temporarily rendered akinetic but whch may be expected to recover provided it remains perfused (17) or 'hibernating' myocardium which is very poorly perfused but sufficiently to remain viable although insufficiently nourished to contract actively (18). It is particularly important to recognize patients with significant volumes of hibernating myocardium who may be at lower risk from revascularization than patients with the same ejection fraction but completely infarcted myocardium and gain more benefit from surgery with recovery of a proportion of resting left ventricular function (19), improvement in symptoms of heart failure as well as from ischaemia, and improve prognosis (20).

Electrocardiography and echocardiography may leave clues of hibernating myocardium with persistent R waves and normal myocardial appearances but radionuclides have the potential to make this diagnosis more reliably. Thallium is extracted by viable but not necessarily contractile myocardium, and not by fibrous tissue. Because hibernating myocardium has by definition, poor perfusion, it takes much longer than usual for thallium to redistribute to hibernating myocardium. As a result images are repeated 24 hours after injection to try and demonstrate viable, hibernating myocardium.

Stunned and hibernating myocardium is the subject of investigation at present so it is likely that definition of viability will become easier and more reliable in future.

Coronary angiography

The non-invasive methods discussed so far detect the functional consequences of ischaemia in terms of myocardial perfusion and left ventricular function. In many patients it may become necessary to define the coronary anatomy either to come to a definite diagnosis or because an intervention is required. At present only coronary angiography is able to demonstrate the anatomy of the entire course of the epicardial coronary arteries.

Coronary angiography is routinely performed from the femoral artery under mild sedation and local anaesthesia. The brachial approach may be used and becomes necessary in patients with severely tortuous iliac vessels or with peripheral vascular disease. In patients who are taking oral anticoagulant drugs the brachial approach has the advantage that the anticoagulant treatment need not be interrupted as the brachial artery is dissected out and is closed by direct suture, minimizing the risk of bleeding. On the other hand, the femoral artery is punctured percutaneously with a fine gauge needle and the vessel cannulated over a guide wire. Haemostasis is achieved by compression.

Coronary angiography is usually accompanied by assessment of left ventricular function with contrast injections in one or two views. Mitral regurgitation, if present, will also be demonstrated. Selective injection of each coronary artery is performed in multiple views to demonstrate each coronary segment in more than one plane.

Coronary angiography is the most reliable method of making a definite diagnosis and is essential before coronary artery surgery or percutaneous transluminal coronary angioplasty (PTCA). It is an invasive investigation and subjects the patient to a substantial radiation dose. Thus, it carries a much higher risk of harming the patient than non-invasive investigations. Coronary angiography should only be performed if the benefit outweighs the potential risk.

The most common complications of cardiac catheterization are related to the arterial entry site. Bleeding and the formation of a small haematoma at the femoral puncture site are quite frequent. Fortunately major haemorrhage and massive haematoma are rare but can cause serious morbidity risking ileofemoral deep venous thrombosis, necrosis of the overlying skin, and serious blood loss if bleeding occurs in the retroperitoneal space. False aneurysms may develop with a small blood-filled space outside the artery in direct connection with the circulation. The incidence is approximately 0.5%. Although some resolve spontaneously there is concern that the aneurysm may expand or rupture. Previously treatment involved closing the arterial puncture site by suture after surgical exposure of the artery. Recently ultrasound with colour-flow Doppler, which had been used only to diagnose false aneurysms, has been increasingly used to treat the aneurysm. The ultrasound probe is positioned over the aneurysm and used to compress the cavity with the colour-flow demonstrating when flow into the cavity ceases. Compression is maintained for repeated 5 minute periods until the cavity is obliterated and flow no longer returns.

Other local complications include dissection of the ileofemoral vessels or brachial artery and occlusive haematoma formation.

Complications involving damage to structures distant from the arterial entry site are usually due to direct damage to the endothelium or embolization of atheroma, blood clot, or air. The most feared complications are cerebrovascular accidents, usually due to embolization, and coronary artery occlusion due to disruption of a coronary arterial atheromatous plaque with dissection of the coronary artery. Inevitably these dissections involve the origin of the right or left coronary arteries. Dissection of the right coronary artery can be managed in the cardiac catheterization laboratory by PTCA and coronary artery stenting, but occlusion of the left coronary artery is usually rapidly followed by cardiac arrest and death unless the patient can be massaged until on cardiopulmonary bypass and the coronary arteries grafted in a very few minutes.

Predictably the risk of complications is higher in the more severely ill patients, so that with good technique, in a modern cathetherization laboratory, the risk of major complication in an elective routine case should be very small (less than 0.2%) (21). As a result, routine coronary angiography is increasingly regarded as suitable to be performed as a day case.

After completion of the procedure the angiogram is studied systematically and reported. A good quality angiogram will reveal evidence of previous left ventricular damage and the extent of coronary artery disease so that decisions can be made about the further management of the patient.

Other modalities

Cross-sectional imaging using CT or MRI can be used to image the cardiovascular system. At present they are poorly suited to assessing patients with coronary artery disease but are useful to study the pericardium and aorta, the latter in patients with aortic dissection or other aneurysms.

The investigation of clinical syndromes

The patient with non-specific chest pain

Chest pain is a common symptom. Although many forms of chest pain may have a benign cause, it is understandable that a diagnosis should be sought expeditiously. The diagnosis of typical effort or classical angina may be made easily but not all angina is typical and it may be difficult to exclude the diagnosis with confidence on clinical grounds. As there is no non-invasive diagnostic investigation, the case for and against the diagnosis must be built up carefully starting with a thorough clinical assessment. A patient history of the presenting complaint together with documentation of risk factors will go a long way to making the case. Physical examination and the resting ECG may well be normal in the early stages of ischaemic heart disease but may offer useful clues if there is evidence of previous left ventricular damage.

In most patients with angina the history is typical but inevitably there will be cases in which there remains uncertainly about the diagnosis. These patients will need further investigation. The logical first step is an ECG exercise test. In many cases this investigation will come down firmly for or against a diagnosis of ischaemic heart disease. Those patients with an equivocal or negative test at a low workload may justify further investigation using a myocardial scintigram and even angiography depending upon the overall clinical picture and, from time to time, the social circumstances of the patient. Little doubt is acceptable in the cases of individuals who carry a heavy responsibility for the well-being of others, for instance HGV and PSV drivers and airline pilots. A false positive result may have unfortunate consequences for the patient and if suspected should be followed up with a myocardial perfusion scintigram or angiography.

Typical angina pectoris

Usually the investigation of patients with stable angina is quite straight forward. Patients with classical effort angina should be assessed thoroughly by clinical examination including documentation of risk factors and their modification. A 12-lead ECG should be recorded, as evidence of previous infarction may strengthen the case for invasive investigation. In patients with limiting symptoms despite adequate medical treatment an exercise test may not be strictly necessary before proceeding to angiography but the information gained from this investigation may help decision-making after the angiogram.

In the case of patients with well controlled symptoms, continuing medical therapy may well be appropriate if they are unlikely to have prognostically important disease. It is in this group of patients that an exercise test may be particularly helpful as those capable of an high workload can be confidently expected to have a good prognosis, whereas those limited at a low workload may have a relatively symptomless ischaemic burden and may justify catheterization for the further assessment of prognosis. As discussed before, patients exercising for more than 6 but less than 9 minutes (stage 3 of the Bruce protocol) are in an intermediate risk group. Radionuclide imaging to assess the functional consequences of ischaemia may be helpful. If the left ventricular ejection fraction responds normally to stress then conservative management may be appropriate but a significant fall in ejection fraction would imply extensive left ventricular ischaemia suggesting that angiography should be recommended.

In patients in whom angiography is justified because of severe symptoms or non-invasive evidence that they are at high risk, this investigation will complete the data on which risk factor stratification and thus management can be decided.

Acute ischaemic syndromes

Patients with a recent, sudden change in their symptoms, presumably due to a change in the anatomy of their coronary artery disease, can be considered as a group as they are at an higher risk of acute myocardial infarction. This group includes patients with recent onset of angina, frankly unstable angina and those with subendocardial infarction and early post-infarction angina. Owing to the unstable nature of their disease, there will be a low threshold for invasive investigation and a high proportion will come to early catheterization. Nevertheless, some individuals will settle on medical therapy and may be managed conservatively if an exercise test is reassuring.

In recent years, there has been increasingly active management of patients with acute myocardial infarction. Such advances have considerably improved the care of these patients, but their management is beyond the scope of this chapter.

Patients with ischaemic left ventricular dysfunction

Since the Coronary Artery Surgery Study (5) and its European equivalent (European Coronary Surgery Study (22)), it has been accepted that patients with impaired left ventricular function and multivessel coronary artery disease benefit prognostically from coronary artery surgery. However, there must be a degree of left ventricular impairment beyond which the risk of surgery, together with the continuing effect of persisting left ventricular damage on prognosis, make surgery ineffective at improving the patient's outlook. In general terms an ejection fraction of 0.20 is considered to be this point. However, in most cases infarcted myocardium contains some viable myocardium mixed in with fibrous tissue. Typically, resting left ventricular function is unchanged by surgery but the revascularized, partially infarcted segment may, under sympathetic stimulation, contribute to an increase in exercise ejection fraction. However, in some individuals the mass of non-contractile but viable myocardium is sufficient that revascularization may result in an improvement in resting ventricular function, strengthening the case of prognostic surgery in these patients with severe myocardial damage (20).

In some individuals ischaemia may render the subtended myocardium akinetic but with the potential to recover a significant proportion of its contractile function. Two expressions of the phenomenon are described in the literature: 'stunning' and 'hibernation'. These differ largely in their chronicity. Stunning is the version when a region of myocardium suffers a sufficiently severe ischaemic insult, short of complete infarction, to prevent it from recovering contractile function for days or weeks. Hibernation is more chronic. Interruption of anterograde flow renders the subtended myocardium akinetic but with sufficient blood flow remaining, perhaps via collaterals, to prevent complete infarction. Recovery of contractile function will depend upon restoration of a more normal degree of coronary blood flow to the hibernating segment.

In the clinical setting, stunning is likely to be encountered in the context of an acute ischaemic event, particularly subendocardial infarction. Recovery should be assured unless there remains the substrate for further ischaemic insults in which case angiography and intervention are likely to be indicated by continuing symptoms or evidence of inducible ischaemia.

Identifying hibernating myocardium is more challenging. The patient is likely to have a long history of ischaemic heart disease with one or more episodes of myocardial infarction. The patient may present with symptoms of a mixture of heart failure and limiting angina. Physical examination may reveal signs of heart failure, a dilated heart with pulmonary congestion on the chest radiograph and a dilated left ventricle with poor contractile function on echocardiography. Although, if hibernating myocardium is present, left ventricular wall thinning and echocardiographic myocardial character may appear less abnormal than expected, this is difficult to quantify and is unreliable. Similarly there will be evidence of previous myocardial infarcted on the electrocardiogram, but R wave height may be surprisingly well preserved. Of course a region of hibernation may occur in the context of relatively well preserved left ventricular function, but its identification only really becomes a clinical issue in the presence of severe left ventricular impairment.

Assuming that the patient is optimally treated medically (if not, suitable treatment should be instituted) a poor prognosis is predictable. Surgery should be considered if this is likely to improve the prognosis. The first aim is to confirm the degree of left ventricular impairment. A radionuclide ventriculogram is the most appropriate investigation as it is more reliable and reproducible than others. An exercise study is worth including as evidence of further deterioration with stress will reinforce the indication for intervention. If the ejection fraction proves to be greater than 0.20 then the benefits of surgery are likely to be outweighed by the risks assuming that the results of subsequent angiography indicate that the patient's vessels are favourable for grafting. If the ejection fraction is less than 0.20 then the presence of significant volumes of hibernation myocardium becomes important.

There are no standardized or recommended methods of demonstrating the presence of hibernating myocardium but various approaches are under evaluation. Of course a prerequisite is that the myocardium has been shown to be akinetic and/or does not show systolic thickening. Beyond that it is necessary to demonstrate evidence of viability. There are currently three main approaches to this problem.

Demonstrating some contractile reserve under sympathetic stimulation

This is usually attempted by stress echocardiography using a β-adrenergic agonist such as dobutamine. Certainly improved wall thickening would suggest viability with contractile potential, but could be argued that this form of stress could increase the degree of ischaemia concealing contractile potential.

Demonstrating collateral flow to the akinetic segment

Epicardial collateralization of the occluded coronary vessel may be visible on angiography but its absence does not exclude collateralization and its presence does not confirm collateral flow to the myocardial capillaries. Myocardial collateralization is a prerequisite for viability. A promising research technique is myocardial contract echocardiography (23). Special 'sonicated' contrast fluid is injected into the contralateral coronary artery during coronary arteriography. If the region that may be hibernating 'lights up' with contrast, then the presence of capillary myocardial col-lateralization is confirmed.

Demonstrating metabolically viable myocardium

Assuming that this is technically possible, this approach appears to be the most logical and is attempted using radionuclide tracers. Radionuclide labelled metabolic substrates, such as glucose, are effective but in practice ^{201}Tl is the most widely used as the others need a reasonably local cyclotron.

As discussed above, thallium may redistribute to hibernating myocardium slowly, so late imaging, 24 hours after the initial injection perhaps with re-injection, is necessary (24). In some cases the volume of myocardium taking up thallium during the early imaging period may be con-siderably better than expected compared to measures of contractile function.

The decision to offer surgical treatment to patients with several left ventricular impairment will depend upon a number of variables including the results of angiography and the technical suitability of the coronary vessels for grafting. Nevertheless, the confident demonstration of hibernating myocardium should predict a better long-term result in this group of patients.

Cardiac assessment of patients undergoing non-cardiac surgery

In an ageing population it is likely that a substantial proportion of patients being assessed for non-cardiac surgery will have incidental heart disease. The presence of severe cardiac disease such as heart failure due to valvular disease, recent myocardial infarction, or unstable angina will increase the risk of surgery (25) but with modern anaesthesia and monitoring techniques the additional risk associated with stable coronary artery disease is quite small (26). Clearly the surgeon and particularly the anaesthetist need to be aware of the possibility of inducible cardiac ischaemia, but in the majority of cases and for most surgical procedures a careful history and physical examination complemented by simple investigations such as an ECG and chest radi-ograph are all that are necessary.

However, there are groups of patients in whom simple clinical assessment may not be enough to identify those who may be at significantly increased risk because of incidental ischaemic heart disease. The largest group of patients in this category is those with aneurysmal or occlusive disease of the abdominal aorta. It is increasingly accepted that some more reliable form of screen-ing of these patients for ischaemic heart disease is desirable. Additional investigations are justified for three reasons. Both ischaemic heart and abdominal aortic disease share the same pathophysiology; atheroma. The incidence of ischaemic heart disease is likely to be very high in patients with peripheral vascular disease. Because these patients are often immobile or are limited by claudication, they may not exercise enough to be aware of angina so may not give a history of effort chest pain. The final reason is the severe cardiovascular stress that occurs during clamping of the aorta which risks acute left ventricular failure or an acute coronary event.

At present there is no consensus over which screening investigation is most appropriate. In the past some units have catheterized all patients and grafted those with severe coronary artery disease (27,28). However, this approach is very expensive and the risks may not be justified if a suitable non-invasive alternative is available.

There is no doubt that inducible cardiac ischaemia does increase the morbidity and possibly mortality of peripheral vascular surgery (29,30). Many of these patients will be unable to complete a satisfactory exercise test because of claudication, so exercise ECG testing is unlikely to be helpful. Thallium scintigraphy using pharmacological stress has been recommended by some authors (31,32).

However, the chief determinant of mortality is the presence of impaired left ventricular function (26). Stress radionuclide ventriculography using dynamic exercise or pharmacological stress using dobutamine is perhaps the most logical technique in this group of patient as it reliably measures left ventricular function and can detect reversible ischaemia. In particular, severe reversible ischaemia will be detected as a fall in ejection fraction with stress. Those patients whose ischaemic heart disease may be treated to reduce the risk of abdominal aortic surgery can be catheterized and the coronary arteries grafted if necessary. The severity of resting left ventricular impairment can be used to plan the aortic surgery. Patients with moderate left ventricular impairment may well be operated on with a minimal excess risk but may well justify more intensive peri- and postoperative monitoring (33). Those with severe left ventricular impairment may well be best managed conservatively as the risk of abdominal aortic surgery will be high and the prognosis from the heart disease may be less favourable than that of the aortic disease (34).

Conclusions

Clinical methods remain the mainstay of the diagnosis of ischaemic heart disease. Non-invasive investigations may help secure the diagnosis but are most valuable in assessing the severity of disease in patients in whom the diagnosis is considered probable so that patients with prognostically important disease can be selected for invasive investigation and possibly revascularization.

References

1. Goldman L. Quantitative aspects of clinical reasoning. In: Wilson JD *et al. Harrison's Principles of Internal Medicine*, 12th edn. New York, McGraw-Hill, 1991, pp. 5–11.
2. Davies MJ, Thomas AC. Plaque fissuring — the cause of acute myocardial infarction, sudden ischaemic death and crescendo angina. *Br Heart J* 1985;**53**:363.
3. Davies MJ, Thomas AC, Knapman PA, Hangartner JR. Intramyocardial platelet anggregation in patients with unstable angina suffering sudden ischemic cardiac death. *Circulation* 1986;**73**:418.
4. Mock MB, Ringqvist I, Fisher LD *et al.* Survival of medically treated patients in the Coronary Artery Surgery Study (CASS) Registry. *Circulation* 1982;**66**:562.
5. Alderman EL, Bourassa MG, Cohen LS *et al.* Ten-year follow-up of survival and myocardial infarction in the randomized coronary artery surgery study. *Circulation* 1990;**82**:1629.
6. Dagenais GR, Rouleau JR, Christen A, Fabia J. Survival of patients with a strongly positive exercise electrocardiogram. *Circulation* 1982;**65**:452.
7. Stables RH, Trotman-Dickenson B. Prospective assessment of the value of a chest radiograph in the performance of diagnostic cardiac catheterisation in adults. *Br Heart J* 1994;**72**:540.

8. Goldman I, Cook EF, Mitchell N *et al*. Incremental value of exercise test for diagnosing the presence or absence of coronary artery disease. *Circulation* 1982;**66**:945.

9. Lim R, Kreidieh I, Dyke L, Thomas J, Dymond DS. Exercise testing without interruption of medication for refining the selection of mildly symptomatic patients for prognostic coronary angiography. *Br Heart J* 1994;**71**:334.

10. Goldschlager N, Selzer A, Cohen K. Treadmill stress tests as an indication of presence and severity of coronary artery disease. *Ann Int Med* 1976;**85**:282.

11. Weiner DA, McCabe C, Hueter DC *et al*. The predictive value of anginal chest pain as an indicator of coronary disease during exercise testing. *Am J Cardiol* 1978;**96**:458.

12. Bogaty P, Dagenais GR, Cantin B *et al*. Prognosis in patients with a strongly positive exercise electrocardiogram. *Am J Cardiol* 1978;**64**:1284.

13. Wilkenshoff U. Stress echocardiography. In: Schmailzl KJG, Ormerod O, eds. *Ultrasound in cardiology* Oxford, Blackwells Science, 1994, pp. 185–213.

14. Adam WE, Tarkowska A, Bitter F, Stauch M, Geffer H. Equilibrium (gated) radionuclide ventriculography. *Cardiovasc Radiol.* 1979;**2**:161.

15. Gill JB, Ruddy TD, Newell JG *et al*. Prognostic importance of thallium uptake by the lungs during exercise in coronary artery disease. *N Engl J Med* 1987;**317**:1485.

16. Kiat H, Berman DS, Maddahi J. Comparison of planar and tomographic exercise thallium — 201 imaging methods for the evaluation of coronary artery disease. *J Am Coll Cardiol* 1989;**13**:613.

17. Braunwald E, Kloner RA. The stunned myocardium: prolonged, post-ischaemic ventricular dysfunction. *Circulation* 1982;**66**:1146.

18. Rahimtoola SH. A perspective on three large multicentre clinical trials of coronary artery bypass surgery for chronic stable angina. *Circulation* 1985;**72**(suppl V):123.

19. Rahimtoola SH. Coronary artery bypass surgery for chronic stable angina — 1981. A perspective. *Circulation* 1982;**65**:225–31.

20. Eitzman D, Al-Aouar Z, Kanter HL *et al*. Clinical outcome of patients with advanced coronary artery disease after viability studies with positron emission tomography. *J Am Coll Cardiol* 1992;**20**:559.

21. Grossman W. In: Braunwald E, ed. *Heart disease. A textbook of cardiovascular medicine*, 4th edn Philadelphia. WB Saunders, 1992.

22. European Coronary Surgery Study Group. Long-term results of prospective randomized study of coronary artery bypass surgery in stable angina pectoris. *Lancet* 1982;**2**:1173.

23. Sabia PJ, Powers ER, Ragosta M, Sarembock IJ, Burwell LR, Kaul S. An association between collateral blood flow and myocardial viability in patients with recent myocardial infarction. *N Engl J Med* 1992;**327**:1825–31.

24. Mori T, Minamiji K, Kurogane H, Ogawa K, Yoshida Y. Rest injected thallium-201 imaging for assessing viability of severe asynergic regions. *J Nucl Med* 1991;**32**:1718.

25. Goldman L, Caldera DL, Nussbaum SR *et al*. Multifactorial index of cardiac risk in non-cardiac surgical procedures. *N Engl J Med* 1977;**297**:845.

26. Dirksen A, Kjoller E. Cardiac predictors of death after non-cardiac surgery evaluated by intention to treat. *British Medical Journal* 1988;**297**:1011.

27. Hertzer NR, Young JR, Kramer JR *et al*. Routine coronary angiography prior to elective aortic reconstruction. Results of selective myocardial revascularisation in patients with peripheral vascular disease. *Arch Surg* 1979;**114**:1336.

28. Hertzer NR, Beven EG, Young JR *et al.* Coronary artery disease in peripheral vascular patients. A classification of 1000 angiograms and results of surgical mamagement. *Ann Surg* 1984;**199**:223.

29. Leppo J, Plaja J, Gionet M, Tumolo J, Paraskos JA, Cutler BS. Noninvasive evaluation of cardiac risk before elective surgery. *J Am Coll Cardiol* 1987;**9**:269.

30. Raby KE, Goldman L, Creager MA *et al.* Correlation between preoperative ischemia and major events after peripheral vascular surgery. *N Engl J Med* 1989;**321**:1296.

31. Boucher CA, Brewster DC, Darling RC, Okada RD, Strauss HW, Pohost GM. Determination of cardiac risk by dipyridamole-thallium imaging before peripheral vascular surgery. *N Engl J Med* 1985;**312**:389.

32. Eagle KA, Coley CM, Newell JB *et al.* Combining clinical and thallium data optimizes pre-operative assessment of cardiac risk before major vascular surgery.

33. Wells PH, Kaplan JA. Optimal management of patients with ischemic heart disease for non-cardiac surgery by complementary anesthesiologist and cardiologist interaction. *Am Heart J* 1981;**102**:1029.

34. Jamieson WRE, Janusz MT, Miyagishima RT, Gerein AN. Influence of ischemic heart disease on early and late mortality after surgery for peripheral occlusive vascular disease. *Circulation* 1982;**66** suppl 1:1–92.

2 Percutaneous intervention in ischaemic heart disease

Adrian P. Banning

Historical perspective

Charles Dotter and Melvin Judkins were the first physicians to attempt to use catheters for a therapeutic purpose when they used a coaxial system of catheters in patients with peripheral arterial disease in 1964 (1). The term 'transluminal angioplasty' was coined but, despite initially encouraging results, application of the technique was limited by problems with puncture site haematoma and distal emboli. Andreas Gruentzig, trained by Zeitler in Germany, continued to refine the angioplasty technique in peripheral arteries and in 1974 he developed a double lumen catheter with a distensible PVC balloon which revolutionized angioplasty. This catheter applied circumferential pressure to the stenosis rather than the axial pressure of the previous catheters and it also created a smaller puncture site, thus reducing procedural complications. By 1976, Gruentzig had successfully miniaturized the catheter and he was performing coronary angioplasty in dogs and in human cadavers. In May 1977, Gruentzig passed a balloon catheter retrogradely from the arteriotomy site during elective coronary artery bypass surgery and inflated the balloon within a human coronary stenosis. No evidence of embolization was detected and follow-up angiography suggested an improvement in the stenosis.

Gruentzig performed the first human percutaneous transluminal coronary angioplasty in Zurich, in September 1977. The technique was the subject of intense interest and in 1978 Gruentzig began live demonstration courses in Zurich. Interest in the technique increased exponentially (2) and in 1993 600 000 coronary procedures were performed worldwide.

Angioplasty procedure

Coronary angioplasty is usually performed from the right femoral artery although some centres prefer either the brachial or radial artery approach as this facilitates early patient mobilization. All patients undergoing angioplasty should be pretreated on the ward with aspirin and then receive intravenous heparin before the procedure (10–15 000 U). An introducer sheath (6–8 French) is inserted using the Seldinger technique and a specially shaped guiding catheter is placed into the coronary ostium. A guide wire(s) is then manipulated through the target stenosis using fluoroscopy. A deflated balloon is passed along the guide wire and into the stenosis where it is inflated for a variable period of time. The balloon is then withdrawn and the angiogram is repeated to assess the result. The balloon inflation may be repeated using either the same balloon

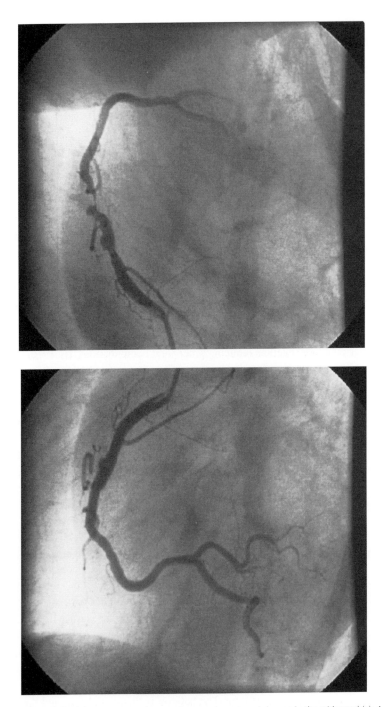

Fig. 2.1 LAO projection of a right coronary angiogram. A severe long stenosis is seen in the mid vessel (a). After multiple balloon inflations the stenosis is no longer flow limiting (b).

at a similar or higher inflation pressure or the balloon may be exchanged for a different sized balloon. Once a satisfactory result is achieved (Fig. 2.1), the balloon, guide wire, and guide catheter are removed. The arterial sheath is removed on the ward when the procedural anticoagulation has diminished. Following angioplasty patients should remain on aspirin lifelong and further attention must be paid to modification of risk factors such as smoking, hypertension, and lipid status.

Indications and results of angioplasty

For patients with three vessel coronary disease and impaired left ventricular function, successful coronary artery bypass grafting has a prognostic benefit and surgery is clearly the treatment of choice. Most patients with good left ventricular function and left main stem stenosis or three vessel coronary disease including a proximal left anterior descending stenosis are also managed surgically.

For patients with single-vessel coronary disease, coronary artery bypass surgery has no prognosis benefit and thus the application of angioplasty designed to relieve symptoms is the obvious treatment for this patient group. In the early days of angioplasty only patients with single-vessel coronary disease and limiting angina despite appropriate medical treatment were considered for treatment. Subsequently randomized studies such as ACME (3) confirmed that following angioplasty patients were less likely to have persistent angina than those allocated to continued medical treatment.

Encouraging clinical experience with angioplasty prompted investigators to compare surgery and angioplasty in broader patient groups, including those symptomatic patients not likely to receive prognostic benefit from bypass surgery. These randomized comparisons (4,5) demonstrated similar symptomatic and prognostic outcomes in both groups but a higher repeat intervention rate in the patients who underwent angioplasty. These studies performed in the present era demonstrated that, for patients with symptomatic angina and no prognostic mandate for bypass surgery, angioplasty was a legitimate treatment alternative.

Technical refinement, particularly coronary stenting, have resulted in a continued broadening of the clinical indications for angioplasty. The stent or surgery (SOS) trial is currently recruiting patients with multivessel coronary disease in a randomized comparison, but the frenetic pace of clinical development in interventional cardiology may result in the results of any such randomized studies being outdated by further technical advances, even before the studies are completed. The pace of change in angioplasty is illustrated by the fact that in 1977 patients with single-vessel disease and good left ventricular function were considered for angioplasty if the lesion was discrete, proximal, non-calcified, and concentric. By 1997 the indications for angioplasty had changed so dramatically that simple and complex lesions throughout the coronary tree both in native vessels and in arterial conduits are now routinely treated with angioplasty. Angioplasty is also used to treat patients with stable and unstable angina and increasingly patients presenting early with myocardial infarction. Even unsupported disease of the left main coronary artery, until recently an absolute contraindication for angioplasty, is now occasionally treated using balloons and stents (6).

The extensive cumulative worldwide experience of angioplasty allows prediction of acute procedural success based on the site of the lesion, its eccentricity, length, and the presence of calcification. Success is less likely with chronic occlusions (>6 months) long lesions and bifurcation stenoses but even non-calcified, concentric, short (<15 mm) narrowings in either the circumflex or right coronary arteries thought to be most suitable for balloon angioplasty may dissect and occlude, so procedural success for any lesion can never be assured.

Pathology of balloon angioplasty injury

The principal mechanisms that are responsible for successful dilation of coronary lesions by angioplasty are plaque compression, plaque fracture, and localized medical dissection and stretching of the arterial wall (7).

When Gruentzig described modern angioplasty, he assumed that compression of the intimal atherosclerotic plaque against the arterial wall with subsequent redistribution of the plaque contents was the principal mechanism by which an increase in luminal area was achieved. However, it is now recognized that particularly in patients with chronic arterial stenoses, where the lesions are predominately fibrocellular and may be calcified, this mechanism contributes a relatively small amount to the increase in luminal area. These 'hard', chronic arterial stenotic lesions are most likely to fracture when pressure is applied, whereas compression and redistribution of the plaque may be more important in the lipid-rich plaques responsible for the acute coronary syndromes.

The major mechanism of successful coronary angioplasty is splitting or fracturing of the atherosclerotic plaque. The creation of clefts of dissection, extending from the lumen for a variable distance into the plaque, enlarges the channel for blood flow, thus reducing obstruction. Studies using intravascular ultrasound have confirmed these findings *in vivo*, and demonstrated that angiography is, at best, a crude method of predicting the extent of plaque disruption following balloon dilatation (8). Predicting angiographically the likely extent of any dissection prior to balloon dilatation is also notoriously difficult. When the dissection cleft extends into the media, an extensive intramural channel can be created which may be visible angiographically. When visible dissection flaps are localized, stable, and do not compromise flow they may be regarded as an acceptable outcome to balloon dilatation. However, when an extensive dissection flap is unstable, it may compromise flow and can cause abrupt closure of the vessel. The presence of an extensive unstable dissection flap generally requires further treatment, often involving either intracoronary stenting or occasionally emergency coronary bypass surgery.

Stretching of the plaque free wall segment may be an additional mechanism by which angioplasty increases luminal diameter, particularly in eccentric stenoses. When stretching is the predominant mechanism of the increase in luminal diameter, the plaque itself may remain unaltered and passive elastic recoil over the ensuing hours will limit any long term procedural benefit.

Complications of angioplasty

The two principal complications of angioplasty are early (abrupt) vessel closure and progressive re-narrowing or re-stenosis.

Abrupt vessel closure

Before intracoronary stenting became accepted practice, abrupt vessel closure occurred in up to 12% (9) of patients treated by balloon angioplasty. The actual rate varied with the definition applied; periprocedural occlusion should be separated from occlusion occurring in the ward after a successful dilatation. Acute occlusion is usually related to the creation of a large intimal flap which compromises blood flow and/or the presence of occlusive intracoronary thrombus (7). As exposed media is highly thrombogenic, both mechanisms are often present simultaneously. As previously discussed, it is often not possible to predict which stenosis is likely to occlude acutely, but clinical studies have highlighted severe long complex lesions and unstable angina as independent risk factors (9).

The management of threatened or actual acute vessel closure has been changed dramatically by the introduction of intracoronary stenting (10). Before stenting, repeat dilatation with prolonged inflation times and the administration of intracoronary thrombolysis were the mainstays of treatment. Balloon expandable intracoronary stents provide a scaffold which can compress the dissection flap against the wall, thus increasing coronary flow and reducing the tendency to thrombosis. In lesions which are unsuitable for stenting because the vessels are small or tortuous or because of the presence of significant proximal disease, emergency bypass surgery remains an alternative.

Re-stenosis after balloon angioplasty

Progressive luminal narrowing occurring after a technically successful balloon dilatation procedure, or 're-stenosis', is the 'Achilles heel' of angioplasty. Although the term implies the return of haemodynamically significant coronary stenosis at the site of a successful angioplasty, the actual definition varies dramatically in different studies and up to 13 different definitions have been proposed (11). Once a lesion is narrowed beyond 50% the risk of developing angina, infarction or sudden death increase substantially (12). Thus in principle, for an angioplasty procedure to be regarded as successful the residual luminal diameter obstruction should be < 50% and a clinically significant recurrent stenosis should obstruct the lumen by > 50%.

Serruys and colleagues (13) have pioneered the use of quantitative angiographic analysis with computer assisted automatic edge detection systems. These systems are highly accurate and very precise (standard deviation 0.2–0.36 mm) and their accuracy has reduced the inter- and intra-observer variability inherent in systems reliant upon visual interpretation (14). Applying quantitative angiographic analysis has dramatically altered the conduct of clinical trials into re-stenosis, and repeat angiography within a predetermined time frame, regardless of symptomatic status, and dedicated core laboratories for angiographic analysis are now considered routine. As angioplasty is constantly being refined and improved, an accurate estimate of an angiographic re-stenosis rate remains controversial but most authors suggest a baseline rate of 30–40%. Reducing the rate of re-stenosis by 10% could save > $300 million per annum in the USA alone. Thus, solving the problem of re-stenosis is of the utmost clinical and financial priority.

A variety of clinical factors have been implicated in the re-stenotic process. Although many studies have tried to link the risk of re-stenosis with the risk of atherosclerosis, differences do appear to exist. Diabetes, unstable angina, and recent onset of symptoms have been identified as risk factors in most studies, but male sex and hypertension are probably less important and serum cholesterol and smoking appear to have little relation to the risk of re-stenosis (reviewed in 15). Re-stenosis is most common when angioplasty is performed in the proximal left anterior descending artery, in saphenous vein grafts, or in vessels that are total occluded with significant collateral circulation (16).

Limited availability of tissue for analysis has hampered investigators studying the pathology of human re-stenosis. The only sources of tissue are postmortem specimens or tissue obtained from directional atherectomy. As already discussed, successful balloon angioplasty is usually associated with cracking of the atherosclerotic plaque and medial dissection. When re-stenosed, the initial underlying plaque can still be clearly identified, but the luminal channels created by the balloon are filled by fibrocellular tissue or neointima. This tissue comprises a loose connective tissue matrix of collagen and acid mucopolysaccharides, interspersed with vascular smooth muscle cells. The smooth muscle cells are often larger than normal, stellate in shape, and are arranged in a haphazard fashion. Capillary ingrowth, scattered lymphocytes, and macrophages are also frequent but lipid and calcium deposits are notably absent.

The process of re-stenosis after angioplasty involves many complex and interlinked biological events. These include formation of thrombus, proliferation of vascular smooth muscle cells, migration, and the synthesis and deposition of extracellular matrix components. Some neointimal growth appears to be almost ubiquitous following angioplasty although it remains unclear why this response to injury in some patients should be so exuberant that it results in luminal encroachment and restriction of blood flow. As Glagov's law states that during the development of an atherosclerotic lesion the luminal dimension is often preserved by compensatory enlargement of the artery (17), it has been proposed that re-stenosis may reflect not only neointima formation but also the chronic failure of the vessel wall to enlarge in response to balloon injury (18). According to this theory, re-stenotic vessels show a smaller overall vessel wall diameter than other arteries, resulting in lumen narrowing independent of the degree of intimal hyperplasia. Clinical support for this theory comes from serial intravascular ultrasound data on patients who have undergone angioplasty which demonstrated that up to 60% of the late luminal loss may reflect late geometric remodelling occurring at 4–12 weeks (19). Insertion of an intracoronary stent limited this late loss and it is proposed that this may be the mechanism by which stents reduce re-stenosis. The actual pathophysiological mechanisms responsible for this phenomenon are unclear, but local wall shear stress and tensile stress conditions inflicted by angioplasty have been implicated.

The incidence of re-stenosis appears to peak at approximately 6 months, and it has therefore been suggested that symptoms developing after this period are likely to reflect new atheromatous disease. This data is supported by findings in serial angiographic and intravascular ultrasound studies which have demonstrated that maximal luminal loss appears to occur between weeks 4–12 and that the lesion thereafter is relatively quiescent (19). In a study by Mata (20) their overall re-stenosis rate was 23%. Of the 34% with angina the angiographic re-stenosis rate was 50%, but in the asymptomatic group only 19% had re-stenosis. Thus, the overall correlation between symptoms and angiographic re-stenosis is poor and recurrent anginal symptoms following angioplasty require angiography to define the aetiology.

When angioplasty is performed to a re-stenosed lesion the risk of subsequent re-stenosis is probably similar to that at the initial dilatation, although there is some evidence that the risk is increased when the occurrence of symptoms and re-stenosis is rapid (16). The risk of re-stenosis does, however, increase with a third dilation and may be as high as 45% for a fourth dilatation (21). Thus repeat angioplasty is a reasonable option for an initial recurrence of symptoms, but recurrence of symptoms following this procedure may require coronary stenting or coronary bypass surgery.

Given the complexity of the biological processes involved in neointima formation, monotherapy directed at blocking the effect of any single mediator is unlikely to be successful. Despite this, a large number of agents have been used experimentally and in clinical trials. It is clear from the accumulated literature that although some agents have been beneficial in rat and rabbit models, results in clinical studies have been disappointing. This lack of concordance in part reflects species differences, but it also reflects differences in experimental and clinical drug concentrations.

High local concentrations of drugs can be achieved using modified catheters but this effect is transient unless the drug can be retained at the site of injury (22,23). Various catheter-based delivery devices have been developed to address these problems including pressure injection directly into the arterial wall using porous balloons (24), low pressure drug delivery via double-skinned perforated balloons (25), hydrogel-coated balloons which apply a thin layer of agent directly on to the vessel wall (26), helical balloons with channels into the coil spaces (27), catheters with tiny delivery needles capable of intramural injection (28), and iontophoresis catheters which electrophoretically drive the drugs into arterial tissues (29). These systems have limited efficiency and some may themselves cause additional arterial injury during the drug delivery process (30).

Systemic agents which have been used unsuccessfully in humans include anticoagulants, antiplatelet agents, calcium channel blockers, angiotensin converting enzyme inhibitors, fish oils, lipid lowering therapy, and anti-proliferative agents.

Anti-platelet agents have been extensively investigated and aspirin therapy is routine after clinical angioplasty. Clinical studies have failed to show any definite benefit from treatment with aspirin alone (dose 80–1500 mg/day) (for review see 16) a thromboxane A_2 receptor antagonist (31) or prostacyclin (32). Some small studies have suggested some benefit from ticlopidine (a pyridine derivative which irreversibly inhibits platelet function) and trapadil (a phosphodiesterase inhibitor which also antagonizes PDGF) but these results have yet to be confirmed in larger studies.

Intracoronary stenting

The first human implantation of a coronary stent was carried out in 1986 when Puel implanted a self-expanding mesh stent or Wallstent. The initial results were disappointing as there was a high rate of in-stent thrombosis and occlusion within the first week of implantation. Complex anticoagulation regimes were devised but these were associated with problems particularly at the site of the femoral artery puncture.

Despite these problems, the increasing awareness of the limitations of balloon angioplasty maintained enthusiasm for the concept of stenting particularly as a 'bail out' procedure to stabilize arterial dissections following angioplasty. Several varieties of stent were developed and increasing clinical experience resulted in modification of post-stent care protocols including early removal of the femoral arterial sheath. Ground-breaking work by Colombo using intravascular ultrasound then demonstrated that many stents were not actually fully deployed following routine stent procedures. He and his co-workers showed that, using high pressure balloon inflation to ensure correct stent deployment against the arterial wall, stenting could be performed with drastically reduced anticoagulation regimes and improved short-term and long-term results. Benchmark studies such as STRESS (33) and BENESTENT (34) then demonstrated that elective stenting could be performed safely with superior results to angioplasty in selected patients groups. These studies supplemented by advances in stent design and availability of ticlopidine revolutionized the procedure and coronary stent implantation is now routinely practised around the world in approximately 60–70% of all coronary interventions.

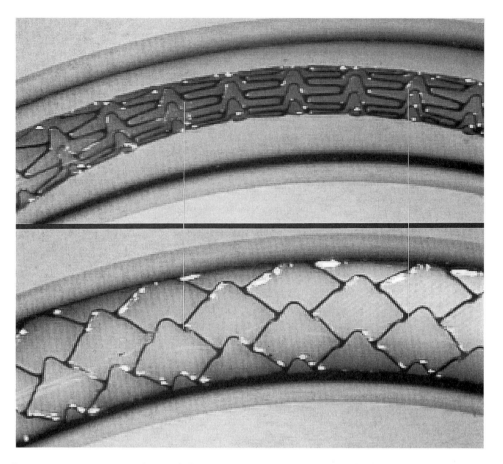

Fig. 2.2 A coronary stent crimped on to a balloon prior to deployment (upper panel). After balloon inflation the stent is expanded revealing its 'cellular' structure of interlinked struts (lower panel). See also colour plate section (Plate 3).

Several varieties of intracoronary stent are available. Most stents are stainless steel but tantalum, nitinol, cobalt alloy, and platinum iridium have been used. Some stents are self-expanding (Wallstent, radius stent) but most are mounted on a collapsed angioplasty balloon and deployed by maximal balloon inflation (Fig. 2.2). The Palmaz Schatz stent used in BENESTENT is a laser cut slotted tube stent and a number of variations of this stent have now been developed (e.g. Nir, Multilink). The other main type of balloon mounted stent is the coiled wire stent based originally on the Gianturo-Rubin stent (Microstent, Cross-Flex). The choice of stent depends on the relative length, strength, and flexibility of the stent. In general the slotted tube stents tend to be less flexible but provide greater radial strength than the coiled wire stents. For long areas of atheroma longer stents may be deployed or multiple stents can be overlapped (Fig. 2.3).

Patients who received a stent should be on aspirin therapy and anticoagulated with heparin during the procedure. Standard post-procedural care involves early removal of the arterial sheath, aspirin and ticlopidine, a potent anti-platelet agent which is given 2–4 weeks following the procedure.

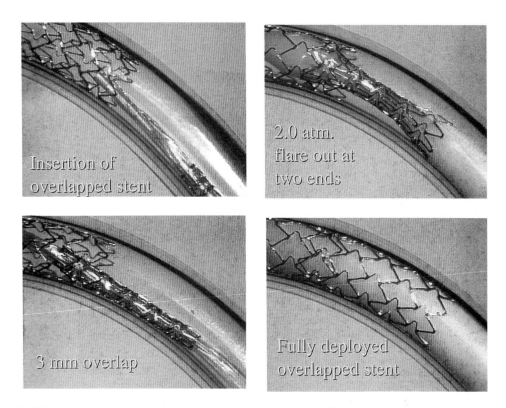

Insertion of
overlapped stent

2.0 atm.
flare out at
two ends

3 mm overlap

Fully deployed
overlapped stent

Fig. 2.3 Schematic representation of the techniques involved in sequential stenting of a long coronary stenosis. See also colour plate section (Plate 4).

Complications of stenting

The principal complications of coronary stenting are thrombotic occlusion, which may occur within the first 24 hours but occasionally can occur 5–7 days after the procedure, and stent restenosis, the incidence of which peaks at 3–4 months.

As discussed earlier the incidence of thrombotic occlusion of stents has been reduced dramatically by the routine use of high pressure balloon inflation following the initial deployment of the stent. This ensures complete expansion of the stent and optimal opposition of the stent struts against the arterial wall. A randomized study has demonstrated that ticlopidine and aspirin are superior to the combination of aspirin and warfarin (35) and this combination of agents has become standard in many centres although some authorities believe that aspirin alone is sufficient if the stent is correctly deployed, particularly in a larger vessels.

Abciximab is a chimeric glycoprotein IIb/IIIb receptor antibody used increasingly in high risk angioplasty particularly when thrombus is suspected angiographically (Fig. 2.4). Both EPILOG and IMPACT II studies have demonstrated dramatic reductions in the incidence of death, myocardial infarction, or urgent revascularization when treatment with glycoprotein IIb/IIIb receptor antibody was compared with placebo (36). Based on these results some centres have even advocated using abciximab before intervention in all patients with an acute coronary syndrome, although in the UK cost is likely to prevent this becoming generally accepted practice.

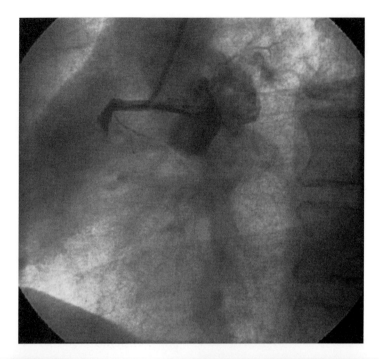

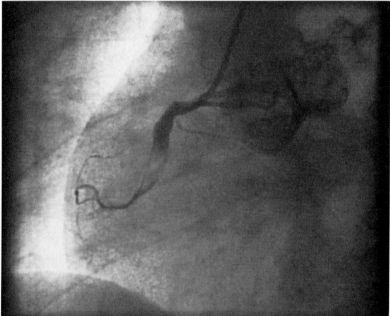

Fig. 2.4 LAO projection of a right coronary angiogram. The vessel is occuded proximally (a). Passage of the guide wire reveals tortuosity of the vessel and extensive filling defects (thrombus) (b). Eventually the distal vessel is reached with the guide wire and multiple balloon inflations are performed. This results in some antegrade flow but multiple filling defects remain (c). Administration of Abciximab and placement of multiple stents results in an excellent angiographic result (d).

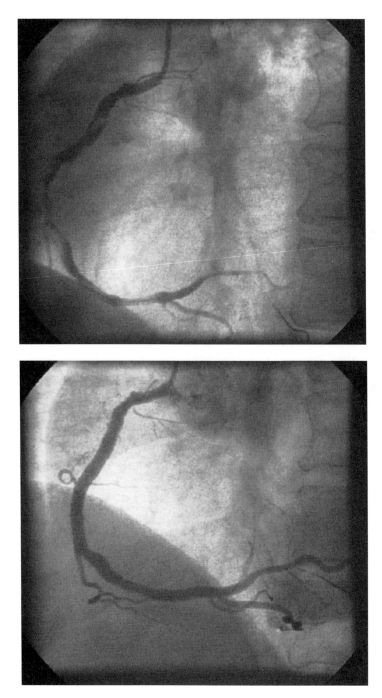

Fig. 2.4 *Continued*

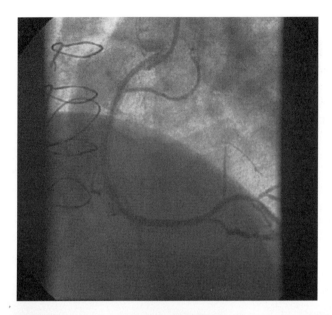

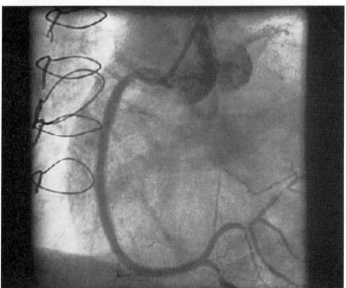

Fig. 2.5 LAO projection of a right coronary angiogram. The vessel has been stented and there is diffuse in stent restenosis (a). Balloon inflation and repeat stenting results in a good angiographic result initially (b). Restenosis recurred 3 months later and the patient required CABG.

As with re-stenosis after simple balloon angioplasty, some renarrowing is ubiquitous and probably inevitable following stent insertion. Neointimal hyperplasia is the consistent pathological finding. There are three angiographic patterns of re-stenosis following insertion of a coronary stent. The infiltration may be diffuse throughout the stent or it may be discrete within the stent or alternatively the lesion may actually be adjacent to the stent (either proximal or distal) and the stent may remain patent. Re-stenosis adjacent to the stent and discrete in-stent re-stenosis can both be treated with reasonable results using further balloon angioplasty.

In contrast, diffuse in-stent re-stenosis has an extremely high rate of recurrence if the lesion is treated by further balloon angioplasty (recurrence rates > 80%) and optimal management of diffuse in-stent re-stenosis has yet to be defined (Fig. 2.5). Mindful of the failures to influence angioplasty re-stenosis with pharmacological treatments, investigators have tended to concentrate on physical manoeuvres such as debulking of the lesion with a Rotablator under intravascular ultrasound guidance (see later) or debulking using laser angioplasty. These treatments are currently being compared in clinical studies but the most dramatic early results have come from the application of intracoronary radiation. Using radiation delivered using a specially adapted guide wire, re-stenosis rates < 10% have been reported (37) although long-term data are not yet available.

The other potential solution for in-stent re-stenosis is to prevent the problem before it occurs using various coatings applied to the stent. Heparin coatings have been used in Benestent II and there are plans to produce stents coated with oligonucleotides and phospholipid. Although most angioplasty companies are currently investigating various stent coatings, it is noteworthy that with current financial constraints any developments must be competitively priced if they are to achieve a significant market share.

Directional coronary atherectomy

Atherectomy relieves luminal obstruction, by shaving atheroma from the wall of the diseased vessel. The excavated tissue is retained in the cutting chamber, thus allowing tissue from actual site of angioplasty to be retrieved for subsequent analysis (38). The technique was pioneered in the pre-stent era to address some of the limitations of balloon angioplasty, but the dramatic results obtainable routinely following stent insertion and unfavourable comparisons between angioplasty and directional coronary atherectomy (CAVEAT, (39) and CCAT, (40)) have restricted widespread clinical application. In current clinical practice ostial lesions, bifurcation lesions, and some very eccentric and shelf-like lesions are thought to be best treated by directional atherectomy. As directional atherectomy is the only interventional technique capable of producing samples for histological analysis its research role may continue beyond its clinical applications.

Rotationary coronary atherectomy

Rotational coronary atherectomy or rotablation involves passage of a rotating burr of various sizes along a guide wire. The technique was developed to treat tough, calcific lesions which could not be treated by balloon angioplasty alone and studies have demonstrated that the burr does preferentially ablate non-elastic atherosclerotic plaque whereas normal arterial wall is deflected away. Unfortunately, re-stenosis remains a problem with this technique but other complications include coronary artery perforation, coronary spasm, and impaired slow coronary flow. Although improvement in technique have generally addressed these shortcomings, cost, the limited numbers of lesions which balloon angioplasty cannot dilate, and the significant technical demands have limited widespread application. Enthusiasts claim that treating diffuse in stent restenosis under intravascular ultrasound guidance may continue to provide a 'niche application' for this technique.

Intravascular ultrasound

Angiography remains the gold standard for assessing the degree of atheromatous disease in the coronary arteries. However, by its very nature, injecting contrast down the lumen of the artery has limitations. These include trying to visualize the complex three-dimensional anatomy of coronary stenoses using a two-dimensional technique, its inability to differentiate between a healthy artery and an diffusely atheromatous artery without lumen compromise, and the inability of a contrast technique to provide information about the tissue composition of coronary stenoses.

Intravascular ultrasound (IVUS) employs a miniaturized ultrasound probe mounted on to a catheter. The probe is passed along the angioplasty guide wire and through any arterial stenoses both before and after angioplasty balloon inflation. The ultrasound images can detail the composition and type of coronary plaque before dilatation and imaging can be repeated immediately following angioplasty allowing the increase in luminal diameter and the mechanism of this increase to be observed (8). Using IVUS the understanding of the pathological processes which occur following balloon inflation has improved and this has permitted investigators to correlate changes observed in pathological specimens with this newer *in vivo* information.

The role of IVUS in routine clinical practice remains controversial. When the technique was originally introduced the imaging catheters were large and cumbersome. This resulted in time-consuming imaging and a small risk of arterial dissection. Technical refinement has reduced the size of the catheters and improved their flexibility and this has significantly reduced the procedural risk of imaging. Scanning can now be performed quickly and safely in expert hands and it is clear that IVUS can provide clinically useful additional information in some cases. This information includes accurate sizing of the artery, particularly in the presence of diffuse arterial disease when determining the reference diameter of the normal vessel may be difficult, and data about the composition of the stenosis which may favour alternative interventional strategies; e.g. in the presence of circumferential calcification artherectomy may preferred to balloon dilation.

As discussed earlier in the chapter many of the insights which IVUS has provided have been applied routinely in interventional procedures, e.g. high pressure balloon inflation of stents. Despite this many interventionists feel that in routine cases, the incremental information provided by IVUS is limited and any potential benefits have to be balanced against the additional cost of the catheters (which are not reusable). Thus at present IVUS remains principally a research tool and a technique employed in unusual cases, e.g. rotablation for in-stent restenosis. Studies are being performed to assess whether routine use of IVUS can reduce the rates of restenosis by optimizing coronary stent insertion. It appears that unless routine IVUS can provide this type of benefit to patients its use will remain restricted for the foreseeable future.

Summary

Percutaneous cardiac intervention is a widely adopted treatment for many patients with coronary artery disease. Many of the initial limitations of angioplasty have been overcome by the advent of coronary stents, and with the use of stents most coronary stenoses can now be tackled percutaneously. Although re-stenosis remains problematic, further advances in stent design including drug-eluting stents and the therapeutic use of radiation are likely to improve long-term results.

References

1. Dotter CT, Judkins MD. Transluminal treatment of arteriosclerotic obstruction: description of a new technique and a preliminary report of its application. *Circulation* 1964;**30**:654.
2. Gruentzig AR, Senning A, Siegenthaler WE. Non-operative dilatation of coronary artery stenoses. Percutaneous transluminal coronary angioplasty. *N Engl J Med* 1979;**301**:61–8.
3. Parisi SJ, Folland ED, Hartigan P (on behalf of the veterans affairs ACME investigators). A comparsison of angioplasty with medical therapy in the treatment of single vessel coronary artery disease. *N Engl J Med* 1992;**326**:10–16.
4. RITA trial participants. Coronary angioplasty versus coronary artery bypass surgery: the randomised intervention treatment of angina (RITA) trial. *Lancet* 1993;**341**:573–8.
5. CABRI (Coronary angioplasty versus bypass revascularisation investigation) *Lancet* 1995;**346**:1179–84.
6. Davies CH, Banning AP, Channon K, Ormerod OJ. Left main coronary stenting for elderly patients unsuitable for bypass surgery. *Int J Cardiol* 1997;**62**:13–18.
7. Waller BF. Pathology of coronary balloon angioplasy and related topics. In: Topol EJ, ed. *Textbook of inteventional cardiology, Philadelphia:* WB Saunders 1990, pp. 395–451.
8. Losordo DW, Rosenfield K, Pieczek A, Baker K, Harding M, Isner J. How does angioplasty work? Serial anaysis of human iliac arteries using intravascular ultrasound. *Circulation* 1992;**86**:1845–58.
9. Ellis SG, Roubin BS, King SB. In hospital cardiac mortality after acute closure after coronary angioplasty: analysis of risk factors from 8,207 procedures. *J Am Coll Cardiol* 1988;**11**:211–16.
9. Mabin TA, Holmes DR, Smith HC *et al.* Intracoronary thrombus: Role in coronary occlusion complicating percutaneous transluminal coronary angioplasty. *J Am Coll Cardiol* 1985;**5**:198–202.
10. Sigwart U, Puel J, Mirkovitch V, Joffre F, Kappenberger L. Intravascular stents to prevent occlusion and restenosis after transluminal angioplasty. *N Engl J Med* 1987;**316**:701–6.
11. Holmes DR, Schwartz RS, Webster MWI. Coronary restenosis: what have we learned from angiography. *J Am Coll Cardiol* 1991;**17**:14B–22B.
12. Harris PJ, Behar VS, Coley MJ, Harrel FE, Lee KL, Peter RH, Kang Y, Roseti RA. The prognostic significance of 50% coronary stenosis in medically treated patients with coronary disease. *Circulation* 1980;**62**:240–8.
13. Serruys PW, Luijten HE, Beatt KJ *et al.* Incidence of restenosis after successful coronary angioplasty: A time related phenomenon. A quantitative angiographic study in 342 consecutive patients at 1, 2, 3 and 4 months. *Circulation* 1988;**77**:361–71.
14. Mancini J. Quantitative coronary angiographic methods in the interventional catherisation laboratory. An update and perspective. *J Am Coll Cardiol* 1991;**17**:23B–33B.
15. Califf RM, Fortin DF, Frid DJ *et al.* Restenosis after coronary angioplasty: an overview. *J Am Coll Cardiol* 1991;**17**:2B–13B.

16. Califf RM, Ohman M, Frid DJ *et al.* Restenosis: the clinical issues. In: EJ Topol ed. *Textbook of inteventional cardiology*, Philadelphia: WB Saunders, 1990, pp. 363–94.

17. Glagov S, Weisenberg E, Zairns CK, Stankunavicius R, Kolettis GJ. Compensatory enlargement of human atherosclerotic arteries. *N Engl J Med* 1987;**316**:1371–5.

18. Post MJ, Borst C, Kuntz RE. The relative importance of arterial remodelling compared with intimal hyperplasia in lumen renarrowing after balloon angioplasty. A study in the normal rabbit and in the hypercholesterolaemic Yucutan micropig. *Circulation* 1994;**89**:2816–21.

19. Mintz GS, Popma JJ, Pichard AD *et al.* Arterial remodeling after coronary angioplasty: a serial intravascular ultrasound study. *Circulation* 1996;**94**:35–43.

20. Mata LA, Bosch X, David PR, Rapold HJ, Corocos T, Bourassa MG. Clinical and angiographic assessments 6 months after double vessel percutaneous transluminal coronary angioplasty. *J Am Coll Cardiol* 1985;**6**:1239–44.

21. Tierstein PS, Hoover C, Ligon B *et al.* Repeat restenosis: efficacy of the third and fourth angioplasty (abstract). *J Am Coll Cardiol* 1987;**9**(2):63A.

22. Kaplan AV. Local delivery: new directions in restenosis. In Topol EJ, Ed. *Restenosis Summit VI*, Cleveland Clinic Foundation, Ohio, USA 1994, pp. 358–63.

23. Lincoff AM, Topol AJ, Ellis SG. Local drug delivery for the prevention of restenosis, fact fantasy and future. *Circulation* 1994;**90**:2070–84.

24. Wolinsky RL, Thung SN. Use of a perforated balloon catheter to deliver concentrated heparin into the wall of the normal canine artery. *J Am Coll Cardiol* 1990;**15**:475–81.

25. Hong MK, Wong SC, Farb A *et al.* Feasibility and drug delivery efficiency of a new balloon angioplasty catheter for performing simultaneous local drug delivery. *Cor Art Dis* 1993;**4**:1023–7.

26. Azrin MA, Mitchel JF, Alberghini TV *et al.* Effect of local delivery of heparin on platelet deposition during in vivo balloon angioplasty using hydrogel-coated balloons (Abstract). *Circulation* 1993;**88**(suppl 1)310A.

27. Hong MK, Wong SC, Popma JJ. A dual purpose angioplasty-drug infusion catheter for the treatment of intragraft thrombus. *Cathet Cardiovasc Diagn* 1994;**32**:193–5.

28. Gonschior P, Deil S, Maier GR, Dellian M, Goetz AE, Hofling B. Feasibility of local drug application with a new catheter (abstract) *J Am Coll Cardiol* 1994 (suppl 1):188A

29. Fernandez Ortiz A, Meyer BJ, Mailmac A *et al.* A new approach for intravascular drug delivery: iontophoretic balloon. *Circulation* 1994;**89**:1518–22.

30. Wolinsky RL. The problems and the promise of local drug delivery. In: Topol EJ, ed. *Restenosis Summit VI*. Cleveland Clinic Foundation, Ohio, USA, 1994, pp. 352–6.

31. Serruys PW, Rutsch W, Heyndrickx GR *et al.* For the CARPORT study group. Prevention of restenosis after percutaneous transluminal angioplasty with thromboxane A_2-receptor blockade. *Circulation* 1991;**84**:1568–80.

32. Gershlick AH, Spriggins D, Davies SW *et al.* Failure of epoprostenol (prostacyclin, PGI_2) to inhibit platelet aggregation and to prevent restenosis after coronary angioplasty: results of a randomised placebo controlled trial. *Br Heart J* 1994;**71**:7–15.

33. Fischman DL, Leon MB, Baim DS *et al.* A randomised comparison of coronary stent placement and balloon angioplasty in the treatment of coronary artery disease. *N Engl J Med* 1994;**331**:496–501.

34. Serruys PW, De Jaegere P, Kiemenenejj F *et al.* A comparison of balloon expandable stent implantation with balloon angioplasty in patients with coronary artery disease. *N Engl J Med* 1994;**331**:489–95.

35. Schomig A, Neumann FJ, Kastrati A *et al.* A randomised comparison of antiplatelet and anticoagulant therapy after the placement of coronary artery stents. *N Engl J Med* 1996;**334**:1084–9.

36. Steinhubl SR, Lincoff M. Antithrombotic therapy with intracoronary stenting. *Heart* 1997;**78**(suppl 2):21–3.

37. Tierstein PS, Massulo V, Jani S *et al.* Radiation therapy following coronary stenting 6 month follow up of a randomised control trial (abstract). *Circulation* 1996;**94**(suppl I):I210.

38. Robertson GC, Hinohara T, Selmon MR, Johnson DE, Simpson JB. Directional coronary atherectomy. In: Topol EJ ed. *Textbook of inteventional cardiology* Philadelphia: WB Saunders, 1990, pp. 563–80.

39. Topol EJ, Leya F, Pinkerton CA, Whitlow PL, Hofling B, Simonton CA. A comparison of directional atherectomy with coronary angioplasty in patients with coronary artery disease: the CAVEAT study group. *N Engl J Med* 1993;**329**:221–7.

40. Adelman AG, Cohen EA, Kimball BP *et al.* A comparison of directional atherectomy with balloon angioplasty for lesions of the left anterior descending coronary artery. *N Engl J Med* 1993;**329**:228–33.

3 Systemic effects of cardiopulmonary bypass

John J. Dunning

Without cardiopulmonary bypass, cardiac surgery as we know it today would not be possible. Yet the very technology which enables the surgeon to perform complex surgery on the heart is itself damaging and exerts effects on the patient which manifest themselves in every system of the body. Although temporary dysfunction of various systems is usual, most of the systemic side effects are well tolerated and rapid postoperative correction is the rule. However, under certain circumstances the systemic effects on one or more organ systems may be more pronounced, resulting in distressing symptoms and iatrogenic conditions which are difficult to correct.

A number of physiologic variables are under direct external control during cardiopulmonary bypass. These include total systemic blood flow, systemic venous and arterial pressure, arterial oxygen and carbon dioxide levels, perfusate haematocrit, and the temperature of both perfusate and patient.

Other parameters are under partial external control with a variable component determined by the patient. These include systemic and pulmonary vascular resistances, pH balance, regional and organ blood flow, and mixed venous oxygen saturation.

This chapter outlines the systemic complications of cardiopulmonary bypass and considers the aetiology of these conditions.

Cardiopulmonary bypass circuit

In order to establish cardiopulmonary bypass the mechanical pump must first be connected to the patient. In most cardiac surgery this is achieved by introducing cannulae directly into the ascending thoracic aorta and the venae cavae via the right atrium.

The aortic cannulation site may lead to physical complications. It is possible to cause aortic dissection either during incautious insertion of a cannula through the vessel wall, or by inadequate closure of the aortotomy at the removal of the cannula. This may leave a weak area which can act as the lead point for dissection. In addition, when cannulating a heavily diseased vessel it is possible to cause displacement of calcified debris which may give rise to thromboembolic complications such as a cerebrovascular accident.

The aortic cannula is usually chosen of a size that will allow a high flow rate with minimal gradient across the cannula, permitting the turbulence caused by the blood flow as it leaves the cannula to be minimized. This again reduces the likelihood of embolic phenomena caused by particulate matter displaced from the aortic wall.

Finally, care must be exercised at the time of connection of the aortic cannula to the primed circuit of the pump to ensure that no air bubbles are introduced to the circuitry since this may also cause cerebral injury.

Once cardiopulmonary bypass is established an aortic cross clamp is applied either once or repetitively to permit coronary artery grafting or valve surgery to be performed. Again care must be exercised during clamping and handling of the aorta since this may lead to embolic phenomena, or even aortic dissection.

Systemic venous blood is usually returned to the pump by means of large cannulae introduced either directly to the two venae cavae, or by means of a large cavoatrial pipe which has two drainage ports: the first is placed in the inferior vena cava, and the second series of holes is located in the right atrium close to the mouth of the superior vena cava. The pipes are selected to be as large as possible to ensure adequate drainage to permit high flow rates and low systemic venous pressure during cardiopulmonary bypass. In particular, congestion of the drainage from the head and neck must be avoided since this may lead to cerebral oedema and injury.

The pipes are usually held in place by purse string sutures introduced in the right atrial free wall – a thin and delicate structure, which may be injured by injudicious movement of the relatively rigid pipes. Postoperative dysrhythmias may result from trauma to the cavoatrial junction as a result of cannulation related injury.

Additional cannulae may be placed in the heart and pericardium to scavenge blood which returns to the heart by collateral circulation. These pipes drain blood by direct suction; they are usually relatively smaller in calibre and may result in direct physical trauma to cellular components of the blood, particularly if the suction is high. Such haemolysis, if excessive, may cause injury to capillary beds in organs such as the kidneys and lungs.

Physiological response to cardiopulmonary bypass

Blood

Within the elements of cardiopulmonary bypass circuits there are many factors which have a direct influence on blood components, both cellular and chemical. It is known that the stress generated within the bypass circuits can cause both immediate and delayed injury to red cells, and that the components must be designed in a way to minimize such injury.

Red blood cells undergo lysis whenever they meet with walls, when they are subjected to turbulence, or whenever there is high shear stress. In order to minimize these effects the walls of pipes and oxygenators must be made as smooth as possible, and the size of textured protrusions on the foreign surface should be smaller in diameter than the cells passing over the surface. Although immediate haemolysis has been commonly accepted as an index of trauma to blood, it has also been demonstrated that autohaemolysis of pumped blood occurs over the following 24 hours [1]. Further experimental work demonstrated that it was not interaction with the walls alone that led to this damage, but also exposure to intermittent positive pressure and sub-haemolytic shear rates [2]. Chemical changes in the structure of the red cell membrane and stimulation of lipid peroxidase systems may be important in the destruction of such injured cells.

It is known that different forms of mechanical pump exert greater or lesser haemolytic effects. Studies using the concentration of plasma free haemoglobin or lactate dehydrogenase as indices of haemolysis have compared the effects of roller head pumps, centrifugal pumps, and impeller pumps for cardiopulmonary bypass. *In vitro* evidence shows that the level of haemolysis induced by the roller pump and the impeller is greater than that caused by a centrifugal pump head (3,4).

However, it is not only red blood cells that are injured by the physical effects of extracorporeal circuits. Platelets are activated, and fragmented by the pumps and the extensive exposure to foreign surfaces, and it has again been demonstrated both in *in vitro* studies and in clinical studies, that different pump heads exert different effects, with the roller head being repeatedly shown as the most damaging.

The effects of the different pump heads are not only seen on the formed elements of blood, but may also contribute to systemic injury in other ways. It has been demonstrated that plastic tube which is exposed to the repeated trauma of a roller pump undergoes a process of spallation, during which particles the size of blood cells are shed, creating the risk of particle embolization and an increased morbidity. Clearly flow rates and duration of bypass will affect the severity of such a hazard (5,6) and the design of circuit components must be to minimize these effects.

Cardiopulmonary bypass causes a systemic inflammatory response which is gradually becoming more completely understood, and in due course this will allow the deleterious effects to be minimized. The blood cells contribute to the generalized inflammatory response to cardiopulmonary bypass, although this response is essentially non-specific. Lymphocytes are part of the specific immune response system and play little part in the inflammatory response. Eosinophil and basophilic granulocytes play little part too. The role of natural killer cells is not clear. Neutrophils activated by complement and other soluble inflammatory mediators play a major role in the response to cardiopulmonary bypass. Their response is characterized by migration, increased adhesiveness, and secretion of cytotoxic substances, including oxygen free radicals.

The activation of complement and sequestration of white cells within the pulmonary circulation has attracted attention (7). It is now known that complement, coagulation, fibrinolytic, and kallikrein cascades are all activated, with activation of leukocytes and impairment of platelet function. The manifestation of these mechanisms as leukocytosis, increased capillary permeability, accumulation of interstitial fluid and resultant organ dysfunction is well recognized (7).

Activation of complement during cardiopulmonary bypass occurs mainly through the alternative pathway (8), although the classical pathway may also be triggered by interaction with protamine-heparin complexes (9). Levels of complement activation products rise dramatically with initiation of bypass and peak at its termination. Levels are related to duration of the bypass procedure and return to normal only after 48 hours. Cardiac and pulmonary dysfunction, renal failure, and bleeding tendencies have all been linked to the level of anaphylatoxins after cardiopulmonary bypass (7).

Acute lung injury is probably not a result of complement activation alone, but the generation of C5a results in the margination and activation of neutrophils, with adherence to the vascular endothelium (10). This may be important at the time of reperfusion. Further products of complement activation may result in neutrophil degranulation and release of interleukin-1β from monocytes. Models of complement activation are accompanied by sequestration of leukocytes in the capillary bed with evidence of endothelial cell injury and similar injury occurs in models of the adult respiratory distress syndrome (11).

Leukocyte populations are also susceptible to change during cardiopulmonary bypass. At the initiation of bypass there is an immediate fall in circulating leukocyte numbers as a result of both haemofiltration and sequestration of cells in the peripheral circuit. Later there is a relative leukocytosis with the replacement of lost mature forms by immature cells from the bone marrow. To some extent hypothermia modulates this response (12,13).

Leukosequestration also occurs within the pulmonary capillary beds, as pulmonary blood flow is reduced with the initiation of bypass. After removal of the aortic cross clamp, neutrophils but not lymphocytes remain sequestered (13). Although these cells may be relatively inactive there is evidence for release of lipid peroxidation products after removal of the aortic cross clamp. This reflects cell membrane injury and offers indirect evidence for an injurious role of sequestered neutrophils (14).

Neutrophils granules contain neutral serine proteases (e.g. elastase) and glycoproteins (e.g. lactoferrin) which have important roles in the inflammatory response and host defence. They may also be relevant in the systemic response to cardiopulmonary bypass. Lactoferrin may influence the production of oxygen free radicals, whereas the capacity for elastase to produce both parenchymal and endothelial injury suggests it may have a role in the capillary and pulmonary changes associated with cardiopulmonary bypass (15–17).

Under normal circumstances injury from elastase is prevented by anti-proteases which are present throughout tissue. However, oxygen free radicals which are released throughout bypass (and which may be neutrophil derived (18)) produce oxidation of antiprotease and slow down the rate of elastase inhibition. In addition, peroxidation products may cause direct injury to lipids and nucleic acid, denaturing cell surface proteins and further enhancing tissue injury (19).

The response of blood-borne components to cardiopulmonary bypass is gradually becoming more completely understood. However, it is also clear that the response is a complex one. With improvements in materials and device design, some of the coarser events have been excluded, and other strategies are evolving to further minimize the systemic response. Anti-inflammatory agents such as corticosteroids, oxygen radical scavengers, monoclonal antibodies directed against specific mediators, inhibitors of neutrophil activation, and complement regulatory proteins may all offer hope for the future reduction of systemically mediated effects of cardiopulmonary bypass.

Temperature

One advantage of extracorporeal circulation is that it is possible to control the temperature of the perfusate accurately. The first effective clinical heat exchanger was introduced by Brown in 1958 (20). Since then temperature has become one of the most important parameters to be selected for each patient undergoing cardiopulmonary bypass.

At low temperatures the basal metabolic activity in organ systems are reduced, thereby reducing their oxygen requirements. This offers a degree of protection against ischaemic injury and since collateral blood returns to the heart during most cardiopulmonary bypass it also prevents premature rewarming of cardiac tissue following cardioplegic arrest. In addition it offers a degree of flexibility allowing for such disasters as pump failures or split pipes, permitting a period of up to 10 minutes of circulatory arrest at 28°C to effect repairs.

The temperature will affect acid-base balance, and after profound hypothermia it is normal to see an acidotic state. Longer rewarming may be required following profound cooling, and if there is not full temperature equilibration a profound temperature after drop may be seen on return to the intensive care area, perhaps with an associated acidosis.

An additional consideration is that enzyme systems are temperature dependent and optimal function is usually only achieved at normal body temperature. This is particularly of concern following profound hypothermia, when the coagulation cascade may be grossly deranged. Additional blood products such as platelets, fresh frozen plasma, and even cryoprecipitate may need to be administered to correct coagulation anomalies.

Kidneys

The incidence of acute renal failure following cardiac surgery varies in reported series from 2.5% to 31% (21,22) with postoperative oliguria running as high as 60%.

The aetiology is multifactorial, with age, preoperative renal function, and combined procedures believed to be significant variables for identifying patients at risk (23). During cardiopulmonary bypass renal perfusion may be impaired by a variety of mechanisms which include low perfusion flow, hypotension, non-pulsatile flow, vasoconstriction induced by pharmacological agents, and microembolic phenomena.

The resultant acute tubular necrosis is a serious systemic complication of cardiopulmonary bypass and there is an observed increase mortality associated with this state (24). Further renal damage may result as a result of excessive haemolysis during bypass. The free haemoglobin precipitates in the renal tubules in the presence of acid urine (25). Others have found that tubular obstruction was a major factor in the continuance of already established renal failure (26).

The debate continues about the management of renal failure in the postoperative period. Many physicians advocate the introduction of dialysis for the oliguric patient as early as 24 hours after surgery, whereas others would advocate waiting for as long as possible. The outcome for established renal failure following cardiac surgery may be poor, but often this reflects other ongoing pathology such as low cardiac output syndromes which are themselves the cause of the renal dysfunction.

Central nervous system

The central nervous system is perhaps the most sensitive organ system in the human body, with relatively minor influences affecting the individual's neuropsychology. It is therefore perhaps not surprising that the effect of cardiopulmonary bypass should be felt by this system. Embolization and hypoperfusion with their resultant hypoxia have always been regarded as the essential aetiological factors in neurological disturbances and manifest themselves in the very obvious signs of strokes. However, with recent psychometric testing it has become evident that cognitive function may also be impaired with alteration of mood and affect, and the assumption is that the mechanism of injury is the same, only differing in degree and distribution.

There are essentially three mechanisms of cerebral injury. The first is that of mechanical injury resulting from emboli. These may be particulate, resulting from traumatization of diseased blood vessels, or gaseous following intra-cardiac entrapment of air. Microemboli are produced by the interactions between blood and the artificial surfaces of the bypass circuit, and also from spallation of plastic pipes as they pass through the roller head of a mechanical pump. Indeed there is growing evidence from transcranial Doppler studies that cerebral microemboli occur in all patients undergoing cardiopulmonary bypass.

The second type of injury results from the physiological variation in blood flow distribution which causes changes in autoregulation of the microvasculature, cellular metabolism and the response to reperfusion (27). The flow produced by cardiopulmonary bypass may be non-physiological for a variety of reasons including an abnormal site for the return of oxygenated blood from the pump, reduced flow rates, non-pulsatile flow, temperature, and pH.

A further physical feature which may influence the cerebral blood flow during cardiopulmonary bypass is the presence of carotid artery disease. There is ongoing debate over the best approach to the treatment of combined carotid disease and cardiac disease. Some surgeons support correction of carotid anomalies prior to cardiac surgery, some as a staged procedure after cardiac surgery, and some advocate combined surgery. With so much disagreement it seems likely that there is no absolute right and wrong. Perhaps the emphasis should be to control the bypass conditions absolutely to maintain high cerebral blood flow irrespective of the carotid vascular state.

In addition, pharmacological agents which may be cumulative in the face of impaired liver and renal function may also lead to altered neurological states.

Deep hypothermic circulatory arrest finds use in neonatal and some adult surgery, since it provides a bloodless operative field, and permits removal of the aortic cross clamp. However, it is a potentially hazardous technique since it leaves the brain (and other organs) ischaemic for the duration of arrest. There continues to be debate over the total safe period of circulatory arrest, despite clinical and experimental studies to elucidate its neurological sequelae. Abnormal neurological function and a reduction of the normal neuronal population have been reported in gerbils after circulatory arrest of more than 45 minutes (28).

In human studies, electroencephalographic changes during and after circulatory arrest, the development of postoperative seizures, and late motor development have all been examined. In one study by Kirklin *et al.*, freedom from major neurological events decreased rapidly when the period of arrest exceeded 50 minutes at 18–20°C (29). Similarly, most clinical studies suggest that intellectual and psychomotor development are unlikely to be impaired if the arrest period is kept less than 60 minutes at 18–20°C (30–32). Further adult studies have suggested that the safe period of circulatory arrest may be prolonged by more profound cooling. Detailed intraoperative electroencephalography has shown that electrical activity may still be present down to nasopharyngeal temperatures of 12–16°C, suggesting more profound cerebral cooling may extend the traditionally accepted period of safe arrest (33).

Other procedures that may improve neurological outcome after cardiac surgery include the use of low flow or intermittent perfusion to prevent the prolonged periods of circulatory arrest. In adult surgery particularly, selective antegrade arterial or retrograde venous perfusion of the brain may also be undertaken (34,35).

Advances in materials science may in the future allow cardiopulmonary bypass without full heparinization, in turn reducing deleterious effects on platelet activation and function, reducing the likelihood of embolic phenomena. Hypothermia remains the mainstay of current cerebral protection, not only by reducing cerebral metabolism, but also by increasing tissue levels of high energy phosphates and intracellular pH, both of which improve the tolerance of ischaemia (35). Possibly beneficial manipulations which require further evaluation include the modification of blood pH, the prevention of hyperglycaemia, the administration of beta-blockers and calcium antagonists, *N*-methyl-D-aspartic acid receptor antagonists, and free radical scavengers (27,35,36)

Despite the potential problems of cardiopulmonary bypass, the great majority of patients are left with no detectable long-term neurological sequelae.

Heart

At the commencement of cardiopulmonary bypass the heart is diseased, and may be dysfunctional. At the termination of the procedure the heart has a new disease, in that the ventricle has now undergone a global ischaemic insult whether a surgical technique using cross clamp fibrillation or cardioplegia has been used. This renders the myocardium unable to utilize efficiently the oxygen with which it is supplied.

A further problem is encountered since the heart becomes oedematous over the first 6–12 hours after bypass, and with this the ventricles become more rigid and less compliant. This effect is particularly marked after prolonged period of bypass, combined with profound hypothermia. Indeed on occasion the swelling may be such that it is impossible to close the sternum immediately without causing compression of the heart and a tamponade syndrome.

Optimal cardiac rate at the end of bypass is also important. The cardiac output in the immediate post-bypass phase is essentially rate dependent, and this may necessitate the use of temporary epicardial pacing in the face of bradycardia and other dysrhythmias.

Low cardiac output may occur and pharmacological intervention become necessary. Such therapy is aimed at increasing myocardial contractility, decreasing the afterload, and increasing substrate. Correction of post-bypass acidosis may also be important. Inotropic support in the post-bypass phase should be utilized early rather than late, and less frequently the use of an intra-aortic balloon pump may be necessary to augment systemic perfusion pressures, while offloading the ventricle. This last measure also improve the diastolic perfusion of the myocardium and encourages the recovery processes in the heart.

Transient intraoperative conduction delays may occur following the ischaemic period. These are again related to purely physical effects such as oedema, or trauma during surgery (particularly valve surgery), but may also be precipitated in the face of electrolyte disturbance such as hypokalaemia and hypomagnesaemia which are relatively common as a result of preoperative diuretic use. Again, temporary epicardial pacing either of both the atria and ventricles, or of the ventricles alone may be necessary.

Perioperative myocardial infarction occurs with an incidence of about 5% (37). Important factors in determining the outcome are the severity of pre-existing coronary artery disease and the duration of cardiopulmonary bypass. The significance of an uncomplicated perioperative infarct is not clear, since long term prognosis does not appear to be changed. However, if the infarct is complicated by congestive cardiac failure, cardiogenic shock, dysrhythmias or cardiac arrest the long-term outcome is poorer.

Lungs

Certain predictable changes occur within the lungs during cardiopulmonary bypass, and these are summarized in Table 3.1. In the majority of patients these changes are not of great significance and do not materially alter the postoperative course. However, the presence of pre-existing pulmonary disease, or congestive cardiac failure with pulmonary oedema, are more likely causes of postoperative respiratory failure.

During cardiopulmonary bypass with full systemic anticoagulation, trauma to the lungs may result in bleeding into the airways with associated loss of surfactant, atelectasis, ventilation/perfusion (V/Q) mismatch, and hypoxaemia. Similarly marked elevations of pulmonary venous pressure during cardiopulmonary bypass may cause haemorrhagic atelectasis with bleeding into peribronchial and perivascular spaces. This vascular leakage results in fulminant pulmonary oedema.

In addition to these mechanisms it is known that the release of inflammatory mediators such as histamine, kinins, and complement also leads to pulmonary injury. However, the advances made in cardiopulmonary bypass technology with modified materials and conversion to membrane oxygenators appears to avoid many of the problems initially seen with bubble oxygenators. In-line arterial filters remove manufacturing debris, platelet aggregates, and particles returned to the oxygenator from the operative field. These factors have combined to make adult respiratory

Table 3.1   Lung changes during cardiopulmonary bypass

Alveolar–arterial oxygen difference	Increased
Physiological shunt	Increased
Respiratory rate	Increased
Airways resistance	Increased
Work of breathing	Increased
Oxygen consumption	Increased
Physiological dead space	Increased
Pulmonary vascular resistance	Increased
Tidal volume	Decreased
Alveolar ventilation	Decreased
Alveolar volume	Decreased
Static compliance	Decreased
Minute ventilation	Unchanged
Respiratory quotient	Unchanged

distress syndrome (ARDS) following cardiopulmonary bypass virtually unknown in patients who do not have pre-existent respiratory pathology.

Respiratory failure without a pre-existent cause is rare, and the normal postoperative course is towards early extubation following limited or no mechanical ventilation, dictated not so much by the patient's respiratory state as by the needs of the chosen anaesthetic technique (38)

Gastrointestinal system

The incidence of abdominal complications following cardiopulmonary bypass is low, occurring in only about 0.5–2% of patients in reported series (39–44). The most common complications are gastrointestinal haemorrhage, acute pancreatitis, and bowel ischaemia. Published series show a decline in the incidence of these complications from 1960 to the present day (45–48) but the mortality due to these complications remains high, ranging from 12% (40) to 67% (44) in different series. When this figure is compared to the in-hospital mortality for patients undergoing cardiac surgery for all conditions (which runs at 3–4%) the size of the problem is realized.

It might reasonably be expected that gastrointestinal haemorrhage is a more frequent complication among patients who have undergone valve surgery and therefore require anticoagulation. The published series from the Cleveland clinic fail to correlate bleeding with specific procedures (49). In contrast, the series from the Mayo clinic find a much higher rate of bleeding in those patients undergoing valve surgery (50).

Several groups have reported gastrointestinal bleeding for which a cause was not found, in association with aortic valve disease, predominantly calcific aortic stenosis (50–52). None of these reports has explained the aetiology of the problem.

The group of patients who bleed most frequently are distinguished by certain clinical features. Patients who have a previous history of gastric or duodenal ulceration are more likely to bleed following cardiopulmonary bypass, particularly if they have a history of previous haemorrhage.

Males are more likely to bleed than females. Longer cardiopulmonary bypass and longer operations predispose to a higher risk of postoperative bleeding (49,50,52). In addition they are the patients who have a higher incidence of other postoperative complications which may increase the likelihood of a bleed from the gastrointestinal tract (50,52).

Acute postoperative bleeding is most commonly caused by multiple gastric and or duodenal ulcers and is followed in frequency by haemorrhagic or erosive enteritis (39,49,50). It has been shown that there is an association between hypoperfusion leading to mucosal ischaemia and gastric erosions (53).

It might be anticipated that patients requiring anticoagulant therapy or administered antiplatelet therapy would be at a higher risk of bleeding, particularly if they have a strong previous history. Although aspirin therapy is known to be an aetiological factor in gastric mucosal ulceration this correlation was not upheld by the studies (50), nor did steroid therapy increase the incidence of gastrointestinal bleeding.

The use of simple antacids has been shown to be effective in reducing the incidence of gastrointestinal bleeding (54); in contrast, the use of cimetidine and ranitidine has not been shown to be effective in reducing bleeding rates. Also this therapy has been shown to be detrimental in terms of altering tracheobronchial pH and therefore the respiratory tract flora, predisposing to nosocomial respiratory tract infections. Sucralfate is perhaps the most effective prophylactic agent and it benefits from the feature that it does not alter gastrointestinal pH, and therefore leaves the flora unaltered (55).

The diagnosis of gastrointestinal complication can be difficult to make in ill patients following cardiac surgery. Often patients require prolonged ventilation and sedation, which clearly makes communication difficult. In addition the symptoms of abdominal pathology may be masked by the use of postoperative analgesia. Consequently, a delay in diagnosis is not uncommon.

Probably the most important aetiological factor in the pathogenesis of abdominal complications is poor visceral perfusion (41–43). It has been suggested that this is at least in part due to long bypass times (41) although in another study there was no significant difference in times between patients who developed gastrointestinal complications and those who did not (39).

The treatment of gastrointestinal bleeding from ulcers has changed dramatically in recent years. With improved endoscopic equipment and techniques it is no longer necessary to perform open surgery at the time of haemorrhage, and many patients can be treated with sclerotherapy at the time of diagnostic endoscopy. In addition the new range of proton pump blocking agents has changed the face of drug therapy for peptic ulceration and provides a useful adjunct to endoscopic therapy, and the use of H_2 antagonists as prophylactic therapy. However, for patients who re-bleed or continue to bleed despite a more conservative approach to management, surgery should be performed without delay. Even though this involves surgery on sick patients, two recent studies have had no mortality attributed directly to laparotomies performed for continued gastrointestinal bleeding (39,44).

Pancreatitis is a commonly reported complication of cardiopulmonary bypass, and covers a spectrum of disease ranging from a mild subclinical condition detectable only by biochemical assay to severe necrotizing haemorrhagic pancreatitis (56). The true incidence is probably higher than expected since many subclinical forms go undetected. However, one postmortem study found evidence of acute pancreatitis in 18% of patients dying following cardiac surgery (57) and a further study found elevated plasma amylase levels in about 25% of patients (58). Low perfusion pressures and low flow states have been implicated as aetiological factors together with microemboli, gallstones, hypothermia, and pre-existent pancreatic disease. Treatment should be conservative in the first instance but early surgery may be necessary for those patients whose condition deteriorates despite appropriate measures (59). Even with awareness of the severity of this complication and the need for early intervention the mortality from pancreatitis remains high (41,43).

The remaining complications of cardiopulmonary bypass are less frequent but carry high mortality. They include acute cholecystitis (mortality 75–85% (41,42)), intestinal infarction and perforation, and colonic pseudo-obstruction.

Intestinal ischaemia may result from poor visceral perfusion during or after surgery and is particularly likely in patients who have pre-existent arterial disease causing partial occlusion of visceral arteries. Once recognized, immediate surgery is necessary for these patients (40,41,47).

In summary, although gastrointestinal complications are not common they carry a significant morbidity and mortality, and early diagnosis and intervention must be the rule.

Liver

Although evidence of hepatic injury is not usually present in the normal convalescent, it is nevertheless recognized that jaundice may occur with an elevated bilirubin level following cardiac surgery (60) in as many as 20% of patients. Although such dysfunction may be related as before to episodes of low flow and low blood pressure during cardiopulmonary bypass, other factors are important including the amount of blood transfused, postoperative hypotension, operative hypoxia, and the use of halothane intraoperatively.

Conclusions

It is clear that the effects of cardiopulmonary bypass are widespread and there is no organ system which is spared from the potentially damaging effects of extracorporeal circulation. There have been tremendous advances in material science which have rendered the hardware less noxious as it has evolved. However, a clear understanding of the systemic side effects of cardiopulmonary bypass is essential to the cardiothoracic surgeon so that he may take measures to further minimize any possible harm. Research continues to elucidate further the mechanisms involved in the systemic inflammatory response, and in turn to develop therapeutic interventions which will further minimize morbidity attributable to 'the pump'.

References

1. Bernstein E, Indeglia R, Shea M, Varco R. Sublethal damage to the red blood cell from pumping. *Circulation* 1967;**35–36**(Suppl 1):226–33.
2. Indeglia R, Shea M, Forstrom R, Bernstein E. Influence of mechanical factors on erythrocyte sublethal damage. *Transactions of the American Society of Artificial Internal Organs* 1968;**14**:264–72.
3. Hoerr H, Kraemer M, Williams J *et al.* In vitro comparison of the blood handling by the constrained vortex and twin roller blood pumps. *Journal of Extra-Corporeal Technology* 1987;**19**:316–21.
4. Stridis E, Chan T. An evaluation of vortex, centrifugal and roller pump systems. In: Thoma H, Schima H, eds. *International workshop on rotary bloodpumps.* Obertauern, Austria, 1988:76–81.

5. Kurusz M, Christman E, Williams E, Tyers G. Roller pump induced tubing wear: Another argument in favour of arterial line filtration. *AmSECT* 1980;**12**:49–59.

6. Orenstein J, Sato N, Aaron B, Buchholz B, Bloom S. Microemboli observed in deaths following cardiopulmonary bypass surgery: silicone antifoam agents and polyvinyl chloride tubing as sources of emboli. *Human Pathology* 1982;**13**:1082–90.

7. Kirklin J, Westaby S, Blackstone E, Kirklin J, Chenoweth D, Pacifico A. Complement and the damaging effects of cardiopulmonary bypass. *Journal of Thoracic and Cardiovascular Surgery* 1983;**86**:845–57.

8. Muller-Eberhard H. Complement. *Annual Review of Biochemistry* 1975;**44**:697–724.

9. Fehr J, Rohr H. In vivo complement activation by polyanion-polycation complexes: evidence that C5a is generated intravascularly during heparin-protamine interaction. *Clinical Immunology and Immunopathology* 1983;**29**:7–14.

10. Charo I, Yuen C, Perez H, Goldstein I. Chemotactic peptides modulate adherence of human polymorphonuclear leukocytes to monolayers of cultured endothelial cells. *Journal of Immunology* 1986;**136**:3412–19.

11. Hosea S, Brown E, Hammer C, Frank M. Role of complement activation in a model of adult respiratory distress syndrome. *Journal of Clinical Investigation* 1980;**66**:375–82.

12. Stahl R, Fisher C, Kucich U *et al*. Effects of simulated extracorporeal circulation on human leukocyte elastase release, superoxide generation, and procoagulant activity. *Journal of Thoracic and Cardiovascular Surgery* 1991;**101**:230–9.

13. Quiroga M, Miyagishima R, Haendschen L, Glovsky M, Martin B, Hogg J. The effect of body temperature on leukocyte kinetics during cardiopulmonary bypass. *Journal of Thoracic and Cardiovascular Surgery* 1985;**90**:91–6.

14. Royston D, Fleming J, Desai J, Westaby S, Taylor K. Increased production of peroxidation products associated with cardiac operations: evidence for free radical generation: *Journal of Thoracic and Cardiovascular Surgery* 1986;**91**:759–66.

15. Ambruso D, Johnston R. Lactoferrin enhances hydroxyl radical production by human neutrophils, neutrophil particulate fractions, and an enzymatic generating system. *Journal of Clinical Investigation* 1981;**67**:352–60.

16. Jochum M, Fritz H. Elastase and its inhibitors in intensive care medicine. *Biomedical Progress* 1990;**3**:55–9.

17. Smedley L, Tonnesen M, Sandhaus R *et al*. Neutrophil-mediated injury to endothelial cells: enhancement by endotoxin and essential role of neutrophil elastase. *Journal of Clinical Investigation* 1986;**77**:1233–43.

18. Fantone J, Ward P. Role of oxygen-derived free radicals and metabolites in leukocyte-dependent inflammatory reactions. *American Journal of Pathology* 1982;**107**:397–418.

19. Hochstein P, Jain S. Association of lipid peroxidation and polymerization of membrane proteins with erythrocyte ageing. *Federation Proceedings* 1981;**40**:183–8.

20. Brown I, Smith W, Emmons W. An efficient blood heat exchanger for use with extra corporeal circulation. *Surgery* 1958;**44**:372.

21. Baht J, Gluck M, Lowenstein J *et al*. Renal failure after open heart surgery. *Annals of Internal Medicine* 1976;**84**:677.

22. Hilberman M, Myers B, Carrier B *et al*. Acute renal failure following cardiac surgery. *Journal of Thoracic and Cardiovascular Surgery* 1979;**77**:880.

23. Corwin H, Sprague S, DeLaria G *et al*. Acute renal failure associated with cardiac operations. *Journal of Thoracic and Cardiovascular Surgery* 1989;**98**:1107.

24. Abel R, Buckley M, Austen W *et al*. Etiology, incidence and prognosis of renal failure following cardiac operations. *Journal of Thoracic and Cardiovascular Surgery* 1976;**71**:323.

25. Clyne D, Kant K, Pesce A *et al*. Nephrotoxicity of low molecular weight serum proteins: physical chemical interactions between myoglobin, haemoglobin, Bence-Jones proteins and Tamm-Horsfell mucoprotein. *Current Problems in Clinical Biochemistry* 1979;**9**:299.

26. Kron I, Joob A, Van Meter C. Acute renal failure in the cardiovascular surgical patient. *Annals of Thoracic Surgery* 1985;**39**:590.

27. Royston D. Interventions to reduce cerebral injury during cardiac surgery: the effect of physiological and pharmacological agents. *Perfusion* 1989;**4**:153–61.

28. Treasure T, Naftel D, Conger K. The effect of hypothermic circulatory arrest time on cerebral function morphology and biochemistry. *Journal of Thoracic and Cardiovascular Surgery* 1983;**86**:761.

29. Kirklin J, Kirklin J, Pacifico A. Deep hypothermia and circulatory arrest. In: Arcinegas E, ed. *Paediatric cardiac surgery*. Chicago: Year Book Medical Publishers, 1985:67–77.

30. Messmer B, Schallberger U, Gattiker R *et al*. Psychomotor and intellectual development after deep hypothermia and circulatory arrest in early infancy *Journal of Thoracic and Cardiovascular Surgery* 1976;**72**:495.

31. Clarkson P, MacArthur B, Barratt-Boyes B *et al*. Development progress after cardiac surgery in infancy using profound hypothermia and circulatory arrest. *Circulation* 1980;**62**:855.

32. Wells F, Coghill S, Caplan H *et al*. Duration of circulatory arrest does influence the psychological development of children after cardiac operations in early life. *Journal of Thoracic and Cardiovascular Surgery* 1983;**62**:823.

33. Coselli J, Crawford E, Beall AJ *et al*. Determination of brain temperatures for safe circulatory arrest during cardiovascular operation. *Annals of Thoracic Surgery* 1988;**45**:638.

34. Usui A, Hotta T, Hiroura M. Retrograde cerebral perfusion through a superior vena caval cannula protects the brain. *Annals of Thoracic Surgery* 1992;**53**:47–53.

35. Swain J, Anderson R, Siegman M. Low flow cardiopulmonary bypass and brain protection: a summary of investigations. *Annals of Thoracic Surgery* 1993;**56**:1490–2.

36. Griepp E, Griepp R. Cerebral consequences of hypothermic circulatory arrest in adults. *Journal of Cardiac Surgery* 1992;**7**:134–55.

37. Roberts A. Perioperative myocardial infarctionand changes in left ventricular performance related to coronary artery bypass graft surgery. *Annals of Thoracic Surgery* 1983;**35**:208.

38. Lichtenthal P, Wade L, Niemyski P *et al*. Respiratory management after cardiac surgery with inhalationa anaesthesia. *Critical Care Medicine* 1983;**11**:603.

39. Egleston C, Gorey T, Wood A, McGovern E. Gastrointestinal complications after cardiac surgery. *Annals of the Royal College of Surgeons* 1993;**75**:52–6.

40. Welling R, Roth R, Albers J, Glaser R. Gastrointestinal complications after cardiac surgery. *Archives of Surgery* 1986;**121**:1178–80.

41. Krasna M, Flancbaum L, Trooskin S *et al*. Gastrointestinal complications after cardiac surgery. *Surgery* 1988;**104**:773–8.

42. Leitman M, Paull D, Barie P. Intra-abdominal complications of cardiopulmonary bypass operations. *Surgery Gynecology and Obstetrics* 1987;**161**:251–4.

43. Moneta GL, Misbach GA, Ivrey TD. Hypoperfusion as a possible factor in the development of gastrointestinal complications after cardiac surgery. *American Journal of Surgery* 1985 May:**149**(5):648–50.

44. Huddy S, Joyce W, Pepper J. Gastrointestinal complications in 4473 patients who underwent cardiopulmonary bypass surgery. *British Journal of Surgery* 1991;**78**:293–6.
45. Harjola P, Siltanen P, Appelqvist P, Laustela E. Abdominal complications after open heart surgery. *Annales Chirurgiae et Gynaecologiae* 1968;**57**:272.
46. Lawhorne T, Davis J, Smith G. General surgical complications after cardiac surgery. *American Journal of Surgery* 1978;**136**:254.
47. Wallwork J, Davidson K. The acute abdomen following cardiopulmonary bypass surgery. *British Journal of Surgery* 1980;**67**:410.
48. Lucas A, Max M. Emergency laparotomy immediately after coronary bypass. *Journal of the American Medical Association* 1980;**244**:1829.
49. Taylor P, Loop F, Hermann R. Management of acute stress after cardiac surgery. *Annals of Surgery* 1973;**178**:1.
50. Welsh G, Dozois R, Bartholomew L, Brown A, Danielson G. Gastrointestinal bleeding after open heart surgery. *Journal of Thoracic and Cardiovascular Surgery* 1973;**65**:738.
51. Williams RJ. Aortic stenosis and unexplained gastrointestinal bleeding. *Archives of Internal Medicine* 1961;**108**:859.
52. Katz S, Kornfeld D, Harris P, Yeoh C. Acute gastrointestinal ulceration with open heart surgery and aortic valve disease. *Surgery* 1972;**72**:438.
53. Kivilaakso E, Silen W. Pathogenesis of experimental gastric-mucosal injury *New England Journal of Medicine* 1979;**301**:364–9.
54. Mead J, Folk F. Gastrointestinal bleeding after cardiac surgery. *New England Journal of Medicine* 1969;**281**:799.
55. Berk J. In: *Handbook of critical care*. 3rd ed. Boston: Little Brown, 1990:43–58.
56. Haas G, Warshaw A, Daggett W, Aretz H. Acute pancreatitis after cardiopulmonary bypass. *American Journal of Surgery* 1985;**149**:508–14.
57. Feiner H. Pancreatitis after cardiac surgery. *American Journal of Surgery* 1976;**131**:684–8.
58. Rattner D, Gu Z-Y, Vlahakes G, Warshaw A. Hyperamylasemia after cardiac surgery: Incidence, significance and management. *American Surgeon* 1989;**209**:279.
59. Rose D, Ranson J, Cunningham J, Spencer F. Patterns of severe pancreatic injury following cardiopulmonary bypass. *American Surgeon* 1984;**199**:168–72.
60. Chu C, Chang C, Liaw Y, Hsieh M. Jaundice after open heart surgery: A prospective study. *Thorax* 1984;**39**:52.

4 Myocardial protection

John Pepper

The concept of placing new grafts to bypass obstructions in coronary arteries is attractively simple. The objective of every operation should be a technically perfect result without producing myocardial damage. Currently only a minority of surgical patients present with normal left ventricular function; most have damaged ventricles but the damage may in part be reversible. Until recently the attention of surgeons had fallen almost exclusively on the myocyte but it is becoming clear that protection of the coronary endothelium and the specialized conduction tissue are also important in the pursuit of a perfect result. From the practical viewpoint the prerequisites for optimal protection are uniform and adequate distribution of a protective agent, excellent visualization of the operative field, a simple technique that does not distract the surgeon, and optimal protection of the brain and kidneys.

The consequences of inadequate myocardial protection are serious but not always immediately obvious. Low cardiac output (a cardiac index of less than 2.0 L min^{-1} m^{-2}) leading to prolonged hospital stay and high costs is a well-known scenario, but more subtle degrees of damage may result in delayed myocardial fibrosis. The long-term outlook for patients with coronary disease is determined in large part by the function of the left ventricle. Demographic changes in recent years have resulted in large numbers of elderly patients and patients with impaired left ventricular function being referred for operative myocardial revascularization [1]. In such patients the margins of functional reserve are narrow and methods of protection have therefore to be focused.

The principal requirement for clinical use of any protection strategy is appropriate testing in the laboratory, preferably in models that bear some resemblance to conditions encountered in clinical practice. Clinical cardioplegia was introduced by Melrose [2] who advocated the use of hypotonic potassium citrate blood to facilitate arrest and provide ideal operating conditions. This basic concept was sound but it was not subjected to the rigorous testing now employed; clinical results were erratic and clinical cardioplegia was abandoned for nearly 20 years. Later studies showed that the problem with the Melrose solution was inappropriate concentration of constituents rather than inappropriate composition. Studies by Buckberg [3] lent full support to the original constituents of the Melrose solution. Nowadays safe concentrations of alkalotic, hypotonic, potassium citrate blood are used by many surgeons whenever the aorta is clamped. The long time lapse between the original introduction of cardioplegia via Melrose and renewed interest in the subject by the studies of Bretschneider [4], Kirsch [5] and Hearse [6] in Europe and Gay and Ebert [7] in the US led to alternative non-cardioplegic techniques to produce a quiet operative field, namely ischaemic arrest and ventricular fibrillation. A further important development during the end of this period was the introduction of coronary artery surgery. This was relatively low risk surgery which began to concentrate the minds of surgeons on the problems of perioperative myocardial damage. Sceptical observers in those early days attributed loss of angina to perioperative infarction. This provided a challenge for coronary surgeons and was a catalyst for a renewed interest in myocardial preservation. Views about myocardial protection among surgeons tend to be polarized, such as 'non-cardioplegia versus cardioplegia', 'antegrade versus retrograde' or 'warm versus cold'. In the following sections these apparent differences will be discussed.

Ischaemia versus ventricular fibrillation

Ischaemia implies an imbalance between oxygen supply and demand. It must be distinguished from hypoxia since the concept includes both a reduction in oxygen supply and an accumulation of the waste products of metabolism. The oxygen supply : demand mismatch is most obvious when blood supply is interrupted at 37°C without cardioplegic arrest and leads to the phenomenon of 'stone heart', which reflects irreversible cardiac contracture due to inadequate protection. Ischaemia stops the heart by interrupting the supply of oxygen needed to produce sufficient ATP for electromechanical coupling. Recent studies of ischaemic preconditioning define some adaptive mechanisms that develop during brief coronary flow interruption (8,9). The physiology of this condition is incompletely understood but appears to be quite species-specific and probably to involve adenosine A_1 receptors (10). Evidence of preconditioning in humans is rather scarce. Deutsch *et al.* (11) studied a small group of patients undergoing angioplasty with a regional 90 second coronary occlusion separated by 5 minutes of reperfusion. The second episode of ischaemia caused less chest pain, less ST elevation, and less myocardial lactate production. The authors concluded that the lessened ischaemic response during the second balloon inflation was evidence that the myocardium had been preconditioned by the first inflation. The fact that cardiac vein flow was lower during the second inflation that the first suggested that this adaptation to ischaemia was not due to an increase in collateral flow. Flameng and colleagues (12) looked at arterial–coronary sinus differences in lactate, inorganic phosphate, and potassium after release of aortic cross clamping in a randomized group of 72 patients undergoing coronary artery bypass grafting. They found that the washout of inorganic phosphate, potassium, and lactate progressively diminished after subsequent brief ischaemic episodes and was attributed to ischaemic preconditioning. In a pilot study Yellon *et al.* (13) reported that the fall in myocardial ATP concentration during the standard duration of cross clamp fibrillation can be dramatically reduced if it is preceded by two 3 minute periods of ischaemia. This pattern of metabolic protection in humans is analogous to the change in myocardial ATP observed in the original preconditioning studies by Murry and colleagues (9). As changes in coronary collateral flow do not complicate the interpretation of these results, the authors argue that this probably represents preconditioning in humans.

This rapidly developing area of investigation may throw light on overlapping areas of interest such as myocardial stunning and hibernation. Recent experimental studies show that brief interruption of regional coronary flow increases tolerance to a subsequent prolonged ischaemic interval, reduced stunning, and limits necrosis. Experimental testing of pre-bypass ischaemia before prolonged aortic clamping with cold cardioplegia shows worsened rather than improved recovery (14). It may be that the mechanisms responsible for ischaemic preconditioning are retarded by deep hypothermia and are effective only with intermittent ischaemia with mild hypothermia as described by Flameng (15) especially when used in conjunction with drugs such as nucleoside transport inhibitors (e.g. lidoflazine) that affect adenosine metabolism, block calcium channels, and hasten asystole.

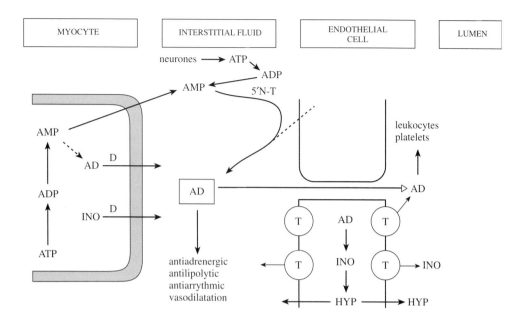

AD = adenosine, INO = inosine, HYP = hypoxanthine

D = diffusion   (T) = Nucleoside transport

Fig. 4.1   Adenosine metabolism: sites of nucleoside action of transport inhibitors.

Recent evidence suggests that adenosine protection of a globally ischaemic heart is mediated by interaction with adenosine A_1 receptors (16). Furthermore, the use of exogenous adenosine either post-ischaemia or as an infusion (16,17) or as an addition to a preservation solution (18,19) results in improved left ventricular function. Adenosine is very labile and disappears fast from its site of production as it is rapidly deaminated or washed out on reperfusion (20). In order to benefit from the properties of adenosine, local concentrations should remain elevated throughout the reperfusion period. Engler and Gruber (21) proposed the following therapeutic approaches for augmenting adenosine:

- Adenosine-regulating agents such as AICA riboside (22)
- specific adenosine agonists
- nucleoside transport inhibition (23,24).

The concept of nucleoside transport inhibition (NTI) is based on the ability of some drugs to inhibit adenosine transport so that adenosine accumulates at the site of production and stays there during the reperfusion phase (Fig. 4.1). The group of drugs lidoflazine, mioflazine, and soluflazine have been shown to be potent and specific nucleoside transport inhibitors (25). Efficient NTI may be an almost ideal tool to exploit the beneficial effects of adenosine because they act on demand — if sufficiently specific they will have effect only if, and as long as, adenosine is produced — and because their action will be restricted to the local ischaemic area exactly where adenosine is produced. There is a dual effect on adenosine metabolism and release. The prolonged accumulation of adenosine in the interstitial space may allow it to reach its receptors to cause vasodilatation and to express anti-adrenergic, anti-lipolytic, and anti-arrhythmic effects. The steady release of adenosine within the lumen of the micro vessels during reperfusion will prevent local aggregation of platelets and activation of leukocytes. Flameng and colleagues (15) have shown in the dog heart that lidoflazine and its analogue, mioflazine, are able to protect the heart against 1 hour of normothermic global ischaemia. The same group have demonstrated enhanced myocardial protection in a group of patients undergoing coronary bypass grafting as evidenced by ATP, creatine phosphate, and myocardial glycogen content, none of which was depressed. Similarly, myocardial ultrastructure was well preserved and functional outcome was excellent.

The avoidance of ischaemia while maintaining a quiet perfused heart undergoing ventricular fibrillation was first introduced by Senning (26). This technique was used extensively until the mid 1970s and continues to provide good results in some centres (27). However, many surgeons abandoned this technique because of the advent of cardioplegia and the demonstration of suben-docardial myocardial necrosis by Taber (28) and Najafi (29). Studies of regional blood flow meas-urement by Buckberg *et al.* (30) explained how this damage occurred. These studies showed that oxygen demand during electrically induced ventricular fibrillation is substantial (31) and that subendocardial perfusion is impaired in a fibrillating heart if the heart is electrically fibrillated (32), or distended (33), or hypertrophied (34), or when perfusion pressure is low. In these canine studies electrically induced fibrillation resulted in ischaemia due to compression of subendocar-dial vessels especially if the ventricle was allowed to distend. Hypothermia reduces the vigour of ventricular fibrillation, thereby limiting the compression of intramyocardial vessels. In clinical practice it has been shown that deep hypothermic (25°C) ventricular fibrillation is an effective method for construction of distal anastomoses when aortic atherosclerosis precludes safe aortic clamping.

To avoid these problems a number of surgeons during the early 1970s developed the tech-nique of intermittent ischaemic arrest in coronary artery surgery (35). The essential features of this method are moderate hypothermia, good systemic venous drainage to ensure an empty heart, and the performance of distal and proximal anastomoses in alternate fashion allowing the heart to beat in a non-working mode during performance of the proximal anastomosis. The increased oxygen demand associated with fibrillation has only ever been demonstrated in canine hearts subjected to continuous electrical fibrillation. In clinical practice a short burst of AC current is used to initiate fibrillation and is then removed. It is important that the left ven-tricle is not allowed to distend especially if there is any degree of hypertrophy and therefore left ventricular venting is recommended if distension begins to develop. The advantages of this technique are its simplicity and low cost as there is no requirement for extra perfusion pumps, heat exchanger, or special cannulae. Furthermore it offers great flexibility allowing the operative plan to be changed (for example, the insertion of an extra graft requiring additional saphenous vein) without an increase in the overall ischaemic time. Generally ischaemic times for distal anastomoses can be kept at 7–12 minutes but extension to 15 minutes is quite acceptable.

The disadvantages of this method are that it is a 'fussy' technique requiring continuous careful observation of the heart by the surgeon. Multiple claming of the aorta in the elderly with athero-sclerotic disease is likely to increase the risk of cerebral emboli. Blauth and others (36) identified atheroembolic causes of stroke significantly more in patients with coronary artery procedures (26%) than in those undergoing valve procedures (9%). A stroke rate of 0.2% overall and 0.7% in the isolated coronary bypass group was significantly less than found in the multiple cross clamped group. If coronary bypass grafting is to be combined with aortic valve replacement it becomes a rather cumbersome technique. Despite widespread use of cardioplegic techniques, pockets of resistance remain and excellent results are produced with this method (12,37,38). In the current era of cost effectiveness and cost acceptability, non-cardioplegic methods in the hands of experienced surgeons are very attractive both in established centres and in new units starting up their coronary artery surgical programme.

Crystalloid versus blood cardioplegia

The rationale for the use of cold cardioplegic myocardial preservation is that it reduces oxygen consumption of the myocardium to such low levels during the ischaemic period of aortic cross clamping that the energy stores are sufficient to maintain cellular structure and the energy-dependent cell membrane pumps that preserve transcellular gradients of sodium, potassium, calcium, and magnesium. Thus myocardial cell viability and function are preserved. During aortic cross clamping myocardial energy is derived primarily from the anaerobic metabolism of myocardial glycogen and glucose. This small energy output is sufficient to maintain myocardial viability during relatively prolonged ischaemia if the energy demands are sufficiently low (4). When the heart is electromechanically quiescent the energy demands are determined primarily by myocardial temperature and to some extent by resting wall tension. At 22°C the oxygen consumption of the myocardium in the electromechanically quiescent heart is around 0.3 mL 100 g^{-1} min^{-1} whereas at 37°C it is around 1.0 mL 100 g^{-1} min^{-1}. By contrast, while the heart at 22°C is beating or electrically fibrillated, oxygen consumption is approximately 2.0 mL 100 g^{-1} (30). Currently the most widely used cardioplegic solution in the UK is the St Thomas' Hospital No. 1 solution developed by Hearse and Braimbridge (6). This solution contains, among other ions, potassium at a concentration of 20 mmol L^{-1}. At this concentration potassium blocks the initial 'fast' or inward sodium current phase of myocardial cell depolarization. Even with such concentrations electromechanical activity can persist or return in the presence of agents such as catecholamines which open the latent 'slow' or inward calcium current phase of myocardial cell depolarization upon which potassium has no effect. When cold cardioplegia is used clinically after establishing cardiopulmonary bypass the aorta is cross clamped and the cold cardioplegic solution (at approximately 4°C) is infused over 2–3 minutes either into the closed aortic root if the aortic valve is competent or directly into the coronary ostia in the presence of aortic regurgitation. Because of non-coronary collateral myocardial blood flow, blood continues to flow into the heart leading to re-warming and resumption of electromechanical activity (39). In clinical practice, therefore, either myocardial temperature is monitored with a septal temperature probe or the heart is reperfused with cold cardioplegic solution every 20–30 minutes. Continuous external cardiac cooling with iced slushed saline is often performed when possible to keep the heart cold.

Although cold cardioplegia has improved the early results of coronary artery surgery, many important details of the technique remain undefined. Methods of delivery vary from uncontrolled bag squeezing to dedicated pumps and heat exchangers with monitoring of aortic root pressure. As we learn more about the relationship between the functional integrity of the coronary endothelium and ventricular performance, it becomes clear that we need to pay attention to aortic pressure during cardioplegic infusion. Cardioplegic agents have been infused in crystalloid solutions (5–7), in crystalloid solutions containing albumin (40) and in blood removed from the oxygenator reservoir (41). Blood exerts an oncotic pressure that varies with the degree of haemodilution, is readily available, has substantial buffering qualities due to the histidine imidazole groups, and provides oxygen. Red blood cells contain endogenous oxygen-derived free radical scavengers (superoxide dismutase, catalase, glutathione) which may reduce free radical mediated injury during reperfusion. The potential disadvantages of blood include poor control of specific ionic composition, its content of undesirable products of the extracorporeal circulation including catecholamines, and its rheological characteristics at low temperatures. Although the oxyhaemoglobin dissociation curve is shifted to the left with hypothermia, substantial unloading of oxygen occurs during hypothermic blood cardioplegic perfusion (31).

In recent years there has been a change in many cardiac units towards the adoption of blood cardioplegia. Is there evidence to support this change or is it just a whim of surgical fashion? Fiendel et al. (42) showed in an experimental model that blood cardioplegia as compared to crystalloid cardioplegia offered superior protection to the myocardium subjected to 4, 5, and 6 hours of arrest. When the blood solution was cooled to 4°C they saw no evidence of sludging or rouleaux formation in electron microscopic biopsies. In another experimental study, Robertson and colleagues (43) compared the distributions of blood and asanguineous solution beyond coronary stenoses. Blood cardioplegia resulted in lower temperatures beyond critical stenoses and required a shorter period to asystole. They reasoned that the decreased viscosity of the asanguineous solution diverted the cardioplegia away from the obstructed vessel and towards the normal coronary bed.

Unfortunately in clinical practice there is a remarkable lack of randomized clinical trials. We have to fall back on observational or retrospective studies with historical controls. In general it appears that an advantage for blood cardioplegia becomes obvious only in patients with impaired ventricular function undergoing extended operations. For example, Shapira et al. (44) found no difference between blood and crystalloid cardioplegia in a group of low risk coronary bypass patients when left ventricular contractility was assessed. However, Cunningham et al. (45) and Singh et al. (46) showed that ATP stores and mitochondrial integrity were better maintained with blood cardioplegia. Iverson and colleagues (47) examined the effects of blood and crystalloid cardioplegia in 237 patients. There was no difference in left ventricular stroke work index or enzyme levels in the group with left ventricular end diastolic pressures (LVEDP) less than 18 mmHg. However, if LVEDP exceeded 18 mmHg blood cardioplegia resulted in small but significantly better stroke work indices and lower enzyme levels. Roberts et al. (48) also demonstrated that blood cardioplegia may provide better protection for patients with low ejection fractions (< 40%) and with prolonged cross-clamp times (> 90 minutes). Daggett et al. (49) in a non-randomized retrospective study of 400 patients concluded on the basis of ECG evidence and clinical outcome that blood cardioplegia provided better myocardial protection than crystalloid cardioplegia. As an alternative to oxygenated blood, the cardioplegic solution may be oxygenated by bubbling oxygen into a crystalloid solution and adding agents to increase oxygen carrying capacity. In experimental studies, Bodenhamer et al. (50) and Hicks et al. (51) used fluorocarbons to increase oxygen carrying capacity and they demonstrated superior protection with these solutions. Gardner et al. (52) used free radical scavengers to increase the oxygen carrying capacity of his solution and claimed to obtain good protection. Ledingham and colleagues (53) using the isolated working rat heart found that oxygenation of St Thomas' Hospital solution resulted in improved preservation as reflected by a more rapid return of sinus rhythm, improved post-ischaemic recovery of aortic flow and reduced leaking of creatinine kinase. Interestingly Illes et al. (54) in an experimental canine study produced strong evidence that the efficacy of blood-based cardioplegic solutions cannot be attributed to a plasma component or to the greater oxygen carrying capacity of the red blood cells. They suggested that other factors such as free radical scavenging, buffering capacity, or oncocity may contribute to metabolic preservation. In support of the concept of free radical scavenging, experimental studies by Julia *et al.* (55) have shown a marked reduction in the beneficial effect of blood cardioplegic reperfusion when endogenous red blood cell glutathione and catalase are blocked pharmacologically.

There has been a trend among cardiac surgeons to adopt polarized position on myocardial preservation. These attitudes are not really helpful. A better approach is to keep a flexible attitude and be prepared to use different methods for different situations. Common to all methods of cardioplegia, however, is the control of reperfusion.

Control of reperfusion

Reperfusion can be given either antegrade or retrograde. While uncertainty persists concerning the adequacy of flow to the right ventricle via the retrograde route, many surgeons prefer to use the antegrade route. Anecdotal information indicates that retrograde perfusion to the right ventricle provides nutrient capillary flow that is only 25% of the left ventricle. During cold cardioplegic perfusion this is less critical as the requirements of the right ventricle are markedly reduced. In present day coronary surgery, where one pedicle arterial graft is invariable and multiple arterial grafts increasingly common, it seems advantageous to at least initiate reperfusion via the retrograde route in order to ensure even distribution to areas particularly in the left ventricle which have been supplied with these pedicled grafts. Suboptimal perfusion may precipitate serious arrhythmias (56) or may cause myocardial stunning (57). Gallinones and Hearse (58) showed that reperfusion with blood produced a different outcome in terms of cardiac function than reperfusion with a crystalloid solution. Specifically there was better recovery of left ventricular function after blood reperfusion.

For antegrade delivery, an aortic root cannula is used because the flow rates of appropriately controlled aortic root perfusion are too large for safe accommodation by a needle. The flow rate during reperfusion is controlled to maintain a constant aortic root pressure and this pressure is monitored via a side arm on the aortic root cannula. Similar pressure monitoring is carried out during retrograde perfusion (Fig. 4.2). Aortic pressure is maintained at 60–70 mmHg mean and coronary sinus pressure at 40–50 mmHg mean. It is important to avoid left or right ventricular distension throughout the reperfusion period in order to reduce wall tension and presumably minimize wasteful energy expenditure by myocytes. This will also serve to minimize any decrease in subendocardial blood flow.

One of the primary goals of reperfusion is to ensure rapid regeneration of the energy charge of the heart (the energy stored in ATP, creatine phosphate, and their metabolites) (59). The rapidity of this process is increased by the maintenance of electromechanical quiescence (60). If this rule is followed Digerness *et al.* (61) showed in the isolated rat heart that this results in improved functional recovery. Buckberg and colleagues which also demonstrated the advantages of an initially hyperkalaemic reperfusion and introduced the technique into clinical cardiac surgery. Its advantages have been confirmed in a randomized trial by Teoh *et al.* (62), although as expected the advantages are difficult to demonstrate in good risk patients (63). The optimal duration of electromechanical quiescence during reperfusion has not been established. The greater the ischaemically induced reduction in the energy charge of the myocytes the longer should be the period during which energy production is channelled to the restoration of energy charge. It is

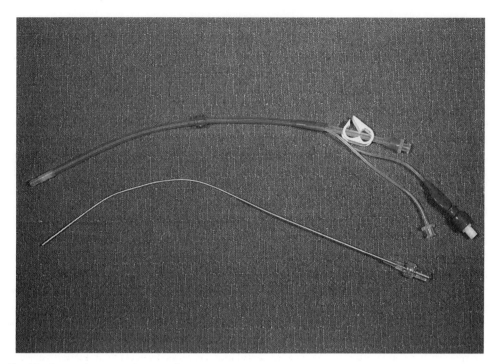

Fig. 4.2 Retrograde coronary sinus cannula.

the author's preference to administer the warm reperfusion (or 'hot shot') in a retrograde manner to ensure even distribution in the presence of pedicled arterial grafts. During the first 2 minutes after removal of the aortic cross clamp aortic pressure is maintained at 30 mmHg. It is then raised to 60–80 mmHg or the patient's preoperative diastolic blood pressure.

After a period of myocardial ischaemia coronary vascular endothelial cells appear to be in a state in which they are easily damaged by high reperfusion pressure (64,65). It is therefore wise initially to have a low coronary perfusion pressure. Conversely there appear to be important disadvantages if the aortic root pressure after the first few minutes is too low. Aldea *et al.* (66) showed that when coronary perfusion pressure is reduced from 70 mmHg to 40 mmHg endocardial flow is severely reduced. Reduction of perfusion pressure to 20 mmHg leads to significantly increased heterogeneity of regional myocardial blood flow. Fontan *et al.* (67) found no difference in outcomes in patients undergoing coronary artery bypass grafting using the technique of controlled aortic perfusion between patients in whom reperfusion pressure was 50 mmHg and those in whom it was 70 mmHg except that electromechanical activity resumed more quickly when reperfusion pressure was 75 mmHg.

Composition of the reperfusate

The reperfusate consists of oxygenated blood to which potassium has been added to achieve a final concentration of 10 mmol L^{-1}. There is no evidence that modifications of the initial reperfusate, other than hyperkalaemia, are advantageous for routine use in cardiac surgery. Fontan *et al.* (68) suggest that it may result in better cardiac performance. In patients with impaired ventricular function there is increasing evidence that more complex reperfusion solutions offer a tangible advantage, especially if the period of global myocardial ischaemia is prolonged. The inclusion of the amino acids glutamate and aspartate in the reperfusion solution could be expected to enhance myocardial recovery because these amino acids are used as substrates during oxidative metabolism and repletion of ATP. This idea was introduced by Rosenkranz and Buckberg (69–72) who showed that they were metabolically and functionally advantageous. Their work has been confirmed by others (73,74).

Acute elevation of the cytosol free calcium in myocytes has been correlated with depletion of ATP and irreversible ischaemic injury (75). Lowering the level of calcium in the reperfusion solution and in the cardioplegic solution reduces reperfusion damage and therefore enhances recovery. When the reperfusate becomes unmodified oxygenated blood, serum calcium becomes normal. It has been proposed that initial reduction of serum calcium is important in avoiding reperfusion injury, but its return to near-normal levels after myocardial recovery enhances cardiac function. After the initial hyperkalaemic phase of reperfusion, electromechanical activity nearly always returns without ventricular fibrillation. There may be a slow idioventricular rhythm and complete heart block but this usually gives way to sinus rhythm. Atrial fibrillation at this stage is uncommon.

It is important for the surgeon not to be impatient at this stage but to ensure that the ventricles remain decompressed. Generally within 15 minutes of the resumption of electromechanical activity the heart has recovered and is capable of supporting the circulation. If this is not the case continuous support on bypass may be required. Present evidence does not support the idea of repeating the hyperkalaemic reperfusion. It is important that aortic root pressure is adequate, that is in the region of 70–80 mmHg mean pressure. α-Agonist drugs such as metaraminol may be required, especially if the patient has been maintained on angiotensin converting enzyme inhibitors in the preoperative period. In the event that a vigorous cardiac contraction does not appear and a modest dose of dopamine has been tried, mechanical support of the circulation by intraaortic balloon pump should be instituted. The adoption of this protocol over the last 2 years has been helpful. In the past uncontrolled reperfusion has led to weak cardiac action with ventricular or atrial fibrillation.

Antegrade versus retrograde cardioplegia

Uniform distribution of cardioplegia is an important prerequisite for effective myocardial protection. This can only be ensured if there is adequate delivery beyond coronary stenoses and obstructions and it becomes more problematic in the presence of diffuse coronary disease.

The limitations of antegrade delivery can be overcome by delivering cardioplegia via the graft or by performing the proximal aortic anastomosis first and administering cardioplegia via the aortic root after each distal anastomosis. There is evidence that giving hyperkalaemic solutions into vein grafts damages the endothelium of the graft (76,77) and the latter technique is cumbersome and unattractive and makes the judgement of the correct graft length difficult. A further objection to complete reliance on antegrade delivery is that adequate and uniform delivery is not achieved in the presence of one or more pedicled arterial grafts. The superior long term results of pedicled internal mammary artery grafts are generally accepted and therefore the overwhelming majority of patients now receive at least one pedicled arterial graft.

Retrograde perfusion of the coronary venous system was first proposed by Pratt (78) and later by Lillehei *et al.* (79). It has several advantages over antegrade delivery, including:

- avoidance of damage to coronary ostia during aortic valve replacement
- exclusion of the need for aortotomy and direct coronary cannulation in the presence of mild aortic regurgitation
- delivery of cardioplegia to jeopardized myocardium
- avoidance of the need to remove retractors during operations on the mitral valve
- retrograde flushing of air emboli from native coronary arteries and of atheromatous debris from patent but diseased vein grafts in re-do operations.

Disadvantages of retrograde cardioplegia include:

- damage to the coronary sinus by excessive infusion pressure or balloon inflation
- displacement of the cannula during retraction of the heart
- uncertainty about adequate perfusion of the right ventricle
- difficulties imposed by uncommon congenital abnormalities such as a left superior vena cava or unroofed coronary sinus (80,81).

The combined techniques of antegrade/retrograde cardioplegia administered alternately but never simultaneously allow benefits to be derived from both routes of delivery. The author's own practice is to give two-thirds of the initial cardioplegic infusion in the antegrade manner and one-third retrograde. Subsequent maintenance doses are given retrogradely after completion of

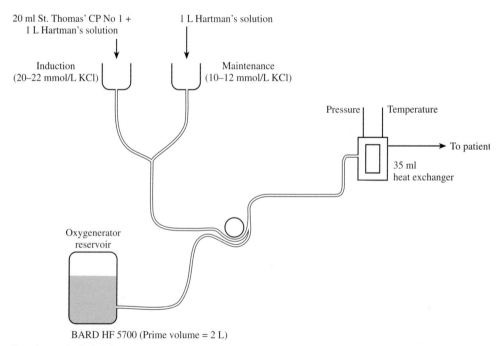

Fig. 4.3 Cardioplegia infusion system.s

each distal anastomosis (Fig. 4.3). Care is taken to observe filling, of the posterior interventricular vein or (if there is a simultaneous aortic valve replacement) to observe retrograde filling of blood in the right coronary ostium. If by these means right ventricular perfusion is judged not to be adequate, antegrade perfusion should be given. Clinical application of this combined strategy has produced satisfying clinical results in patients (82–84).

Warm versus cold

Hypothermia in cardiac surgery has a long pedigree, going back to the early studies of Bigelow (85) and Shumway (86). These two authors were among the first to recognize that hypothermia is a way of limiting ischaemic injury especially without cardioplegia. It continues to play an important role in the non-cardioplegic technique of intermittent ischaemic arrest. Increasingly the value of cardiac hypothermia is being questioned. Hypothermia produces favourable effects by

- reducing the rate of myocardial metabolism and oxygen consumption
- reducing the rate of the process leading to death of myocytes
- promoting electro-mechanical quiescence.

But there is no favourable effect on coronary endothelium or coronary vascular resistance or on the rate of recovery of ischaemically damaged myocardium. Hypothermia probably has several adverse effects, including oedema due to inactivation of the sodium/potassium ATP pump (87), alteration of platelets and leukocytes (88), altering membrane stability (89), and reducing calcium flux leading to contracture if the beating heart is rapidly cooled by perfusing it with cold non-cardioplegic blood (90). This latter effect can be offset by warm blood cardioplegic induction before profound myocardial cooling (91).

Myocardial energy requirements are determined principally by cardiac electromechanical work and secondarily by temperature. As discussed earlier in this chapter, attempts to lower myocardial temperature below 15°C have very little effect on myocardial oxygen balance. Indeed, the administration of large volumes of crystalloid cardioplegia into hearts with diffuse coronary disease will serve largely to produce haemodilution, myocardial oedema, and hyperkalaemia. A recent prospective randomized trial showed superior recovery of right ventricular function in patients with coronary artery disease receiving cold blood cardioplegic solution without topical cooling when the right ventricular temperature averaged 18–20°C versus < 15°C (92). Profound topical cooling may also make postoperative arrhythmias more frequent (93), increased the prevalence of phrenic nerve injury (94) and produce epicardial thermal injury if ice chips are used (95). A preoccupation with myocardial hypothermia can distract the surgeon from other important aspects of myocardial management such as the control of reperfusion.

Intermittent reinfusions of cold cardioplegia at 10–20 minute intervals maintain arrest and hypothermia and the use of blood brings additional protection, partly because of its ability to maintain oxygen delivery, replenish oxygen levels, lessen myocardial oedema, and remove accumulated metabolites. The cold ischaemic periods provide optimal operating conditions for technical precision and delay recovery of electromechanical activity when the cardioplegic solution is washed away by non-coronary collateral flow.

Warm blood cardioplegic induction

Operations on ischaemic hearts or in patients with advanced left or right ventricular hypertrophy or in patients with hibernating myocardium pose extra problems in myocardial protection. Depletion of energy reserves of glycogen are common in such hearts. They are less tolerant of ischaemia during aortic cross clamping, cannot support cell metabolism when blood supply is interrupted and use oxygen inefficiently during reperfusion (96). The studies of Rosenkranz (97) show that a brief (i.e. 5 minutes) infusion of a warm blood cardioplegic induction results in myocardial oxygen uptake in energy depleted hearts but markedly exceeds basal requirements and improves tolerance to prolong the aortic clamping. Enrichment of the cardioplegic solution with amino acid precursors of the Krebs cycle intermediates (glutamate and aspartate) has been shown experimentally to replenish substrates depleted during ischaemia (98), improve oxygen utilization, and further improve the benefits of subsequent blood cardioplegia (97). In the future other beneficial additives are likely to be defined. This area of metabolic enhancement will be further discussed.

Warm blood cardioplegic reperfusion

Reperfusion injury can be defined as the functional metabolic and structural alteration caused by reperfusion after a period of temporary ischaemia, in the present context, global ischaemia. Reperfusion damage is characterized by

- intracellular calcium accumulation
- explosive cell swelling with reduction of post-ischaemic blood flow and reduced ventricular compliance
- inability to use delivered oxygen even when coronary flow and oxygen content are sufficient
- oxygen-derived free radical damage including neutrophil adherence and activation.

The surgeon is in an advantageous position to control conditions of reperfusion after global ischaemia, a situation quite different to that of the interventional cardiologist dealing with reperfusion following the relief of regional ischaemia. This area has been extensively studied by Buckgberg's group from whom the following principles of controlled reperfusion have emerged:

- re-oxygenation to start aerobic metabolism for energy production to repair cellular injury
- re-warming the reperfusate to 37°C to optimize the rate of metabolic recovery (98)
- delivery of the reperfusate over time rather than dose to maximize oxygen use (99)
- lowering oxygen demands by maintaining cardioplegia to channel available oxygen towards reparative processes (100)
- replenishing substrate to optimize aerobic/energy production (101)
- making pH alkalotic to counteract tissue acidosis and optimize enzyme function (100)
- temporarily reducing ionic calcium available to enter the cell (101)
- inducing hyperosmolarity and decreasing perfusion pressure to minimize reperfusion oedema and endothelial damage (64,102).

In addition, neutrophil depletion (103), calcium channel blocking drugs (101), and oxygen-derived free radical scavenging drugs (104) may also limit reperfusion injury damage and may be used more routinely in the future.

The benefits of combining warm and cold blood cardioplegia are most obvious in the haemo-dynamically compromised patient (e.g. with cardiogenic shock) who undergoes revascularization in order to correct left ventricular pump failure. This approach offers the possibility of both a metabolic and a mechanical correction. The published perioperative mortality rate with standard cold cardioplegic techniques is 30–70% in patients with peri-infarction cardiogenic shock (105). Buckberg and colleagues have reported their uncontrolled clinical studies in which a combination of warm induction, multidose cold cardioplegia, and warm reperfusion has been used. The results are impressive, showing a reduction in the operative mortality to less than 10% in patients with post-infarction cardiogenic shock who undergo early revascularization (106).

Continuous versus intermittent cardioplegia

Concern about the adverse consequences of hypothermia and of intermittent ischaemia led sur-geons at the University of Toronto to suggest the use of continuous warm blood cardioplegia without hypothermia. Under his technique the patient and the heart are maintained at 37°C and cardioplegic delivery is virtually continuous (107). The concept is attractive on theoretical grounds as it avoids ischaemia completely. Unfortunately the concept is unproved and is very dependent upon uniform and adequate distribution of the cardioplegic solution.

There are practical difficulties associated with continuous antegrade perfusion as it is difficult to maintain aortic valve competence when the heart is retracted for circumflex grafts. Although retrograde delivery, as recommended by Salerno (108), can circumvent some of these problems, severe cardiac damage can occur if the catheter becomes dislodged and goes unnoticed for any length of time. Continuous cardioplegia can result in large volumes of cardioplegic solution being administered with consequent systemic hyperkalaemia and serum potassium levels in excess of 8 mmol L^{-1}. Normothermic myocardial injury can easily occur if the cardioplegic infusion has to be stopped in order to achieve a bloodless surgical field. Electromechanical activity tends to recur rapidly as non-coronary collateral flow washes out the cardioplegic solution. By contrast the use of hypothermia will delay the return of electromechanical activity. There are other disturbing and unanswered questions about this technique. Will cerebral complications increase during per-fusion with non-pulsatile flow where mean perfusion pressure is lower? Will there be more fatal perfusion accidents due to the very limited time available at 37°C for the extracorporeal circula-tion to be stopped and the problem corrected before cerebral damage occurs?

A recent report by the Warm Heart Investigators (109) goes some way towards answering these questions. This was a large trial conducted at three hospitals in Toronto in 1372 patients undergoing coronary revascularization. They compared 37°C cardioplegia with systemic nor-mothermia to conventional hypothermic cardiac surgery. In the 'cold' group cardioplegia was administered at 5–8°C with systemic hypothermia at 25–30°C. The 30 day mortality was 2.5% in the 'cold' group and 1.4% in the warm group. The failure to detect a difference in primary outcome results accompanied by conflicting secondary outcome measurements (no difference in mean peak CK–MB, but a lower area under the CK–MB time activity curve in the warm group) may reflect a study population who were low risk. In their original communication, Lichtenstein *et al.* (110) reported the benefits of warm heart surgery in a patient with an ischaemic time >3.5 hours. In contrast, the majority of patients in the current study were good risk (mean age of 62 years, 80% with ejection fractions greater than 40%, 74% elective status, and 96% first time operations). In such a patient population most methods of myocardial protection work well.

However, it is reassuring to find that warm heart surgery was not associated with any increase in the rates of stroke. Warm heart surgery has technical difficulties of its own and it is noteworthy that 8% of patients crossed from the warm to the cold group because of continued cardiac activity or flooding of the operative field.

It seems more likely at the time of writing that warm cardioplegic infusions will be used chiefly as adjuncts to an essentially hypothermic cardioplegic technique.

Metabolic enhancement

Until recently the attention of investigators in myocardial protection has been almost exclusively directed to the myocyte. More attention needs to be given to the effects of both ischaemia and reperfusion on the coronary endothelium and conduction tissue. We and others have investigated the relationship between left ventricular function and the functional integrity of the endothelium (111). As we learn more about the functional morphological aspects of silent ischaemia we may be able to apply this knowledge to improve our handling of the coronary endothelium during cardiac surgery. An increasing number of agents have been and are being investigated. Aspartate and glutamate have already been considered. Others include allopurinol (112), co-enzyme Q_{10} (113), and adenosine (16).

Co-enzyme Q_{10} is a naturally occuring component of mitrochondria which transports electrons between flavoproteins and cytochromes during oxidative phosphorylation. This co-enzyme is a potent antioxidant against lipid peroxidation in the myocardial mitochondrial membrane *in vitro*; it therefore has a membrane stabilizing effect. Experimental and clinical studies utilizing Q_{10} in cardioplegia and intravenous infusions prior to reperfusion, as well as oral pretreatment before surgery, have demonstrated a reduction in post-ischaemic ventricular dysfunction (114,115). Pretreatment with allopurinol in experimentally induced ischaemia may reduce infarct size and the incidence of arrhythmias and may improve myocardial function (116). This beneficial action has been attributed to the ability of allopurinol to interfere with the production or actions of oxygen derived free radicals. Recently evidence for the generation of free radicals in cardiac surgery has been reported (117–119). Furthermore, allopurinol has been reported to improve clinical results after cardiac surgery (120–122). In a careful prospective randomized trial of 20 low risk coronary artery surgical patients no benefit in terms of clinical result or myocardial damage as assessed by cardiac troponin T or CK-MB fraction was found (123). It remains unknown whether a benefit might have been demonstrated in a group of patients with acute ischaemia and impaired left ventricular function. The major energy sources for the myocardium under normal conditions are fatty acids and, to a lesser extent, glucose. Under ischaemic conditions the heart switches to anaerobic glycolysis until lactate accumulates and amino acids become an important source of energy.

Recently there has been increased interest in the functional abnormalities in coronary endothelium associated with reperfusion. Van Benthuysen and colleagues (124) in an experimental model of reperfusion injury noted a marked increase in coronary vascular resistance. They concluded that augmented reactivity to vasoconstrictors and a loss of vasodilator function secondary to endothelial injury was the most likely explanation for reperfusion injuries. A number of other studies (125–128) with isolated epicardial coronary arteries have shown that ischaemia and reperfusion caused a marked time-dependent impairment in the ability of vessels to respond to endothelium-dependent agents such as acetylcholine and substance P. Tsao (126) suggested that oxygen-derived free radical mediated injury affecting the release of endothelium derived relaxation factor (EDRF) is primarily responsible for impaired vascular reactivity. Morphological damage to the endothelial cell precedes myocyte necrosis. Endothelial damage occurred in the endothelial cell itself rather than the vascular smooth muscle. If reperfusion does lead to an early impairment of EDRF production by the endothelial cell, the tendency to platelet deposition and aggregation will be increased. Furthermore, quiescent arteries will tend to show an exaggerated constrictive response to platelets. The reduced ability of contracted coronary arteries to relax in response to aggregated platelets could lead to localized vasoconstriction at the site of endothelial injury. This could explain the observed tendency of reperfused myocardium to increased vascular tone of coronary spasm.

There is increased interest in the possibility of drug control of post-ischaemic coronary vascular competence. Potential sites of action include endothelium based receptors, vascular smooth muscle, myocytes, and blood-borne elements such as leukocytes and platelets. Babbitt (16) suggested that adenosine may improve the pathogenesis of ischaemia and reperfusion injury in several ways:

- by replenishment of ATP and endothelial cells
- by arteriolar vasodilatation which will allow an increased oxygen supply and a reduced effect of mechanical obstruction by platelets and leukocytes
- by inhibition of platelet aggregation and thromboxane release
- by reduced leukocyte adherence.

Leukocytes themselves are likely to be major players in reperfusion injury. Possible mechanisms of action include:

- a source of oxygen-derived free radicals leading to reduced control of vascular tone in the coronary bed
- physical obstruction of capillaries
- release of cytokines and proteases, some of which will be cytotoxic.

Strong evidence of a role for neutrophils is provided by Litt *et al.* (129) in which neutrophil depletion, achieved by filtration, was associated with a decrease in tissue injury even when the depletion occurred only at the time of reperfusion. A number of agents have been associated with decreased leukocyte accumulation and a reduction in infarct size, e.g. prostacyclin (130), adenosine (129) and use of a monoclonal antibody against the CD18 integrin of neutrophils. This monoclonal antibody has been shown experimentally to attenuate the influx of neutrophils and to reduce infarct size (130). It is likely that at least some of these agents will appear in clinical trials within the next few years.

Although intraoperative myocardial damage from inadequate protection has decreased progressively, this complication remains the leading cause of death and morbidity after coronary artery surgery. Demographic changes have brought older and sicker patients forward for myocardial revascularization. An individual surgeon needs to have a portfolio of techniques available for different situations and to avoid a rigid adherence to only one strategy for the whole spectrum of coronary surgery, whether in isolation or combined with other procedures. Progress can only be maintained if we keep an open-minded approach to the data available as we strive to avoid intraoperative damage while producing a technically perfect result.

References

1. Califf RM, Harrel FE, Lee KL *et al*. Changing efficacy of coronary revascularisation. Implications for patient selection. *Circulation* 1988;**78** (supplement I):185–91.
2. Melrose DG, Dreyer B, Bentall HH, Baker JBE. Elective cardiac arrest *Lancet* 1955;**2**:21–22.
3. Buckberg GD, Brazier JR, Nelson RL, Goldstein SM, McConnell DH, Cooper N. Studies of the effects of hypothermia on regional myocardial blood flow and metabolism during cardiopulmonary bypass. I. The adequately perfused beating, fibrillating and arrested heart. *J Thorac Cardiovasc Surg* 1977;**3**:87–94.
4. Bretschneider HJ, Hubner G, Knoll D. Myocardial resistance and tolerance to ischaemia: Physiological and biochemical basics. *J Cardiovasc Surg* 1975;**16**:241–60.
5. Kirsch U, Rodewald G, Kalmar P (1972) Induced ischaemic arrest. *J Thorac Cardiovasc Surg*1972;**63**:121–30.
6. Hearse DJ, Stewart DA, Braimbridge MB. Cellular protection during myocardial ischaemia. *Circulation* 1976;**54**:193–202.
7. Gay WA, Ebert PA. Functional, metabolic and morphologic effects of potassium-induced cardioplegia. *Surgery* 1973;**74**:284–90.
8. Cohen MV, Liu GS, Downey JM. Pre-conditioning by a brief coronary occlusion, preserves wall motion in ischaemia/reperfusion. *Circulation* 1990;**82**(suppl III):271.
9. Murry CE, Jennings RB, Reimer KA. New insights into potential mechanisms of ischaemic pre-conditioning. *Circulation* 1991;**84**:442–5.
10. Liu GS, Thornton J, Van Winkle DM, Stanley AWH, Olsson RA, Downey JM. Protection against infarction afforded by pre-conditioning is mediated by A_1 adenosine receptors in rabbit heart. *Circulation* 1991;**84**:350–6.
11. Deutsch E, Berger M, Kussmane WG. Adaptation to ischaemia during percutaneous transluminal coronary angioplasty: Clinical, haemodynamic and metabolic features. *Circulation* 1990;**82**:2044–51.
12. Flameng W, Borges M, Van der Gusse GJ *et al*. Cardioprotective effects of lidoflazine in extensive aortocoronary bypass grafting. *J Thorac Cardiovasc Surg* 1983;**5**:758–68.
13. Yellon DM, Alkhulaifi AM, Pugsley WB. Pre-conditioning the human myocardium. *Lancet* 1993;**342**:276–7.
14. Bolling SF, Olzanski DC, Childs KF, Gallagher KP. Does cardiac 'pre-conditioning' result in enhanced post-ischaemic functional recovery? *Surg Forum* 1991;**42**:239–42.
15. Flameng W, Xhonneux R, Van Belle H. Cardioprotective effects of mioflazine during one hour normothermic global ischaemia in the canine heart. *Cardiovasc Res* 1984;**18**:528–37.
16. Babbitt DG, Virmani R, Forman BM. Intracoronary adenosine administered after reperfusion limits vascular injury after prolonged ischaemia in the canine model. *Circulation* 1989;**80**:1388–99.
16. Lasley RD, Rhee JW, Van Wylen DGL. Adenosine A_1 receptor mediated protection of the globally ischaemic isolated rat heart. *J Mol Cell Cardio* 1989;**22**:39–47.
17. Ledingham S, Katayana O, Lachno D, Yacoub MH. Beneficial effect of adenosine during reperfusion following prolonged cardioplegic arrest. *Cardiovasc Res* 1990;**24**:247–53.
18. Wyatt DA, Ely SW, Lasley RD. Purine enriched asanguine cardioplegia provides superior myocardial protection. *Surg Forum* 1987;**38**:265–7.

19. Petsikas D, Ricci MA, Baffour R. Enhanced 24 hours *in-vitro* heart preservation with adenosine and adenosine monophosphate. *J Heart Transplant* 1987;**9**:114–18.
20. Van Belle H, Goossens F, Wijnants J. Formation and release of purine metabolites during hypoprofusion, anoxia and ischaemia. *Am J Physiol* 1987;**252**:H886–93.
21. Engler RL, Gruber HE. Adenosine: An autocoid. In: Jennings RB *et al*., eds., *The heart and cardiovascular system*, 2nd edn New York: Raven Press, 1992, pp. 1745–64.
22. Gruber HE, Hoffer ME, McAllister DR *et al*. Increased adenosine concentration in blood from ischaemic myocardium by AICA riboside: effects on flow, granulocytes and injury. *Circulation* 1989;**80**:1400–11.
23. Van Belle H, Goossens F, Wijnants J. Biochemical and functional effects of nucleoside transport inhibition in the isolated cat heart. *J Mol Cell Cardiol* 1989;**21**:797–805.
24. Van Belle H, Xhonneux R, Flameng W. Oral pre-treatment with mioflazine completely changes the pattern and remarkably prolongs the accumulation of nucleosides in ischaemic and reperfused myocardium. *Basic Cardiol* 1986;**81**:407–16.
25. Van Belle H. In vivo effects of inhibitors of adenosine uptake. In: Paton DM, ed., *Adenosine and adenosine nucleotides, physiology and pharmacology*. London: Taylor & Francis, 1988, pp. 251–8.
26. Senning A. Ventricular fibrillation during extracorporeal circulation. *Acta Chir Scand* 1951;**171**:8–72.
27. Akins CW, Block PC, Palacios IF. Comparison of coronary artery bypass grafting and percutaneous transluminal coronary angioplasty as initial treatment strategies. *Ann Thorac Surg* 1989;**47**:507–15.
28. Taber RE, Norales AR, Fine G. Myocardial necrosis and the post-operative low cardiac output syndrome. *Ann Thorac Surg* 1967;**4**:12–18.
29. Najafi H, Henson D, Dye WS. Left ventricular haemorrhagic necrosis. *Ann Thorac Surg* 1969;**7**:550–7.
30. Buckberg GD, Fixler DE, Archie JP, Hoffman JIE. Experimental subendocardial ischaemia in dogs with normal coronary arteries. *Circulation Research* 1972;**30**:67–81.
31. Buckberg GD. Recent progress in myocardial protection during cardiac operations. In: Magoon DC, ed., *Cardiac Surgery*, 2nd edn. Philadephia: FA Davis, 1987, pp. 291–319.
32. Hottenrott C, Maloney JV, Buckberg GD. Studies of the effects of ventricular fibrillation on the adequacy of regional myocardial flow. 1. Electrical versus spontaneous fibrillation. *J Thorac Cardiovasc Surg* 1974;**68**:615–25.
33. Hottenrott C, Buckberg GD. Studies of the effects of ventricular fibrillation on the adequacy of regional myocardial flow. 2. Effects of ventricular distension. *J Thorac Cardiovasc Surg* 1974;**68**:626–33.
34. Hottenrott CE, Towers B, Kurkji HD, Maloney JV, Buckberg G. The hazard of ventricular fibrillation in hypertrophied ventricles during cardiopulmonary bypass. *J Thorac Cardiovasc Surg* 1973;**66**:742–53.
35. Brazier JR, Cooper N, McConnell DH, Buckberg GD. Studies of the effects of hypothermia on regional myocardial blood flow and metabolism during cardiopulmonary bypass. IV: Topical atrial hypothermia in normothermic beating hearts. *J Thorac Cardiovasc Surg* 1977;**73**:102–9.
36. Blauth CI, Cosgrove DM, Webb BW *et al*. Atheroembolism from the ascending aorta. *J Thorac Cardiovasc Surg* 1992;**103**:1104–12.

37. Pepper JR, Lockey E, Cankovic-Darracott S, Braimbridge MV. Cardioplegia versus intermittent ischaemic arrest in coronary bypass surgery. *Thorax* 1982;**37**:887–92.

38. Bonchek LI, Burlingame MW, Vazales BE, Lindy EF, Gassmann CJ. Applicability of non-cardioplegic coronary bypass in high-risk patients. *J Thorac Cardiovasc Surg* 1992;**103**:230–7.
    Braimbridge MV, Chayer J, Bitensky *et al.* (1977). Cold cardioplegia or continuous coronary perfusion. *J Thorac Cardiovasc Surg* 1977;**74**:900–6.

39. Brazier J, Hottenrott C, Buckberg G. Non-coronary collateral myocardial blood flow. *Ann Thorac Surg* 1975;**19**:426–35.

40. Conti VR, Bertranou EG, Blackstone EH, Kirklin JW. Cold cardioplegia versus hypothermia for myocardial protection. *J Thorac Cardiovasc Surg* 1978;**76**:577–89.

41. Follette DM, Mulder DG, Maloney JV, Buckberg GD. Advantages of blood cardioplegia over continuous coronary perfusion or intermittent ischaemia: experimental and clinical studies. *J Thorac Cardiovasc Surg* 1978;**76**:604–19.
    Follette DM, Steed DL, Foglia RP, Buckberg DG. Advantages of intermittent blood cardioplegia over intermittent ischaemia during prolonged hypothermic aortic clamping. *Cardiovasc Surg* 1976;**58**:1–200.

42. Feindel CM, Tait GA, Wilson GJ, Klenent P, MacGregor DC. Multi-dose blood versus crystalloid cardioplegia: Comparison by quantitative assessment of irreversible myocardial injury. *J Thorac Cardiovasc Surg* 1984;**87**:585–95.

43. Robertson JM, Buckberg GD, Vinten-Johansen J, Leaf JD. Comparison of distribution beyond coronary stenosis of blood and asanguineous cardioplegic solutions. *J Thorac Cardiovasc Surg* 1983;**86**:80–6.

44. Shapira N, Kirsch MM, Jochim K, Behrendt DM. Comparison of the effect of blood cardioplegia to crystalloid cardioplegia on myocardial contractility in man. *J Thorac Cardiovasc Surg* 1980;**80**:647–55.

45. Cunningham JN, Adams PX, Knapp EA *et al.* Protection of ATP, ultrastructure and ventricular function after aortic cross-clamping and reperfusion: clinical use of blood potassium cardioplegia. *J Thorac Cardiovasc Surg* 1979;**78**:708–20.

46. Singh AK, Farrugia R, Teplitz C, Karlson KE. Electrolyte versus blood cardioplegia: Randomised clinical and myocardial ultrastructural study. *Ann Thorac Surg* 1982;**33**:218–27.

47. Iverson LIH, Young JN, Ennix CL *et al.* Myocardial protection: A comparison of cold blood and cold crystalloid cardioplegia. *J Thorac Cardiovasc Surg* 1984;**87**:509–16.

48. Roberts AJ, Moran JM, Sanders JH. Clinical evaluation of the relative effectiveness of multi-dose crystalloid and cold blood potassium cardioplegia in coronary artery bypass surgery: a non-randomised matched pair analysis. *Ann Thorac Surg* 1982;**33**:421–33.

49. Daggett WM, Randolph JD, Jacobs M *et al.* The superiority of cold oxygenated dilute blood cardioplegia. *Ann Thorac Surg* 1987;**43**:397–402.

50. Bodenhamer RM, De Boer LWV, Geffin GA *et al.* Enhanced myocardial protection during ischaemic arrest: oxygenation of a crystalloid cardioplegic solution. *J Thorac Cardiovasc Surg* 1983;**85**:769–80.

51. Hicks GL, Arnold W, De Wall RA. Fluorocarbon cardioplegia and myocardial protection. *Ann Thorac Surg* 1983;**35**:500–3.

52. Gardner TJ, Stewart JR, Casale AS. Reduction of myocardial ischaemic injury with oxygen-derived free radical scavengers. *Surgery* 1983;**94**:423–9.

53. Ledingham SJM, Braimbridge MV, Hearse DJ. Improved myocardial protection by oxygenation of the St Thomas' Hospital cardioplegic solutions. *J Thorac Cardiovasc Surg* 1988;**95**:103–11.

54. Illes RW, Silverman NA, Krukenkamp IB, Yusen RD, Chausow DD, Levitsky S. The efficacy of blood cardioplegia is not due to oxygen delivery. *J Thorac Cardiovasc Surg* 1989;**98**:1051–6.

55. Julia PL, Buckberg DG, Acar C, Partington MT, Sherman M. Studies of controlled reperfusion after ischaemia. XXI. Reperfusate composition: Superiority of blood cardioplegia over crystalloid cardioplegia in limiting reperfusion damage. Importance of endogenous oxygen free radical scavengers in red blood cells. *J Thorac Cardiovasc Surg* 1991;**101**:303–13.

56. Manning AS, Hearse DJ. Reperfusion-induced arrhythmias: Mechanisms and prevention. *J Cell Mol Cardiol* 1984;**16**:497–518.

57. Kloner RA, De Boer LWV, Dorsee JR *et al.* Prolonged abnormalities of myocardium salvaged by reperfusion. *Am J Physiol* 1981;**241**:H591–9.

58. Gallinones M, Hearse DJ. The consequences of asanguineous versus sanguineous reperfusion after long-term preservation of the heart. *Eur J Cardiothoracic Surg* 1990;**4**:273–7.

59. Atkinson DE. The energy charge of the adenylate pool as a regulatory parameter. Interaction with feedback modifiers. *Biochemistry* 1968;**7**:4030–4.

60. Danforth WH, Naegle S, Bing RJ. Effect of ischaemia and re-oxygenation of glycolytic reactions and adenosine triphosphate in heart muscle. *Circ Res* 1960;**8**:965–71.

61. Digerness SB, Tracy WG, Andrews NF, Bowdoin B, Kirklin JW. Reversal of myocardial ischaemic contracture and the relationship to functional recovery in tissue calcium. *Circulation* 1983;**68**(suppl, II):34–40.

62. Teoh KH, Christakis GT, Weisel RD. Accelerated myocardial metabolic recovery with terminal warm blood cardioplegia. *J Thorac Cardiovasc Surg* 1986;**91**:888–95.

63. Roberts AJ, Woodhall DD, Knauf DG. Coronary artery bypass graft surgery: clinical comparison of cold blood potassium cardioplegia, warm cardioplegic induction and secondary cardioplegia. *Ann Thorac Surg* 1985;**40**:483–8.

64. Okamoto F, Allen BS, Buckberg GD, Gugyi H, Leaf J. Studies of controlled reperfusion after ischaemia. Reperfusate conditions XIV: importance of ensuring gentle versus sudden reperfusion after relief of coronary occlusion. *J Thorac Cardiovasc Surg* 1986;**92**:613–20.

65. Sawatari K, Kadoba K, Bergner BA, Mayer JE. Influence of initial reperfusion pressure after hypothermic cardioplegic ischaemia on endothelial modulation of coronary tone in neonatal lambs. Impaired coronary vasodilator responce to acetyl choline. *J Thorac Cardiovasc Surg* 1991;**101**:777–82.

66. Aldea GS, Austin RE, Flynn AE, Coggins DL, Husseini W, Hoffman JIE. Heterogeneous delivery of cardioplegic solution in the absence of coronary artery disease. *J Thorac Cardiovasc Surg* 1990;**99**:345–53.

67. Fontan F, Madonna F, Naftel DC. The effect of reperfusion pressure on early outcomes after coronary artery bypass grafting: a randomised trial. *J Thorac Cardiovasc Surg* 1993;**106**:989–94.

68. Fontan F, Madonna F, Naftel DC. Modifying myocardial management in cardiac surgery: A randomised trial. *Eur J Cardiothorac Surg* 1992;**6**:127–37.

69. Lazar HL, Buckberg GD, Manganaro AM. Reversal of ischaemic damage with amino acid substrate enhancement during reperfusion. *Surgery* 1980;**80**:702–9.

70. Lazar HL, Buckberg GD, Manganaro AM, Becker H. Myocardial energy replenishment of secondary blood cardioplegia with amino acids during reperfusion. *J Thorac Cardiovasc Surg* 1980;**80**:350–9.

71. Rosenkranz ER, Buckberg GD, Laks H, Mulder DG. Warm induction of cardioplegia with glutamate-enriched blood in coronary patients with cardiogenic shock who are dependent on inotropic drugs and intra-aortic balloon support. *J Thorac Cardiovasc Surg* 1983;**86**:507–18.

72. Rosenkranz ER, Okamoto F, Buckberg GD. Advantages of glutamate-enriched cold blood cardioplegia in the energy-depleted hearts. *Circulation* 1982;**66**:suppl II,151–5.

73. Choong YS, Gavin JB. l-Aspartate improves the functional recovery of explanted hearts stored in St Thomas's Hospital cardioplegic solution at 4°C. *J Thorac Cardiovasc Surg* 1990;**99**:510–17.

74. Gharagozloo F, Melendez FJ, Hein RA *et al.* The effect of amino acid l-glutamate on the extended preservation ex vivo of the heart for transplantation. *Circulation* 1987;**76**:suppl V, 65–70.

75. Steenbergen C, Murphy E, Watts JA, London RE. Correlation between cytosolic free calcium, contracture, ATP and irreversible ischaemic injury in perfused rat heart. *Circ Res* 1990;**66**:135–46.

76. Olinger GN, Boerboom LE, Boncheck LI, Hutchinson LB, Kissebah AH. Hyperkalaemia in cardioplegic solutions causing increased cholesterol accumulation in vein grafts. *J Thorac Cardiovasc Surg* 1983;**85**:590–4.

77. Mankad PS, Chester AH, Yacoub MH. Role of potassium concentration in cardioplegic solutions in mediating endothelial damage. *Ann Thorac Surg* 1991;**51**:89–93.

78. Pratt FH. The nutrition of the heart through the vessels of the Thebesius and coronary veins. *Am J Physiol* 1898;**1**:86–94.

79. Lillehei CW, De Wall RA, Gott VL. The direct vision correction of calcific aortic stenosis by means of a pump-oxygenator and retrograde coronary sinus perfusion. *Dis Chest* 1956;**30**:123–32.

80. Menasche P, Piwnica A. Retrograde cardioplegia through the coronary sinus. *Ann Thorac Surg* 1987;**44**:214–16.

81. Chitwood WR Jr. Retrograde cardioplegia: Current methods. *Ann Thorac Surg* 1992;**53**:352–5.

82. Diehl JT, Eichlorn EJ, Konstam MA *et al.* Efficacy of retrograde coronary sinus cardioplegia in patients undergoing myocardial revascularisation: A prospective randomised trial. *Ann Thorac Surg* 1988;**45**:595–602.

83. Loop FD, Higgins TL, Randa R, Pearce G, Estafanous FG. Myocardial protection during cardiac operations: Decreased morbidity and lower cost with blood cardioplegia and coronary sinus perfusion. *J Thorac Cardiovasc Surg* 1992;**104**:608–18.

84. Buckberg GD, Drinkwater DC, Laks H. A new technique for delivering anterograde/retrograde blood cardioplegia without right heart isolation. *Eur J Cardiothoracic Surg* 1990;**4**:163–8.

85. Bigelow WG, Lindsay WK, Greenwood WF. Hypothermia. Its possible role in cardiac surgery. *Ann Thorac Surg* 1950;**13**:849–56.

86. Shumway NE, Lower RR. Hypothermia for extended periods of anoxic arrest. *Surg Forum* 1959;**10**:563–4.

87. Kaijser L, Jansson E, Schmidt W, Bomfin V. Myocardial energy depletion during profound hypothermic cardioplegia for cardiac operations. *J Thorac Cardiovasc Surg* 1985;**90**:896–900.

88. Teoh KH, Christakis GT, Weisel RD. Dipyridamole reduces myocardial platelet and leukocyte deposition following ischaemia and cardioplegia. *J Surg Res* 1987;**42**:36–44.

89. Neeling JR, Whitmer JT, Rovetto MJ. Effective coronary blood flow on glycolytic flux and intracellular pH in isolated rat hearts. *Circ Res* 1975;**37**:733–40.

90. Rebeyka IM, Hanam SA, Borges MR *et al*. Rapid cooling contracture of the myocardium: the adverse effect of pre-arrest cardiac hypothermia. *J Thorac Cardiovasc Surg* 1990;**100**:240–9.

91. Williams WG, Rebeyka IM, Tibshirani RJ *et al*. Warm induction of blood cardioplegia in the infant. A technique to avoid rapid cooling myocardial contracture. *J Thorac Cardiovasc Surg* 1990;**100**:896–901.

92. Mullen JC, Birnbaum PL, Weisel RD. Profound cardiac hypothermia for myocardial protection. *J Thorac Cardiovasc Surg* 1993;**105**:421–7.

93. Weisel RD. Discussion of Gundry SR, Sequeira, Coughlin TR, McLaughlin JS: Post-operative conduction disturbances — a comparison of blood and crystalloid cardioplegia. *Ann Thorac Surg* 1989;**47**:384–90.

94. Allen VS, Buckberg GD, Rosenkranz ER *et al*. Topical cardiac hypothermia in patients with coronary disease: an unnecessary adjunct to cardioplegic protection and cause of pulmonary morbidity. *J Thorac Cardiovasc Surg* 1992;**104**:626–631.

95. Speicher CE, Ferrigan L, Wolfson SK, Yalav EH, Rawson AJ. Cold injury of myocardium and pericardium in cardiac hypothermia. *Surg Gynae Obstet* 1962;**114**:659–65.

96. Lazar HL, Buckberg GD, Manganaro AM. Myocardial energy replenishment and reversal of ischaemic damage by substrate enhancement of secondary blood cardioplegia with amino acids during reperfusion. *J Thorac Cardiovasc Surg* 1980;**80**:350–9.

97. Rosenkranz ER, Buckberg GD, Laks H, Mulder DG. Warm induction of cardioplegia with glutamate-enriched blood in coronary patients with cardiogenic shock who are dependent on inotropic drugs and intra-aortic balloon support. *J Thorac Cardiovasc Surg* 1983;**86**:507–18.

98. Lazar HL, Buckberg GD, Manganaro A. Limitations imposed by hypothermia during recovery from ischaemia. *Surg Forum* 1980;**31**:312–15.

98. Tixier D, Matheis G, Buckberg GD, Young HH. Donor hearts with impaired haemodynamics: Benefit of warm substrate enriched blood cardioplegia induction during cardiac harvesting. *J Thorac Cardiovasc Surg* 191;**102**:207–14.

99. Allen BS, Okamoto F, Buckberg GD, Bugyi H, Leaf J. Studies of controlled reperfusion after ischaemia XII: Considerations of reperfusate 'duration' versus 'dose' on regional, functional, biochemical and histochemical recovery. Studies of controlled reperfusion after ischaemia: Reperfusate conditions. *J Thorac Cardiovasc Surg* 1986;**92**:594–604.

100. Follette DM, Fey K, Buckberg GD *et al*. Reducing post-ischaemic damage by temporary modification of reperfusate calcium, potassium, pH and osmolarity. *J Thorac Cardiovasc Surg* 1981;**82**:221–38.

101. Allen BS, Okamoto F, Buckberg GD *et. al*. Studies of controlled reperfusion after ischaemia IX: benefits of marked hypokalaemia and diltiazem on regional recovery. *J Thorac Cardiovasc Surg* 1986;**52**:564–572.

102. Okamoto F, Allen BS, Buckberg GD, Young H, Bugyi H, Leaf J. Studies of controlled reperfusion after ischaemia. Reperfusate composition XI: interaction of marked hyperglycaemia and marked hyperosmolarity in allowing immediate contractile recovery after four hours of regional ischaemia. *J Thorac Cardiovasc Surg* 1986;**92**:583–93.

103. Engler RL, Schmid-Schonbein GW, Pavelec RS. Leukocyte capillary plugging in myocardial ischaemia and reperfusion in the dog. *Am J Pathol* 1983;**111**:98–111.

104. Emerit I, Fabiani J-N, Ponzio O, Murday A, Lunel F, Carpentier A. Clastogenic factor in ischaemia-reperfusion injury during open-heart surgery: Protective effect of allopurinol. *Ann Thorac Surg* 1988;**46**:619–24.

105. Berg R, Selinger SL, Leonard JJ. *Surgical management of acute myocardial infarction in cardiac surgery*, Philadelphia: FA Davis, 1992, pp. 61–74.

106. Allen BS, Rosenkranz ER, Buckberg GD *et al*. Studies on prolonged acute regional ischaemia VI: myocardial infarction with left ventricular power failure: a medical/surgical emergency requiring urgent revascularisation with maximal protection of remote muscle. *J Thorac Cardiovasc Surg* 1989;**98**:691–703.

107. Lichtenstein SV, Ashe KE, Elati H, El Dalati H. Warm heart surgery. *J Thorac Cardiovasc Surg* 1991;**101**:269–74.

108. Salerno TA, Houck JP, Barrozo CA *et al*. Retrograde continuous warm blood cardioplegia: A new concept in myocardial protection. *Ann Thorac Surg* 1991;**51**:245–7.

109. Warm Heart Investigators. Randomised trial of normothermic versus hypothermic coronary bypass surgery. *Lancet* 1994;**343**:559–63.

110. Lichtenstein SV, El Dalati M, Panos A, Slutsky AS. Long cross-clamp times with warm heart surgery. *Lancet* 1989;**1**, 1443.

111. Amrani M, O'Shea J, Allen N. *et al*. Role of basic release of nitric oxide on coronary flow and mechanical performance of the isolated rat heart. *J Physiol* 1992;**456**:681–87.

112. Chambers DJ, Braimbridge MB, Hearse DJ. Free radicals and cardioplegia: Allopurinol and oxypurinol reduce myocardial injury following ischaemic arrest. *Ann Thorac Surg* 1987;**44**:291–7.

113. Greenburg S, Frishman WH. Co-enzyme Q_{10}: a new drug for cardiovascular disease. *J Clin Pharmacol* 1990;**30**:596–601.

114. Okamoto F, Allen BS, Buckberg GD, Leaf J, Bugyi H. Reperfusate composition: Supplemental role of intravenous and intracoronary co-enzyme Q_{10} in avoiding reperfusion damage. *J Thorac Cardiovasc Surg* 1986;**92**:573–80.

115. Tanaka J, Tominaga R, Yoshitoshi M *et al*. Co-enzyme Q_{10}: the prophylactic effect on low cardiac output following cardiac valve replacement. *Ann Thorac Surg* 1982;**33**:145–9.

116. Stewart JR, Crute SL, Loughlin V, Hess ML, Greenfield LJ. Prevention of free radical-induced myocardial reperfusion injury with allopurinol. *J Thorac Cardiovasc Surg* 1985;**90**:68–72.

117. Cavarocchi NC, England MD, Schaff HV *et al*. Oxygen free radical generation during cardiopulmonary bypass: correlation with complement activation. *Circulation* 1986;**74** (suppl III):130–3.

118. Bolli R, Jeroudi MO, Patel BS *et al*. Marked reduction of free radical generation and contractile dysfunction by antioxidant therapy begun at the time of reperfusion. Evidence that myocardial 'stunning' is a manifestation of reperfusion injury. *Circ Res* 1989;**65**:607–22.

119. Ferrari R, Alfieri O, Curello S *et al*. Occurrence of oxidative stress during reperfusion of the human heart. *Circulation* 1990;**81**:201–11.

120. Johnson WD, Kayser KL, Brenowitz JB, Saedi SF. A randomised controlled trial of allopurinol in coronary bypass surgery. *Am Heart J* 1991;**121**:20–4.

121. Rashid MA, William-Olsson G. Influence of allopurinol on cardiac complications in open heart operations. *Ann Thorac Surg* 1991;**52**:127–30.

122. Tabayashi K, Suzuki y, Nagamine S, Ito Y, Sekino Y, Mohri H. A clinical trial of allopurinol (Zyloric) for myocardial protection. *J Thorac Cardiovasc Surg* 1991;**101**:713–18.

123. Taggart DP, Young V, Hooper J *et al*. Lack of cardioprotective efficacy of allopurinol in coronary artery surgery. *Br Heart J* 1994;**71**:177–81.

124. Van Benthuysen KM, McMurtry IF, Horwitz LD. Reperfusion after acute coronary occlusion in dogs impairs endothelium-dependent relaxation to acetyl choline and augments contractile reactivity in vitro. *J Clin Invest* 1987;**79**:265–74.

125. Pearson PJ, Schaff HV, Vanhoutte PM. Acute impairment of endothelium-dependent relaxation to aggregating platelets following reperfusion injury in canine coronary arteries. *Circ Res* 1990;**67**:385–93.

126. Tsao PS, Lefter AM. Time course and mechanism of endothelial dysfunction in isolated ischaemic- and hypoxic-perfused rat hearts. *Am J Physiol* 1990;**259**:H1660–6.

127. Dauber IM, Van Benthuysen KM, McMurty IF. Functional coronary microvascular injury evidence as increased permeability due to brief ischaemia and reperfusion. *Circ Res* 1990;**60**:986–98.

127. Litt MR, Jeremy RW, Weisman HF, Winkelstein JA, Becker LC. Neutrophil depletion limited to reperfusion reduces myocardial infarct size after 90 minutes of ischaemia. Evidence for neutrophil-mediated reperfusion injury. *Circulation* 1989;**80**:1816–27.

128. Mehta JL, Lawson DL, Nichols WW. Atenuated coronary relaxation after reperfusion: Effects of superoxide dismutase and TxA$_2$ inhibitor. *Am J Physiol* 1989;**257**:H1240–6.

128. Johnson G, Furlan LE, Aoki N. Endothelium and myocardial protecting actions of taprostene, a stable prostacyclin analogue, after acute myocardial ischaemia and reperfusion in cats. *Circ Res* 1990;**66**:1362–70.

129. Olafsson B, Forman MB, Puett DW *et al*. Reduction of reperfusion injury in the canine preparation by intracoronary adenosine: Importance of the endothelium and the 'no reflow' phenomenon. *Circulation* 1987;**76**:1135–45.

130. Ma XL, Tsao PS, Vierman GE. Neutrophil-mediated vascoconstriction and endothelial dysfunction in low-flow perfusion — reperfused cat coronary artery. *Circ Res* 1991;**69**:95–106.

5   Myocardial reperfusion injury

Robert C. Gorman and Timothy J. Gardner

Early in the history of cardiac surgery, it was recognized that some patients who underwent technically successful operations suffered from a syndrome of low cardiac output in the early postoperative period. It was also apparent that the perioperative mortality was increased in these patients. Autopsy and clinical studies in the late 1960s and early 1970s documented that myocardial necrosis (particularly in the subendocardial region) was common after cardiac surgery. This intraoperative loss of myocytes was believed to be the cause of the low cardiac output syndrome. The fact that myocardial necrosis occurred in patients with normal coronary arteries suggested that better intraoperative protection of the myocardium would improve operative results.

Laboratory and clinical research activity over the last 15 years has led to techniques for prolonging myocardial tolerance to ischemia during cardiac surgery. It has become apparent that postoperative myocardial dysfunction is a result of the deleterious effects initiated by a period of global ischemia and exacerbated by reperfusion. Ischemia and reperfusion may cause an irreversible cell necrosis or, if less severe, may result in a reversible depression of myocardial function. The latter phenomenon has been termed myocardial stunning. Myocardial injury due to ischemia and subsequent reperfusion may be viewed as a continuum. At one extreme, a period of ischemia may cause minimal disturbance of myocyte physiology and will result in normal function irrespective of the condition during reperfusion. At the other end of the spectrum, there are cells that are so severely damaged by ischemia that cell death is assured no matter how the reperfusion conditions are modified. Between these extremes, there is myocardium in which metabolic function has been adversely affected by ischemia but may be resuscitated if reperfusion injury is minimized.

Presented in this chapter is a detailed review of the functional, metabolic, and structural alterations that occur within the myocardium during an ischemic insult and subsequent reperfusion. Strategies to minimize reperfusion damage to myocytes and endothelial cells are also discussed. A brief review of the basic concepts of myocardial preservation during ischemia is provided; however, a detailed presentation of this topic is given in chapter 4.

Ischemic injury

Pathophysiology of myocardial ischemia

Myocyte injury

Cessation of blood flow to the myocardium causes biochemical derangements that result in changes in myocyte morphology. These structural changes lead to cell death if blood flow is not re-established. Decreased oxygen and metabolic substrate supply, as well as accumulation of metabolic by-products, are immediate consequences of ischemia. Within seconds, there is conversion from aerobic to anaerobic glycolysis. The anaerobic metabolism of glucose yields less than 10% of the ATP associated with aerobic metabolism. Thus ATP and glycogen stores are rapidly depleted. Protons, lactate, and inorganic phosphates accumulate intracellularly. Low levels of intracellular ATP as well as acidosis act to inhibit function of the Na^+/K^+ ATPase, resulting in a loss of intracellular K^+ and accumulation of Na^+. All these factors act to quickly decrease myocardial contractility and predispose the myocyte to injury upon reperfusion. The biochemical changes that occur during early ischemia do not result in cell ultrastructural changes, and reperfusion at this point ultimately results in restoration of normal myocyte function.

With continued ischemia, ATP levels fall further, as does the total adenosine nucleotide pool. ATP is degraded to ADP, AMP, inosine, and ultimately hypoxanthine. Protons, lactate, and inorganic phosphates continue to accumulate, leading to an increase in intracellular osmolarity. These osmotically active molecules act to draw fluid intracellularly, resulting in cellular swelling and increased stress on the plasma membrane. Other than cell swelling, ultrastructural changes at this point are minimal. Although the plasma membrane remains intact, elevated levels of lysophosphoglycerides indicate that alterations in the cell membrane phospholipid bilayer have begun to occur.

If ischemia is allowed to continue beyond 30–40 minutes, metabolic and morphologic changes begin to occur rapidly. Lysophosphoglyceride levels continue to rise, indicating ongoing compromise of the plasma membrane, α_2-adrenergic receptor density increases, and the Ca^{2+} accumulating activity of the sarcoplasmic reticulum is progressively impaired. Ultrastructural changes after 60 minutes of ischemia include swelling of the myocyte, mitochondria, and sarcoplasmic reticulum. Frank discontinuities in the plasma membrane develop and allow free diffusion of water, electrolytes, and macromolecules through a once semipermeable membrane. At this point, cellular death is assured irrespective of reperfusion conditions.

In addition to the morphologic changes that result from ischemia, there are biochemical sequelae of ischemia that potentiate reperfusion injury. Most significantly, elevated levels of adenosine metabolites (xanthine, hypoxanthine, and inosine) coupled with ischemia-induced conversion of xanthine dehydrogenase to xanthine oxidase set the stage for oxygen free radical production when oxygen supply is re-established. Ischemia also reduces intracellular levels of naturally occurring antioxidants, which further compounds the propensity for free radical formation during reperfusion.

Endothelial injury

The endothelial cells of the myocardial microvasculature are also adversely affected by ischemia. Structural changes appear minimal during the ischemic period itself. However, with reperfusion endothelial cell swelling and separation occur. Platelet and neutrophil aggregates also develop. These factors lead to microvascular occlusion and tissue edema that act to prolong ischemia even after reperfusion. This situation has been termed the no-reflow phenomenon and is discussed in more detail subsequently.

Strategies for myocardial protection during Ischemia

The adverse effects of ischemia and reperfusion are initiated by an imbalance in the cellular supply and demand for oxygen as well as metabolic substrates. The inability to clear the injurious

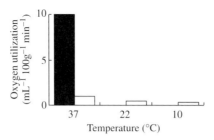

Fig. 5.1 Myocardial oxygen utilization during cardiopulmonary bypass. Black bar indicates beating (working) heart; white bars indicate arrest.

products of anaerobic metabolism also contributes to cell injury. Circumstances that reduce myocardial energy demand mitigate the effects of ischemia and extend the interval during which ischemia may be tolerated. Myocardial energy requirements are determined most importantly by the amount of electromechanical work performed, and to a lesser extent by the temperature. Normothermic cardiac arrest decreases myocardial oxygen consumption by 90%. Cooling of the myocardium to 22°C results in an additional 7% decrease in oxygen demand (Fig. 5.1). Diastolic cardiac arrest with hyperkalemic solution and hypothermia are well-accepted clinical techniques to prevent ischemic injury during cardiac surgery. Various algorithms for implementing these concepts have been developed and are discussed in detail elsewhere in this text.

Recent studies have suggested myocardial protection during ischemia may be improved by providing metabolic substrates both prior to ischemia and during ischemia. Enrichment of cardioplegic solution with Kreb's cycle intermediaries (aspartate and glutamate) in experimental preparations provide additional substrate to support anaerobic metabolism and prevent further reduction in the myocardial energy charge during ischemia. This strategy may be important for myocardial protection in the high-risk patient who comes to surgery with an energy-depleted myocardium due to severe unstable angina, failed angioplasty, shock, or hypertrophy.

Reperfusion injury

The restoration of blood flow after a period of myocardial ischemia has been shown to cause cellular injury that was not present during circulatory interruption. Major features of reperfusion injury include explosive cell swelling, intracellular and mitochondrial calcium accumulation, an impaired ability to utilize oxygen, disruption of cellular enzyme activity, and loss of normal cell membrane function.

Intensive laboratory investigation over the last 20 years has determined that injury induced by myocardial reperfusion is a complex multifactorial process. Oxygen free radicals and activated neutrophils, which abound with reperfusion, have been demonstrated to be major contributors to myocardial injury. These factors, as well as alteration in arachidonic acid metabolism and transmembrane ion homeostasis, act together and potentiate myocardial injury. The result is a self-perpetuating chain reaction of destructive events that may lead to lethal perturbations of myoctye and endothelial cell function.

An understanding of the pathophysiology of this process allows modification of post-ischemic conditions to reduce the degree of injury to the myocardium. Familiarity with this topic is important for the cardiac surgeon, since the potential for clinically significant reperfusion injury exists during all cardiac operations in which the coronary circulation is temporarily interrupted.

Oxygen free radical-induced injury

The generation of oxygen free radicals has been clearly established as a fundamental process in the development of reperfusion injury in many organs including the heart. Free radicals are molecules in which an unpaired electron exists in the outer shell of a molecule, rendering it highly chemically reactive. If two free radicals react, both are eliminated. If a free radical reacts with a non-radical, other free radicals must be produced. This characteristic enables these highly reactive species to participate in rapid self-perpetuating chain reactions. Free radical species commonly found in biologic systems include superoxide ($\cdot O_2$), hydroxyl radical ($\cdot OH$), hydrogen peroxide (H_2O_2), and hypochlorous acid. These compounds are injurious to proteins, sugars, and nucleic acids.

The myocardium is constantly exposed to small quantities of oxygen free radicals as a result of mitochondrial electron transport, prostaglandin synthesis, catecholamine oxidation, and activated neutrophils. Normally, free radicals are degraded safely by a variety of naturally occurring antioxidant systems. Metabolic changes that occur during ischemia and cardiopulmonary bypass greatly enhance the production of free radicals at the time of reperfusion, when an ample supply of oxygen becomes available. Perturbations in adenosine metabolism, activation of neutrophils, and non-cellular radical formation combine to potentiate myocardial injury during reperfusion. An ischemia-induced decrease in antioxidant activity further exacerbates cell injury.

Adenosine metabolism

As previously discussed, sustained myocardial ischemia leads to breakdown of ATP, ultimately resulting in high cellular levels of xanthine and hypoxanthine. In the non-ischemically injured myocardium, these compounds are metabolized via xanthine dehydrogenase with nicotinamide adenine dinucleotide (NAD) being used as the electron acceptor (equation 1).

$$\text{Hypoxanthine} + \text{NAD}^+ + H_2O$$
$$\text{xanthine dehydrogenase} \rightarrow \text{xanthine} + \text{NADH} + H^+ \tag{1}$$
$$\text{Hypoxanthine} + 2O_2 + H_2O$$
$$\text{xanthine oxidase} \rightarrow \text{xanthine} + 2O_2 + 2H^+ \tag{2}$$
$$\text{xanthine} + 2O_2 + H_2O$$
$$\text{xanthine oxidase} \rightarrow \text{uric acid} + 2O_2 + 2H^+ \tag{3}$$

During reperfusion, xanthine dehydrogenase is converted to xanthine oxidase by an enzyme activated by elevated intracellular Ca^{2+} levels. This enzymatic alteration modifies xanthine and hypoxanthine metabolism so that oxygen is used as the electron receptor and superoxide free radicals are formed (equations 2 and 3).

Thus increased levels of ATP metabolites due to ischemia and an increase in xanthine oxidase activity (itself a result of reperfusion-induced Ca^{2+} accumulation) combine to produce significant quantities of free radicals (Fig. 5.2).

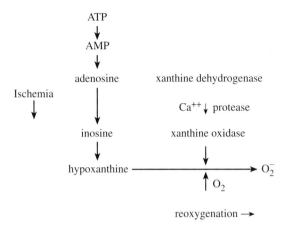

Fig. 5.2   Mechanism for ischaemia induced production of superoxide.

Free radicals and neutrophils

Oxygen free radicals are formed and utilized by neutrophils normally as part of their armamentarium for host defense. Stimulation of neutrophils results in an immediate 'respiratory burst' that develops superoxide, hydrogen peroxide, and hypochloric acid. Cardiopulmonary bypass is a massive inflammatory stimulus that results in a generalized activation of the complement cascade. The resulting formation of C3a, C5a and other chemoattractants activates neutrophils, which subsequently release oxygen radicals. Neutrophils contribute to reperfusion injury by other mechanisms which will be discussed subsequently.

Non-cellular free radical production

Oxygen-derived free radicals may also be created via extracellular inorganic reactions involving iron ions (equation 4).

$$Fe^{2+} + H_2O_2 \rightarrow Fe^{3+} + OH + H^+ \tag{4}$$

Iron-containing products released by hemolysis during cardiopulmonary bypass may facilitate free radical production via this mechanism.

Depletion of protective antioxidants

Endogenous mechanisms exist to control both the production of free radicals and radical mediated damage. Superoxide dismutase catalyzes the reduction of superoxide to the less reactive hydrogen peroxide. Hydrogen peroxide can then be reduced to water by catalase, glutathione peroxidase, or glutathione. The tissue concentration of these antioxidant enzyme systems is depleted during ischemia, thereby decreasing the natural defense mechanisms against oxygen radicals.

Mechanism of free radical injury

During the early reperfusion period, the introduction of abundant supplies of oxygen combined with the previously described ischemia-induced changes in myocardial metabolism results in an explosive production of free radicals. Oxygen radicals react readily via peroxidation reactions with cell membrane lipids. Lipid peroxidation, once initiated, is a process that proceeds as a self-perpetuating chain reaction. Peroxidation alters function of phospholipid bilayers throughout the myocyte. The once semipermeable cell membrane develops frank discontinuities which lead to cell swelling and loss of essential intracellular macromolecules. The sarcoplasmic reticulum ability to accumulate Ca^{2+} is disturbed and contributes to the elevated intracellular Ca^{2+} levels seen with reperfusion. Normal mitochondrial electron transport is also altered as the mitochondrial membrane is disrupted. Thus oxygen free radicals exert their negative effects by a generalized attack on the phospholipid bilayer that is important for many aspects of normal myocyte function.

Calcium-induced injury

Cellular calcium (Ca^{2+}) homeostasis is markedly altered during myocardial reperfusion. Intracellular Ca^{2+} concentration may increase fivefold during uncontrolled reperfusion. Elevated levels of cytosolic Ca^{2+} adversely affect several aspects of normal cell function and are major contributors to myocyte reperfusion injury.

During an ischemic period, cellular Ca^{2+} concentrations change little. With reperfusion, there is a massive influx of Ca^{2+} and decreased uptake by the sacroplasmic reticulum. Both factors contribute to the elevated Ca^{2+} concentration.

Several mechanisms have been proposed to be responsible for the observed loss of Ca^{2+} homeostasis with reperfusion (Table 5.1). Perturbation of plasma membrane Ca^{2+} transport processes appears to be primarily responsible for the net influx of calcium ions. However, Ca^{2+} influx mediated by α-adrenergic receptors and changes in cell phospholipid bilayers due to free radical damage also may contribute to Ca^{2+} accumulation with the myocyte.

Alteration in Ca^{2+} transport systems

Normal myocyte Ca^{2+} homeostasis is maintained by three transport processes: Ca^{2+} channels, Na^+/Ca^{2+} exchangers, and Ca^{2+}-ATP-ase pump. Ca^{2+} channels in normal myocytes allow Ca^{2+} influx during generation of the action potential. Theoretically, these channels could contribute to Ca^{2+} accumulation. Most investigators, however, have failed to demonstrated a reduction in Ca^{2+} overload when calcium channel blockers were given during ischemia or with reperfusion. The Ca^{2+} channel appears to be inactivated during reperfusion and likely does not account for cytosolic Ca^{2+} overload.

The Ca^{2+}-ATP-ase pump normally functions to promote efflux Ca^{2+} from the myocyte against a concentration gradient. Plasma membrane Ca^{2+}-ATP-ase activity is reduced during ischemia and

Table 5.1 Mediators of intracellular calcium accumulation during ischemia and reperfusion

Decreased ATP-dependent ion pump activity (Na^+/K^+, Ca^{2+})
Activation of concentration-dependent ion exchangers (Na^+/H^+, Na^+/Ca^{2+})
Adrenergic receptor-mediated Ca^{2+} influx
Free radical induced membrane Ca^{2+} inophores

further inhibited by reperfusion. This leads to a reduction of Ca^{2+} efflux and contributes to the net Ca^{2+} uptake of reperfusion.

Probably the most important mechanism contributing to the cytosolic Ca^{2+} accumulation during reperfusion is the increased activity of the Na/Ca^{2+} exchanger. This system can act to shuttle Ca^{2+} and Na^+ ions in either direction depending on transmembrane concentration gradients. This exchanger is not dependent on ATP and has been shown to remain functional during ischemia and reperfusion. The increased activity of this ion transport mechanism is a direct result of an elevated intracellular Na^+ concentration that occurs during ischemia and early reperfusion.

Cellular Na^+ sequestration during ischemia and reperfusion is most likely due to an increased activity of the Na^+/H^+ exchanger. The intracellular acidosis that develops with ischemia is a potent stimulus for Na^+/H^+ exchange. In addition, intracellular Na^+ accumulation is further increased by this mechanism during reperfusion as phospholipids from the cell membrane are released. These phospholipids increase the production of diacyl glycerol and protein kinase C, both of which have been shown to stimulate the Na^+/H^+ exchanger.

Cellular Na^+ concentration during early reperfusion is also substantially enhanced by the ATP depletion that occurs during ischemia. Lack of ATP leads to an inhibition of Na^+/K^+ ATPase resulting in a reduced ability to extract intracelleluar Na^+.

Thus, the intracellular accumulation of Na^+ during ischemia and early reperfusion, coupled with a reperfusate containing an abundance of Ca^{2+}, leads to an intense stimulation of the $Na+/Ca^{2+}$ exchanger and a subsequent large rise in cellular Ca^{2+} concentration.

Adrenergic receptor-mediated Ca^{2+} influx

Both α-and β-adrenergic receptors are upregulated during myocardial ischemia as are endogenous catecholamines. Stimulation of the α_1-receptor leads to activation of the Na^+/H^+ exchanger and contributes to elevated intracellular Na^+ levels. Ca^{2+} accumulations occur via the Na^+/Ca^{2+} exchanger as described previously. β-Adrenergic stimulation also contributes to Ca^{2+} accumulation; however, the mechanism is less clear. One possibility is that β-adrenergic mediated hydrolysis leads to disruption of normal plasma membrane functions.

Oxygen free radical-induced Ca^{2+} accumulation

As discussed previously, significant quantities of oxygen free radicals are formed as a result of ischemia and reperfusion. Free radicals increase cell permeability to Ca^{2+} and decrease uptake by the sacroplasmic reticulum. Oxygen radical-induced lipid peroxidation results in the development of substances within the plasma membrane that possess specific ionophoric properties for Ca^{2+} ions. The permeability of the peroxidized plasma membrane is higher for Ca^{2+} than for any other mono- or divalent cation. Reduction in active accumulation of Ca^{2+} by the sacroplasmic reticulum is probably the result of a similar mechanism.

Mechanism of Ca^{2+}-induced injury

The increased availability of cytosolic Ca^{2+} as a result of reperfusion triggers a chain of destructive events that contribute to myocyte injury (Fig. 5.3). Calcium accumulation causes further depletion in myocardial energy charge as Ca^{2+} dependent ATP-ases are stimulated, leading to wastage of already scarce high-energy phosphates. Cytosolic proteases and phospholipases are

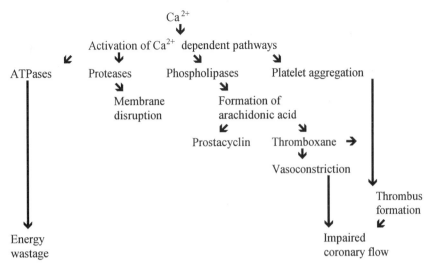

Fig. 5.3 Consequences of loss of calcium homeostasis during postischaemic reperfusion.

also activated, resulting in further injury to cell membranes. Phospholipases also accelerate arachidonic acid metabolism, producing eicosanoids that act to potentiate vasoconstriction, platelet aggregation, and thrombin formation. Calcium also contributes to the conversion of xanthine dehydrogenase to xanthine oxidase, thereby further increasing oxygen free radical production. Finally, cytosolic Ca^{2+} sequestration induces an increase in actin–myosin cross-bridge cycling, which produces myocardial contraction and rigor.

Leukocyte mediated injury

The polymorphonuclear neutrophil has emerged as important contributors to myocardial reperfusion injury. Rapid neutrophil accumulation is observed in reperfused myocardium, with the degree of leukocyte infiltration closely correlating with the extent of injury. Suppression or removal of neutrophils from the reperfusate is associated with a reduction in postischemic injury.

Neutrophils are capable of producing oxygen free radicals and enzymes when presented with an appropriate stimulant. Activated neutrophils produced superoxide, hydrogen peroxide, hydroxyl radical, and hypochlorous acid in a metabolic event referred to as the respiratory burst. Several proteolytic enzymes are also released during degranulation of activated neutrophils. These mechanisms act normally to provide protection against invading micro-organisms.

Ischemic myocardium and cardiopulmonary bypass are potent stimulators of the complement cascade. As a result of complement activation, C3a and C5a are produced in large quantities. These soluble factors are strong chemoattractants for neutrophils and are primarily responsible for their accumulation in ischemic myocardium. Reperfusion allows ready access of neutrophils to previously ischemic tissues. Therefore sequestration of activated neutrophils is accentuated by three factors: myocardial ischemia, cardiopulmonary bypass, and reperfusion.

The mechanism of neutrophil-induced myocardial injury appears to be a direct result of specific neutrophil–endothelial interactions that are currently being elucidated. Briefly, as neutrophils enter a region of reperfused myocardium, there are C5a and IL-8 induced changes in cellular adhesion molecules. Upregulation of L-selectin causes the neutrophil transition to the rolling

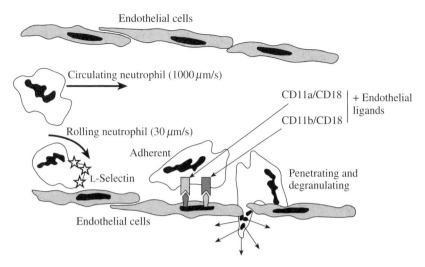

Fig. 5.4 The process of primary and secondary neutrophil adhesion.

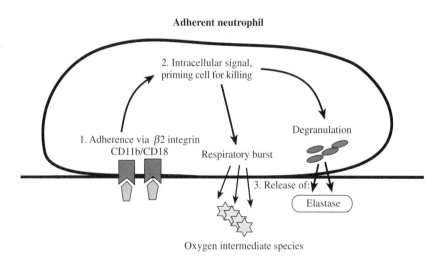

Fig. 5.5 Proposed mechanism for neutrophil degranulation after endothelial cell coupling.

state. This is referred to as primary adhesion (Fig. 5.4). At the same time, C5a increases expression of the cell surface adhesion molecules CD11a/CD18 and CD11b/CD18. These molecules bind with the endothelial cell surface molecules ICAM-1 and ICAM-2. This coupling induces the respiratory burst and neutrophil degranulation (Fig. 5.5). In addition to myocyte injury, the coupling of neutrophils to endothelial cells leads to direct injury to the endothelial cells and mechanical obstruction of the myocardial microvasculature. A better understanding of the mechanism of neutrophil–endothelial adhesion and development of techniques to inhibit it may help to reduce some of the deleterious effects of reperfusion.

Eicosanoids and myocardial reperfusion injury

Eicosanoids are a family of compounds derived from the metabolism of arachidonic acid that are produced in virtually all tissues. Arachidonic acid can give rise to three distinct groups of metabolites: prostaglandins, leukotrienes, and expoxides. Of these, the prostaglandins are most abundantly synthesized and have been most widely studied in reperfusion injury models. Elevated levels of free arachidonic acid in the reperfusion period appears to be a potent stimulus for prostaglandin synthesis. The enhanced eicosanoid synthesis in postischemic reperfused myocardium is the result of activation of the enzyme phospholipase A_2 within the cell membrane. Activation of this enzyme has been associated with an increased activity of the Na^+/H^+ exchanger which, as discussed previously, occurs during ischemia and early reperfusion. It has been proposed that as protons are transported from the cell by the exchanger, an optimum pH is achieved for activation of the enzyme leading to the production of arachidonic acid and its metabolites.

The hypothesis that prostaglandins contribute to postischemic myocardial injury is supported by the fact that inhibitors of their synthesis (non-steroidal anti-inflammatory drugs) reduce reperfusion injury. In addition, the introduction of exogenous prostaglandins reverses the protective effects of prostaglandin synthesis inhibition. Of the nonsteroidal anti-inflammatory drugs, ibuprofen is of particular benefit, resulting in a 70% post-ischemic contractile recovery compared to 11% in control animals using an isolated rat heart model. Aspirin and indomethacin were also effective in this model, increasing recovery to 35% and 40%, respectively.

The ubiquitous nature of prostaglandins coupled with the complex mechanism underlying the deleterious effect of reperfusion currently makes it difficult to describe the precise means by which these eicosanoids contribute to post-ischemic myocardial injury. However, recent studies such as those cited above do suggest that continued research is warranted and may ultimately add to the growing armamentarium available to the cardiac surgeon to reduce the detrimental results of myocardial reperfusion.

Endothelial cell injury and the no-reflow phenomenon

Successful reperfusion of ischemic myocardium depends on an intact microvasculature. Reperfusion of ischemic myocardium has been associated with a generalized capillary 'shutdown' that may result in infarct extension when blood flow is re-established. Prolonged ischemia despite reperfusion has been termed the no-reflow phenomenon. Endothelial cell injury is minimal during ischemia, being almost exclusively initiated by reperfusion. Endothelial cells of the large coronary arteries are minimally affected; however, capillary endothelial structure and function are profoundly disturbed from the beginning of reperfusion.

The capillary failure associated with reperfusion is precipitated by several factors, including endothelial morphologic changes, neutrophil and platelet aggregations, extravascular compression, and plasma extravasation. Endothelial morphologic changes that occur with reperfusion initiate the no-reflow phenomenon. Endothelial cells swell and develop intraluminal projections which act to obstruct the capillary. Large separations between cells occur, exposing the basement membrane and underlying smooth muscle. Endothelial separation leads to increased tissue edema, platelet and fibrin aggregation, and red cell and neutrophil extravasation, as well as exposure of arteriolar smooth muscle to vasoactive substances. All these factors tend to promote capillary occlusion and myocyte injury. The adhesion between activated neutrophils and endothelial cells that occurs during reperfusion (discussed previously) can contribute to microvascular occlusion. Activated neutrophils act to physically obstruct the capillary and release substances injurious to endothelial cells. Extravascular compression of capillaries due to tissue edema can further compromise microvascular reperfusion. Edema results from myocyte swelling and extravasation into the intracellular space. Fluid extravasation into the intracellular space is dependent on the degree of 'capillary leak' as well as the initial reperfusion pressure. A gradual restoration of coronary perfusion pressure has been associated with better preservation of postischemic blood flow than an abrupt return of coronary pressure to systemic levels. In summary, the no-reflow phenomenon is initiated by reperfusion-induced morphologic changes in the endothelium that leads to microvascular occlusion due to luminal obstruction as well as extraluminal compression.

Strategies for minimizing reperfusion injury

As discussed previously, reperfusion injury is characterized by massive cell swelling and intracellular calcium accumulation that result from structural and metabolic abnormalities initiated by a period of ischemia and exacerbated by the restoration of blood flow. Studies have demonstrated that careful control of reperfusion conditions can minimize the extent of irreversible injury in myocardium jeopardized by ischemia. The cardiac surgeon is in the unique position to precisely alter the composition and delivery of the reperfusate to maximize recovery of reversibly injured myocytes. An improved understanding of the pathophysiology of reperfusion injury (Table 5.2) has led to the development of clinically useful strategies to prevent it (Table 5.3).

Table 5.2   Mediators of myocardial reperfusion injury

Oxygen free radicals
Calcium ions
Adrenergic receptors
Arachidonic acid and its metabolites
Glycolytic products
Osmotic factors
Intracellular ionic derangements
Loss of membrane integrity

Table 5.3   Factors demonstrated to reduce myocardial reperfusion injury

Free radical scavengers and antioxidants
Calcium channel blockers
Adrenergic receptor blockers
Cyclo-oxygenase inhibitors
Na^+/H^+ Exchange inhibitors (i.e. amiloride)
Cardioplegic solutions
Reduction of glycolytic products

Maintenance of electromechanical silence

Postischemic myocardial performance has been shown to be improved by continued electro-mechanical quiescence during the first 5–10 minutes of reperfusion. Oxygen uptake is similar during the period, whether the heart is fibrillated or arrested. Consequently, there is a relative increase in oxygen availability in the arrested heart. It is hypothesized that this allows a more rapid repletion of myocardial ATP stores and normalization of ion homeostasis. Electro-mechanical arrest during early reperfusion may also permit better and more homogeneous blood flow throughout the heart.

Treatment of myocardial acidosis

The intracellular accumulation of protons that results from the anaerobic metabolism of glucose during ischemia disrupts several aspects of normal cellular homeostasis and potentiates Ca^{2+} accumulation. Experimental studies have demonstrated that maintenance of the reperfusate pH at 7.8 results in better myocardial performance and less edema. Tris (hydroxylmethyl) aminomethane has been found to be better than ionic buffers because it is more effective at a pH of 7.8 and readily enters cells, thereby functioning as both an intra- and extracellular buffer. The addition of blood to the reperfusate also adds additional buffering capacity due to presence of plasma proteins which contain histidine and imidazole groups.

Protection from oxygen free radicals

Much evidence has been accumulated that implicates oxygen-derived free radicals as a major source of cell injury during reperfusion. This has stimulated interest in the use of compounds that can prevent the accumulation of these toxic species. Superoxide dismutase and catalase are two enzymes that have been studied most extensively for their antioxidant properties. Several studies have demonstrated the salutary effects of both of these compounds in limiting infarct size after a period of ischemia and reperfusion. These enzymes, however, have two distinct disadvantages. They are confined to the extracellular space and they have very short half-lives ($t_{1/2}$ = 15 minutes). The latter may limit the efficacy greatly since there is evidence that oxygen radicals are formed for hours to days after reperfusion. Conjugation of superoxide dismutase with a polyethylene glycol polymer greatly extends the enzyme's half-life and may improve protection from free radicals. Xanthine oxidase inhibitors such as allopurinol have also been shown to protect against reperfusion injury when administered prior to restoration of blood. Efficacy of these compounds is maximized when continued for at least 24 hours. Iron chelators such as deferoxamine (desfemixamine) given just prior to reperfusion appear to limit cell injury by limiting the extracellular oxygen radical production which is catalyzed by free iron ions. The addition of blood to the reperfusate introduces an abundant source of naturally occurring free radical scavengers which have been shown to be of benefit clinically.

Activated neutrophils have been shown to be a significant source of injury during reperfusion. Most of the injury is the result of free radical formation. Leukocyte filtration and prevention of neutrophil endothelial adhesion have been demonstrated in experimental and clinical studies to reduce reperfusion injury considerably.

Reduction of intracellular calcium accumulation

Intracellular Ca^{2+} accumulation is a hallmark of reperfusion injury. Elevated myocyte Ca^{2+} causes multiple disturbances in normal cellular function which have been discussed previously. Reduction of the Ca^{2+} concentrations in the initial reperfusate to 1.0 meq/l improves postischemic myocardial performance. Further reduction in Ca^{2+} concentrations results in as much postischemic myocardial depression as reperfusion with normocalcemic blood. The deleterious effects of extreme hypocalcemia are known as the calcium paradox, and it is probably the result of direct membrane damage.

Pretreatment with calcium channel blockers prior to ischemia and reperfusion can reduce myocardial injury. The mechanism by which these drugs are beneficial remains unclear; however, they probably do not significantly reduce intracellular Ca^{2+} concentrations. They may act by preserving ATP stores by a reduction in myocardial contractility and preserving normal Na^+/K^+ ATP-ase activity.

Finally, postischemic myocyte Ca^{2+} sequestration may be reduced by preventing the rapid accumulation of Na^+ that drives Ca^{2+} entry. Preliminary studies using the Na^+/H^+ exchanger inhibitor amiloride have demonstrated a reduction in myocardial reperfusion injury.

Substrate replenishment

Several studies have indicated that providing metabolic substrates such as glutamate and aspartate in the reperfusate promotes metabolic and functional recovery. The benefit may be due to a more rapid repletion of myocardial energy change. Restoration of normal ATP stores after ischemia injury also may be delayed due to a reduced level of adenosine. As mentioned previously, adenosine is metabolized to inosine during ischemia. Addition of adenosine to the reperfusate has been suggested to accelerate restoration of normal ATP levels.

Prevention of myocardial edema

Myocardial edema may exacerbate reperfusion by increasing coronary vascular resistances and decreasing ventricular compliance. The endothelial injury associated with reperfusion greatly enhances the extravasation of plasma water and proteins. Increasing the osmolarity of the reperfusate to 360 osm using mannitol has been demonstrated to be beneficial in experimental preparations.

Control of the initial reperfusion pressure has also been demonstrated to reduce myocardial edema and the associated no-reflow phenomenon.

Recommended further reading

Allen BS, Okamoto F, Buckberg GD *et al*. Immediate functional recovery after six hours of regional ischaemia by careful control of conditions of reperfusion and composition of the reperfusate; XV, Studies of controlled reperfusion after ischaemia. *J Thoracic Cardiovas Surg* 1986;**92**:621–35.

Ambrosio G, Weisfeldt ML, Jacobus WE, Flaherty JT. Evidence for a reversible oxygen radical mediates component of reperfusion injury. *Circulation* 1987;**75**:282–91.

Ambrosio G, Weissman HF, Mannion JA, Becker LC. Progressive impairment of regional myocardial perfusion after initial restoration of post-ischaemic blood flow. *Circulation* 1989;**80**:1846–54.

Babior BM. Oxygen-dependent microbial killing by phagocytes. *N Engl J Med* 1978;**298**:659–69.

Bernard M, Menasche P, Pietri S *et al*. Cardioplegic arrest superimposed on evolving myocardial ischaemia; improved recovery after inhibition of mydroxyl radical generation by peroxidase or deferoxamine — a ^{31}P NMR study. *Circulation* 1988;78 (Suppl. III):III–164.

Bolli R. Oxygen derived free radicals and post-ischaemic myocardial dysfunction ('stunned myocardium'). *J Am Coll Card* 1998;**12**(1):239–49.

Bolling SF, Bies LE, Bove EL *et al*. Augmenting intracellular adenosine improves myocardial recovery. *J Thor Cardiovas Surg* 1990;**99**:469–74.

Botenhamer RM, DeBoer LWV, Geggin GA *et al*. Enhanced myocardial protection during ischaemic arrest: oxygenation of a crystalloid cardioplegic solution. *J Thoracic Cardiovas Surg* 1983;**85**:769–78.

Bourtillon PD, Poole-Wilson PA. The effects of verapamil, quiescence and cardioplegia on calcium exchange and mechanical function in ischaemic rabbit myocardium. *Circulation Res* 1982;**50**:360–8.

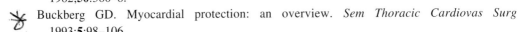Buckberg GD. Myocardial protection: an overview. *Sem Thoracic Cardiovas Surg* 1993;**5**:98–106.

Chambers DE, Parks DA, Patterson G *et al*. Xanthine oxidase: a source of free radical damage in myocardial ischaemia. *J Mol Cell Card* 1985;**17**:145–152.

Chemnitius JM, Sasaki Y, Bureger W, Bing RJ. The effects of ischaemia and sarcolemnal function in perfused canine hearts. *J Mol Cell Card* 1985;**17**:1139–50.

Chenowith DE, Cooper SW, Hugli TE *et al*. Complement activation during cardiopulmonary bypass: evidence for generation of C3a and C5a anaphylatoxins. *N Eng J Med* 1981;**304**:497–503.

Chi L, Tamura Y, Hoff PT *et al*. Effect of superoxide dismutase on myocardial infarct size in the canine heart after six hours of regional ischaemia and reperfusion administration of myocardial salvage. *Circulation Res* 1989;**64**:665–75.

Corr PB, Chayman JA, Kramer JB. Increased β-adrenergic receptors in ischaemic cat myocardium: a potential mediator of electrophysiologic derangements. *J Clin Invest* 1981;**67**:1232.

Curtis WE, Gillinov AM, Wilson IC. Inhibition of neutrophil adhesion reduces myocardial infarct size. *Ann Thor Surg* 1993;**56**:1069–73.

Digerness SB, Kirklin JW, Naftel DC *et al*. Coronary and systemic vascular resistance during reperfusion after global myocardial ischaemia. *Ann Thor Surg* 1988;**46**:447–55.

Downey JM. Free radicals and their involvement during long-term myocardialal ischaemia and reperfusion. *Ann Rev Physiology* 1990;**52**:487–504.

Elliot MJ, Finn AHR. Interaction between neutrophils and endothelium. *Ann Thor Surg* 1993;**56**:1503–8.

Engler RL, Schmid-Schonbein GW, Pavelec RS. Leukocyte capillary plugging in myocardial ischaemia and reperfusion in the dog. *Am J Path* 1993;**111**:98–111.

Ferrari R, Ceconi C, Curello S *et al*. Oxygen mediated myocardial damage during ischaemia and reperfusion: Role of the cellular defences against oxygen toxicity. *J Mol Cell Card* 1985;**17**:937.

Flynn PJ, Becker WK, Vercelloti GM *et al*. Ibuprofen inhibits granulocyte responses to inflammatory mediators: a proposed mechanism for reduction of experimental myocardial infarct size. *Inflammation* 1984;**8**:33–44.

Freeman DA, Carpo JD. Biology of disease: free radicals and tissue injury. *Lab Invest* 1982;**47**:412–26.

Hearse DJ. Reperfusion of ischaemic myocardium. *J Mol Cell Card* 1977;**9**:605.

Hess ML, Okabe E, Ash P, Kontos HA. Free radical mediation of the effects of acidosis on calcium transport by cardiac sarcoplasmic reticulum in whole heart homogenate. *Card Res* 1984;**18**:149–57.

Huant WH, Askari A. Regulation of Na+K+ ATPase by organic phosphate: pH dependence and physiological implications. *Biochem Biophy Res Comm* 1984;**123**:438–43.

Ikeda U, Arisaka H, Takavasu T *et al*. Protein kinase C activation aggregates hypoxic myocardial injury by stimulating Na+/H+ exchange. *J Mol Cell Card* 1988;**20**:493–500.

Jennings RB, Reimer KA, Hill ML *et al*. Total ischaemia in dog hearts *in vitro*: comparison of high energy phosphates production, utilization and depletion. *Cir Res* 1981;**49**:892.

Jewett SL, Eddy LJ, Hochstein P. Is the auto-oxidation of catecholamines involved in ischaemia-reperfusion injury? *Free Rad Bio Med* 1989;**6**:323–6.

Karmazyn M. Ischaemia and reperfusion injury in the heart; cellular mechanism and pharmacological intervention. *Can J Phys Pharm* 1991;**69**:719–30.

Karmazyn M. Synthesis and relevance of cardiac eicosanoids with particular emphasis on ischaemia and reperfusion. *Can J Phys Pharm* 1989;**67**:912–21.

Kirklin JW, Westaby S, Blackstone EH *et al*. Complement and the damaging effects of cardiopulmonary bypass. *J Thoracic Cardio Surg* 1983;**86**:845–57.

Kloner RA, Granote CE, Jennings RB. The 'no reflow' phenomenon after temporary coronary occlusion in the dog. *J Clin Invest* 1974;**54**:1496–1508.

Kontos HA, Wei EP, Ellis EF *et al*. Appearance of superoxide radical in cerebral extracellular space during increased prostaglandin synthesis in cats. *Cir Res* 1985;**57**:142–51.

Krause SM, Hess ML. Characterization of cardiac sarcoplasmic reticulum dysfunction during short-term, normothermic global ischaemia. *Cir Res* 1984;**18**:149–57.

Lazar HL, Buckberg GD, Manganaro AM, Becker H. Myocardial energy replenishment of secondary blood cardioplegia with amino acids during reperfusion. *J Thor Cardio Surg* 1980;**80**:350–8.

Lefer AM, Polansky EW, Bianchi CP, Narayan S. Influence of verapamil on cellular integrity and electrolyte concentrations of ischaemic myocardial tissue in the cat. *Basic Res Card* 1979;**74**:555–67.

Linden J, Brooker G. Properties of cardiac contraction in zero sodium solutions: intracellular free calcium controls slow channel conductance. *J Mol Cell Card* 1980;**12**:457–78.

Lucchesi BR. Modulation of leukocyte mediated myocardial reperfusion injury. *Ann Rev Phys* 1990;**52**:561–76.

Lucchesi BR, Werns SW, Fantone JC. The role of the neutrophil and free radicals in ischaemic myocardial injury. *J Mol Cell Card* 1989;**21**:1241–51.

Matskui T, Shirato C, Cohen WV *et al*. Oxpurinol limits myocardial infarct size without pretreatment. *Can J Card* 1990;**6**:123–9.

McCord JM. Oxygen-derived free radicals in post-ischaemic tissue injury. *N Eng J Med* 1985;**312**:159–63.

McCord JM, Fridovich I. Superoxide dismutase: an enzymatic function for erythrocuprein. *J Bio Chem* 1969;**244**:6049–55.

Nakamishi K, Lefer DJ, Johnstone WE, Vintin-Johansen J. Transient hypocalaemia during the initial phase of reperfusion extends myocardial necrosis after two hours of coronary occlusion. *Coronary Artery Dis* 1991;**2**:1009–21.

Nakamishi K, Vintin-Johansen J, Lefer DJ *et al*. Intracoronary L-arginine during reperfusion improves regional function and reduces infarct size. *Am J Phys* 1992;**263**:H1650–H1658.

Naslund U, Haggmark S, Johansson G *et al*. Superoxide dismutase and catalase reduce infarct size in a porcine myocardial ischaemia/reperfusion model. *J Mol Cell Card* 1986;**11**:1077–84.

Nayer H. The role of calcium in the ischaemic myocardium. *Am J Path* 1981;**102**:262–9.

Nayler WG, Ferrari R, Williams A. Protective effects of pretreatment with verapamil, nifidiquine and propranolol on mitochondrial function in ischaemic and reperfused myocardium. *Am J Card* 1980;**46**:242–8.

Nayler WH, Elz JS. Reperfusion injury: Laboratory artifact or clinical dilemma? *Circulation* 1986;**74**:215–21.

Nishida M, Kuzuys T, Hoshida S *et al*. Polymorphonuclear leukocytes induced vasoconstriction in isolated canine coronary arteries. *Circ Res* 1990;**66**:253–60.

Nishizuka S. The role of protein kinase C in cell surface signal transduction and tumour promotion. *Nature* 1984;**308**:693–8.

Pryor WA. The role of free radical reactions in biological systems. In: *Free radicals in Biology*, WA Pryor (ed). Academic Press, San Diego, Calornia, 1–25.

Quillen JE, Sellke FW, Brooks LA, Harrison DG. Ischaemia-reperfusion impairs endothelium-dependent relaxation of coronary microvessels but does not affect large arteries. *Circulation* 1990;**82**:586–94.

Roy RS, McCord JM. Superoxide and ischaemia: conversion of xanthine dehydrogenase to xanthine oxidase. In: *Oxyradicals and their scavenger systems*; Vol 2, *Cellular and molecular aspects*, R Greenwald and L Cohen, eds: Elsevier Science New York, N.Y. 145–53, 1983.

Rozenkranz ER, Buckberg GD, Laks H *et al*. Warm induction of cardioplegia with warm glutamate enriched blood in coronary patient in cardiogenic shock who are dependent on inotropic drugs and intra-aortic balloon support. *J Thor Card Surg* 1983;**86**:507–18.

Sharma AD, Saffitz JE, Lee BI *et al*. Alpha-adrenergic mediated accumulation of calcium in reperfused myocardium. *J Clin Invest* 1983;**72**:802–18.

Shen AC, Jennings RB. Kinetics of calcium accumulation in acute myocardial ischaemic injury. *Am J Path* 1972;**67**:441–52.

Shlafer M, Myers CL, Adkins S. Mitochondrial hydrogen peroxide generation and activities of glutathione peroxidase and superoxide dismutase following global ischaemia. *J Mol Cell Card* 1987;**19**:1195–1206.

Sperelakis N, Regulation of calcium slow channels of cardiac muscle by cyclic nucleotides and phosphorylation. *J Mol Cell Card* 1988;**20** (Suppl. II):75–106.

Tamura Y, Chi L, Driscoll EM *et al*. Superoxide dismutase conjugated to polyethylene glycol provides sustained protection against myocardial ischaemia/reperfusion injury in canine heart. *Cir Res* 1988;**63**:944–59.

Tan LR, Waxman K, Clark L *et al*. Superoxide dismutase and allopurinol improve survival after an animal model of haemorrhagic shock. *Am Surg* 1993;**59**:79–83.

Tani M. Mechanism of Ca^{2+} overload in reperfused myocardium. *Ann Rev Phys* 1990;**52**:543–9.

Vane JR, Auggard EE, Botting RM. Regulatory function of the vascular endothelium. *N Engl J Med* 1990;**323**:27–31.

Vinten-Johansen J, Lefer DJ, Nakanishe K *et al.* Controlled coronary hydrodynamics of reperfusion reduces infarct size and improves segmental systolic and diastolic function. *Cor Art Dis* 1992;**3**:1081–93.

Walsh LH, Tormey JM. Subcellular electrolyte shifts during *in vitro* myocardial ischaemia and reperfusion. *Am J Phys* 1998;**255**:H917–H928.

Watts JA, Koch CD, LaNoue KF. Effects of Ca^{2+} antagonism on energy metabolism: Ca^{2+} and heart function after ischaemia. *Am J Phys* 1980;**238**:H909–916.

Wearns S, Shea M, Kitsos S *et al.* Reduction in the size of infarction by allopurinol in the ischaemic reperfused canine heart. *Cir* 1986;**73**:518–24.

Wilson IC, Gardner TJ, DiNatale JM *et al.* Temporary leukocyte depletion reduces ventricular dysfunction during prolonged postischaemic reperfusion. *J Thor Card Surg* 1993;**106**:805–12.

6 Anaesthesia for coronary artery bypass surgery

R.O. Feneck and F. Duncan

Although the first coronary artery bypass graft operation was performed by Sabiston in 1962 (1), delay in publishing the report has led to some confusion as to who carried out the first successful procedure. Garret (2), Favaloro (3), and Johnson (4) have all been credited as pioneers of the technique. However, others rapidly followed and by the end of the 1970s coronary artery bypass graft (CABG) surgery was commonly undertaken in hospitals throughout the world, and was certainly the most common major surgical procedure requiring admission to an intensive care unit for postoperative care. The early literature on cardiac anaesthesia is a little clearer. Keown published the first monograph on cardiac anaesthesia in 1956 (5), and Wynands published the first article on anaesthesia for myocardial revascularization in 1967 (6). However, one of the most influential early papers was that of Lowenstein *et al.* in 1969 (7) describing the human cardiovascular responses to large doses of intravenous morphine. Such data led to the development of opioid based anaesthesia, allowing for hypnosis and a profound level of analgesia without cardiovascular depression. Since that time there has been an enormous contribution to the published literature on anaesthesia for CABG surgery. However, despite this apparent progress, many issues remain unresolved.

The development of anaesthesia for coronary artery surgery has led to the identification of anaesthetic techniques that are appropriate to each patient, from the point of view both of the surgical procedure and of the clinical status of the individual patient. In that regard, adult cardiac anaesthesia has had to remain flexible over the last 30 years as the nature of the patients presenting for surgery has changed considerably.

For example, in the 1960s the majority of cardiac surgery patients were undergoing valve replacement surgery. From the anaesthetic point of view, the main haemodynamic problem was one of impending cardiac failure, and anaesthetic techniques were developed where the primary haemodynamic goal was to preserve ventricular function. Such techniques included the use of opioids including morphine (7,8) and later fentanyl and its congeners as the main agents (9–11). Patients presenting for CABG surgery in the early 1970s were quite different. These patients, in the main, had well preserved ventricular function. The main haemodynamic concern lay in the danger of developing myocardial oxygen imbalance and ischaemia, particularly as a result of an increase in myocardial oxygen demand, which may occur if a patient develops a hyperdynamic circulation (hypertension and tachycardia) during periods of intense surgical stimulation. In these patients, anaesthetic techniques where the main goal was the preservation of myocardial contractility were not so appropriate, and techniques that included a reduction in cardiac work were felt to be more closely matched to the needs of the patient (12,13).

In the last 10 years demographic changes and the advent of interventional cardiological techniques including percutaneous transluminal coronary angioplasty (PTCA) have meant that patients presenting for CABG surgery are both older and less fit, often with significantly impaired left ventricular function (14–16). More recently, therefore, anaesthetic techniques have had to balance the preservation of myocardial contractility with the prevention of myocardial oxygen imbalance. In addition, the variable arrhythmogenic effects of different anaesthetic drugs and techniques have necessitated further refinement.

Factors promoting safe cardiac anaesthesia

General anaesthesia has been described as a triad of hypnosis, analgesia, and muscle relaxation (17). The relative importance of each of these three components will vary, depending on the nature of the patient and on the surgical procedure. For example, body surface surgery requires little muscular relaxation and patients may receive a volatile anaesthetic and breathe spontaneously through an anaesthetic circuit. Patients undergoing body cavity surgery usually require neuromuscular blockade either to facilitate surgical access or to permit adequate artificial lung ventilation or both. Intravenous anaesthetic drugs produce a level of unconsciousness that allows for surgical procedures to be undertaken, but unless some analgesic drug has been given, the intraoperative course and most certainly the postoperative course will not be smooth and the patient will be in pain. Conversely, patients who are given only intravenous analgesic drugs such as opioids, even in very large doses, will be free of pain but may be conscious during surgery. Volatile anaesthetic agents, on the other hand, are more complete anaesthetic agents. They provide unconsciousness and analgesia, and also some degree of muscle relaxation, although this is more commonly seen with the older agents and at higher dosage.

None of these observations is controversial, and if these were the only considerations then anaesthesia for CABG or indeed for any form of surgery would be simple. However, anaesthetic drugs and muscle relaxants have numerous effects on the circulation, including arteriolar vasodilatation and venodilatation, vagolysis, depression of myocardial contractility and effects on intracardiac conduction and arrhythmogenesis. Some agents are more effective than others at obtunding the physiological and hormonal response to surgery. With some agents the haemodynamic responses seen are in part dependent on the state of the autonomic nervous system, and with one agent, ketamine, the haemodynamic response seen is affected both quantitatively and qualitatively by the state of the autonomic nervous system (18,19).

It is because of these numerous and varied haemodynamic side effects of anaesthetic agents that anaesthesia for CABG surgery is more complex than simply rendering the patient unconscious and adequately oxygenated. Safe cardiac anaesthesia requires in addition that the myocardial oxygen balance is preserved, that there is no undue myocardial depression leading to cardiac failure, and that significant arrhythmia is avoided. These factors are explored in more detail below.

Myocardial oxygen balance

Myocardial oxygen balance is the matching of myocardial oxygen supply with myocardial oxygen demand. A number of factors have been shown to influence myocardial oxygen balance, and these are shown in Fig. 6.1.

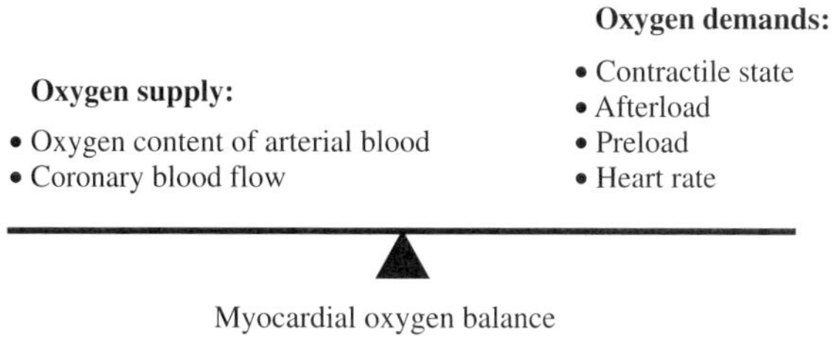

Oxygen demands:
- Contractile state
- Afterload

Oxygen supply:
- Preload
- Heart rate

- Oxygen content of arterial blood
- Coronary blood flow

▲

Myocardial oxygen balance

Fig. 6.1 Factors affecting myocardial oxygen balance.

From the supply side of the equation, it is clear that myocardial oxygen supply is limited by the oxygen carrying capacity of the blood and the coronary blood flow. Oxygen carrying capacity will be enhanced by a high degree of saturation, and by an appropriate level of haemoglobin. It is clear that the level of haemoglobin required is itself a balance between rheological considerations and oxygen carrying requirements. A number of studies have concluded that a haemoglobin level of 8 g/dL or a haematocrit level of 25–28% is an acceptable balance in the early postoperative period (20,21), although this is still controversial. Coronary blood flow is subject to numerous physiological and pharmacological factors. Experimental and human data have shown that coronary blood flow occurs both during ventricular systole and diastole, the major part being in diastole (22). Thus the driving pressure perfusing the normal coronary vasculature is mean aortic diastolic pressure. For adequate perfusion of the ventricular myocardium, the coronary driving pressure has to overcome any compressive forces acting on the subendocardium which may occur as a result of a raised ventricular end-diastolic pressure. A high left ventricular end-diastolic pressure will therefore act as a force limiting subendocardial perfusion.

Since coronary flow occurs mostly during diastole, the time for coronary flow will be limited by the duration of diastole. As heart rate increases, the duration of systole is minimally reduced whereas the duration of diastole is reduced by approximately 65% if the heart rate increases from 60 to 120 beats/minute. Tachycardia has reduced coronary blood flow by up to 50% in patients recovering from CABG surgery (23). Furthermore, again in studies of patients undergoing CABG surgery, tachycardia is one of the few haemodynamic factors to correlate with outcome (24). This may also be due to the fact that tachycardia causes an increase in myocardial oxygen demand as well as a reduction in supply, and because those patients who do not demonstrate a tachycardia are frequently those taking beta-blockers. These drugs will reduce myocardial oxygen consumption by regulating blood pressure, contractility, and heart rate.

The anaesthetic consequences of these observations are not marked. Tachycardia and systemic hypotension are generally avoidable in all but the sickest patients using modern anaesthetic drugs. Tachycardia is also prevented by continuing treatment with beta-blockers on the morning of surgery. The development of ultra-short-acting beta-blockers such as esmolol allows for the use of intraoperative beta-blockers to control heart rate with little theoretical risk of ongoing beta-blockade and myocardial depression causing difficulties in weaning from cardiopulmonary bypass.

However, there are two further important observations concerning anaesthesia and coronary blood flow. The first concerns the effects of anaesthetic agents on coronary blood flow in the diseased myocardium.

Anaesthetic agents have been shown to have differing effects on the autoregulation of coronary blood flow (Fig. 6.2). Enflurane and halothane cause little change from the awake state, whereas

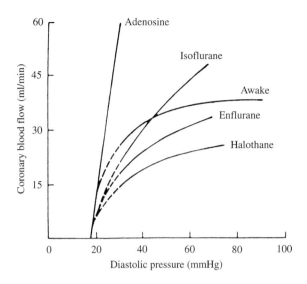

Fig. 6.2 Schematic presentation of the relationship between coronary blood flow and aortic diastolic pressure under the conditions shown. Adenosine, a potent coronary, vasodilator, abolishes the autoregulatory phenomenon. Coronary blood flow appears more pressure dependent with isoflurane than with the other anaesthetic agents (reproduced from reference 25).

isoflurane clearly causes a leftward shift to the curve (25). The effect of this is to make coronary blood flow more dependent on coronary perfusion pressure, increasing the similarity of effect with that of adenosine. This latter agent is a potent coronary vasodilator capable of abolishing coronary autoregulation, resulting in a linear pressure/flow relationship. Studies in experimental animals and in humans have confirmed that isoflurane is a significant coronary vasodilator, but less potent that adenosine (26,27). It has long been known that although coronary vasodilators are effective in treating angina, they may also be responsible for precipitating angina. This is even true of nifedipine and other dihydropyridine calcium channel blockers. There may be a number of causative mechanisms involved, but one that has been postulated is that of 'coronary steal syndrome'.

Coronary steal is dependent on a particular variant of coronary vascular anatomy, in which an area of myocardium is supplied by collateral vessels. In one vessel, coronary occlusion due to atheroma is virtually or actually complete, leading to a state of maximal coronary vasodilatation distal to the stenosis. In another vessel, there is a flow limiting coronary stenosis of at least 50%. In this situation, coronary vasodilatation may lead to a reduction in total coronary blood flow distal to the flow-limiting stenosis. This is particularly true if coronary vasodilatation is accompanied by a significant reduction in coronary perfusion pressure, associated with systemic hypotension (Fig. 6.3). Coronary steal may occur between different areas of the myocardium (collateral steal) or between the subendocardial and subepicardial layers of the left ventricle (transmural steal). In either situation, the effect of coronary vasodilatation is to divert blood to the non-ischaemic area and away from the potentially ischaemic area. In fact true steal necessarily involves luxury or overperfusion of the non-ischaemic area as well as underperfusion of the ischaemic area.

How common is coronary steal-prone anatomy in patients who present for CABG surgery? Buffington reviewed 16 249 angiograms in the Coronary Artery Surgery Study (CASS) registry and found that 23% of patients had coronary anatomy that would make them at theoretical risk

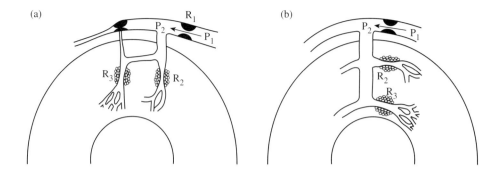

Fig. 6.3 (a) Collateral steal. The vascular bed R_3 is maximally vasodilated and dependent on collateral flow from R_2. Pharmacological vasodilation of the arterioles in R_2 increases the flow across R_1 and reduces the perfusion pressure at P_2. If R_3 cannot dilate further, the result will be a luxury perfusion at R_2 and flow reduction at R_3. (b) Transmural steal. The subendocardium R_3 has less vasodilator reserve, and may be at greater risk than the subcardium R_2 where flow autoregulation may be preserved (reproduced from Epstein S.E., Cannon R.O., Talbot T.L. Hemodynamic principles in the control of coronary blood flow. *American Journal of Cardiology* 1985;**46**:4E–10E).

from coronary steal (28). However, a much greater degree of flow-limiting stenosis is necessary in the collateral vessel if a coronary vasodilator much weaker than adenosine is used. If one assumes that a critical stenosis needs to be present (i.e. >90%) then the proportion of the CASS registry patients susceptible to ischaemia by an anaesthetic-related steal-inducing mechanism drops to 12% (28).

Early studies of isoflurane in humans suggested a useful haemodynamic profile, including systemic (but little pulmonary) vasodilatation, a small fall in blood pressure, reflex tachycardia, and good preservation of cardiac output (29). Anxieties were raised, however, by the later studies of Reiz (30) and Moffitt (31) who both identified ischaemic episodes in patients anaesthetized with isoflurane. They suggested the possibility of a coronary steal syndrome as a causative mechanism. It should be said that these workers used very sensitive markers of ischaemia, detecting the conversion from aerobic to anaerobic cardiac metabolism following coronary sinus catheterization, as well as confirmatory ECG changes. However, a further large scale study failed to demonstrate any adverse effect on outcome in patients anaesthetized with isoflurane as the primary agent (32).

How can we reconcile these differences? Firstly, it may be that other haemodynamic changes are important. Further detailed studies have shown that isoflurane is not implicated in myocardial blood flow redistribution when haemodynamics, and in particular systemic blood pressure, are well controlled (33,34). In the Reiz study (30), coronary perfusion pressure was reduced by 35% using isoflurane; in the Moffitt study (31), systemic blood pressure was reduced by 30% as a haemodynamic target of the study. Others have noted that even carefully controlled laboratory studies have difficulty in producing coronary steal when blood pressure is well maintained (35).

There is no doubt that coronary flow redistribution is more easily induced experimentally by adenosine and even by nifedipine than by isoflurane (36). Adenosine is more likely than isoflurane to induce ischaemia by this mechanism. This may be explained in part by the different potencies that the two drugs have as coronary vasodilators, and also by the fact that, in contrast to adenosine, isoflurane causes a mild degree of myocardial depression thereby reducing myocardial oxygen demand and thus causing less imbalance in the myocardial oxygen supply/demand ratio. This has led to the suggestion that inhaled anaesthetics are less likely to induce coronary steal-induced ischaemia than intravenous coronary vasodilators simply because the anaesthetics cause a degree of protective myocardial depression (37,38). However, in transferring this theoretical argument to the operating room, one must take account of the fact that too much myocardial depression will have obvious adverse consequences, and that hypotension is itself involved in the coronary steal mechanism.

Furthermore, the role of adverse alterations in heart rate cannot be overlooked. A review of the effect of isoflurane anaesthesia and the incidence of ischaemia showed coincidentally that the patients who developed ischaemia were the patients with the highest heart rates (39). Other large scale studies of general anaesthesia have shown that isoflurane is the primary anaesthetic most likely to be associated with significant tachycardia (40). It is possible, therefore, that when considering the relationship between isoflurane anaesthesia and ischaemia, too much attention has been paid to the concept of coronary steal syndrome, and not enough attention to simple haemodynamic parameters such as hypotension and tachycardia.

Should we use isoflurane, or indeed any other anaesthetic drug with coronary vasodilatory properties, in patients undergoing CABG surgery? There is no doubt that isoflurane is widely used for CABG patients in current clinical practice, and that such outcome studies as exist suggest that there is no adverse effect on outcome associated with its use (32,41).

Others have added caveats that isoflurane should be used in low dosage and that hypotension should be avoided, and even that isoflurane is best avoided altogether in some patients (42), but the same could be said of every other anaesthetic. However, it would be quite wrong to assume that isoflurane is no different from other volatile anaesthetics. At the time of writing, it was hard to disagree with Moffitt's conclusion that enflurane remains the preferable volatile agent in CABG patients (39). However, whatever the theoretical merits isoflurane is clearly established as the volatile agent of choice for CABG surgery. Whether it will be supplemented by the newer agents seroflurane and desflurane remains to be seen.

More recently, interest has been directed to the effect that anaesthetics and other drugs may have on modulating the balance of vasodilatation induced by endothelium-derived relaxation factor (EDRF) and vasoconstriction induced by α-adrenergic agonism, and the resultant effect on coronary vascular tone (43). Interest in this area has largely been stimulated by the observation that a high proportion of ischaemic episodes in CABG patients are silent, in that they neither involve symptoms of angina in the awake patient nor are provoked by any degree of haemodynamic disturbance in the anaesthetized patient. This would suggest that such ischaemic episodes must be related to local alterations in myocardial oxygen balance rather than more global changes, and that such alterations may be caused by reductions in myocardial blood flow, in turn caused by alterations in coronary vascular tone mediated in part through sympathetic activation. Certainly there is evidence that some anaesthetics may affect the balance of coronary vascular tone, but the relevance of these early data to the clinical situation is not yet clear. However, there is no doubt that increasing anaesthetic interest is being directed toward the concept of improving or maintaining myocardial oxygen supply area, in contrast to the 1980s when the major effort was concerned with controlling myocardial oxygen demand (44).

The factors provoking myocardial oxygen imbalance by an increase in myocardial oxygen demand and consumption have been well described (45), and control of these factors has been an important part of the care of CABG patients. Systemic vasoconstriction may cause a rise in blood pressure and in left ventricular wall stress and left ventricular work, leading to an increase in oxygen consumption. Such an increase in afterload is not uncommon, particularly following surgical stimulation such as sternotomy or manipulation of the aorta. The enhanced sympatho-adrenal response that results from this may also give rise to an increase in heart rate and an increase in myocardial contractility, both factors that are known to increase myocardial oxygen consumption. This process may also cause an increase in venoconstriction, and an increase in left ventricular end-diastolic pressure, which will also cause an increase in contractile force via the Frank-Starling mechanism, and hence increase oxygen consumption.

Control of those factors influencing myocardial oxygen consumption has been an important goal in cardiac anaesthesia, and a number of strategies have been developed which are widely accepted. Heavy sedative premedication (46) and the continuation of anti-anginal medication right up to the time of surgery have been shown to help prevent the intraoperative development of hypertension and tachycardia (47–49). The development of opioid-based anaesthetic techniques, often using analgesic drugs in high dosage, has meant that the haemodynamic effects of intense surgical stimulation have been effectively obtunded without producing an unacceptable degree of haemodynamic depression in the periods of surgery when stimulation is less intense (10,50). The use of volatile anaesthetic agents in low dosage and in combination with opioid drugs has given greater flexibility in the control of the depth of anaesthesia and in intraoperative haemodynamic control. Also, the intraoperative use of nitrates and beta-blockers has further allowed for close haemodynamic control to be maintained.

The principles of the preservation of myocardial oxygen balance described above are relevant to every patient undergoing CABG surgery. However, the relative importance of differing aspects will vary dependent on each individual patient. For those elective surgical patients with large proximal coronary stenoses and well preserved left ventricular function, control of myocardial oxygen imbalance particularly through preventing increases in oxygen demand will be the main consideration. For those patients with left main stem stenosis, preservation of myocardial oxygen supply and the prevention of a reduction in coronary perfusion pressure may be crucial. In those patients requiring urgent or emergency surgery, close haemodynamic control thereby preserving supply and controlling demand will be essential. However, many of the current population of CABG patients are now both older and less fit than previously, and as a result may be at significant risk from developing perioperative heart failure. This raises another set of issues which are discussed below.

Cardiac failure and undue myocardial depression

There is a large amount of data to suggest that pre-existing poor ventricular function is a significant risk factor in patients undergoing CABG surgery. Data from the original CASS study group (51), and data from numerous other authors (52–57) have all identified the presence of signs of poor ventricular function and/or cardiac failure as being associated with a poor outcome. Data from patients undergoing non-cardiac surgery also suggests that patients who have either clinical signs of heart failure, or poor left ventricular function identified by an appropriate test such as echocardiography or cine-ventriculography, are at significantly greater risk from a poor outcome (58,59).

The impact that anaesthesia may have on the patient with pre-existing cardiac failure may be considerable, since many anaesthetic agents are known to reduce myocardial contractility. In both human and experimental studies, halothane and enflurane have been shown to cause myocardial depression in normal and abnormal myocardium (60–63). Myocardial depression has also been noted with isoflurane, but the consensus is that this agent is less of a myocardial depressant than enflurane or halothane (61,64,65). The newer agent desflurane appears to be similar to isoflurane in its effects (66), but data from sevoflurane studies suggests that it is less myocardial depressant than other agents in current use (67). Although the evidence is relatively controversial, the consensus is that nitrous oxide has myocardial depressant effects which are distinct from any effect of relative hypoxia (68,69). The potency of the myocardial depressant effect with volatile agents appears to be related to the agent (halothane = enflurane > isoflurane = desflurane), the dosage, and the state of resting myocardial function.

The intravenous induction agents have been extensively studied, and the barbiturates, including thiopentone, have been shown to cause a dose-dependent reduction in contractility (70). The benzodiazepines, including diazepam, lorazepam, and midazolam, have been shown to be better tolerated than barbiturates both in sedative and anaesthetic dosage (71–74), and for that reason have become popular agents for induction of anaesthesia in cardiac surgery patients. The haemodynamic effects of propofol have been compared to most other induction agents in cardiac surgery patients. Propofol produces both vasodilatation and myocardial depression (75,76), although the contribution of depression of contractility to the overall haemodynamic effect remains controversial. However, an anaesthetic maintenance infusion of propofol appears to be well tolerated, and propofol/fentanyl anaesthesia appears to be similar to enflurane/fentanyl anaesthesia (77), a technique described by Moffitt and Sethna as the technique of choice for CABG patients (39).

However, it is also clear that anaesthetics do not adversely affect haemodynamics by simply reducing myocardial contractility; they may also cause a significant reduction in vasomotor centre activity and hence in vasomotor tone. This combination of a reduction in contractility, and a loss of vasomotor tone, thereby causing a reduction in preload and in coronary perfusion pressure, may be catastrophic in a patient who has severe underlying myocardial dysfunction.

The main advances in the anaesthetic management of the patient with cardiac failure came about as a result of the observation that the use of high doses of opioids including morphine had little adverse effect on haemodynamics. Previously, patients for coronary revascularization often had well preserved ventricular function, and therefore cardiac failure was not the main risk. However, such patients are also prone to developing myocardial oxygen imbalance perioperatively, and it was noted that high dose opiate anaesthesia could obtund the haemodynamic consequences of surgical stimulation without the risk of undue myocardial depression, even in those patients who had significantly impaired left ventricular function. It therefore became a valuable method of anaesthesia, particularly in those patients who did have significantly impaired left ventricular function, and in whom cardiac failure was a significant risk. However, even in these patients, factors such as prolonged postoperative respiratory depression may militate against the use of high dose opiate anaesthesia for any but the sickest patients. Recently a new fentanyl analogue, remifentanil, has been introduced into clinical practice. This compound has a unique route of metabolism for opioids, being inactivated by whole body esterases. The duration of action is therefore ultra-short, and not influenced by the duration of the infusion. Current experience suggests that remifentanil is safe and effective in patients with poor LV function.

Of the anaesthetic agents, ketamine is unique in that it does not produce a reduction in vasomotor tone or haemodynamic depression. Although its effects are dependent on the presence of an intact sympatho-adrenal response (18), intravenous ketamine may produce an increase in heart rate, blood pressure, and cardiac output (78). Its use is particularly valuable in patients with haemorrhagic hypotension, and it is often felt to be the anaesthetic agent of choice for emergency re-sternotomy for haemorrhage, or cardiac tamponade (79).

Significant arrhythmias

Since the earliest days it has been clear that anaesthesia and surgery may cause a wide variety of arrhythmias. However, repeated studies have shown that these arrhythmias are mostly benign and self-limiting, often terminating at the end of surgery and after discontinuing the anaesthetic. There are many arrhythmogenic factors that occur during anaesthesia and surgery, including alterations in fluid balance and biochemistry, modulations in autonomic nervous system activity, the activation of neuroendocrine responses, the direct effects that anaesthetic drugs may have on intracardiac conduction, and numerous others (80). In addition, in CABG surgery the effects of mechanical stimulation of the heart and the effects of the surgery itself may be arrhythmogenic.

Clearly therefore, surgery in general and cardiac surgery in particular should be considered arrhythmogenic, but fortunately such arrhythmias are rarely significant or long lasting. It is outside the scope of this chapter to discuss in detail mechanisms of arrhythmia under anaesthesia or to identify ways in which anaesthetic agents may minimize or potentiate arrhythmogenicity. However, there are a number of simple tenets.

The first is that volatile agents are in general more arrhythmogenic than intravenous anaesthetics, especially opiates. These arrhythmias are more usually supraventricular than ventricular, and are usually bradyarrhythmias. Halothane has been shown to reduce the sinoatrial nodal frequency and to impair conduction across the atria and may therefore be likely to promote atrioventricular junctional bradycardia (81,82). Enflurane may act similarly, although it is unlikely to sensitize the myocardium to catecholamines or to provoke ventricular ectopy in the manner of halothane (83). Isoflurane has less arrhythmogenic potential generally than these other two agents (84). The opioids all have the potential for causing bradyarrhythmias, particularly during induction of anaesthesia when the rate of rise of plasma concentration may be rapid. In practice this potential adverse effect is often offset by the opposing vagolytic effects of muscle relaxants.

Although junctional bradycardia may be benign in patients with normal hearts, the loss of sinus rhythm in a patient with poor left ventricular function may be haemodynamically significant. The volatile anaesthetics, and particularly enflurane and halothane, may induce arrhythmias in a dose dependent fashion, but there have been reports of anaesthetic drugs having anti-arrhythmic effects also (85). However, this apparent contradiction serves only to highlight the multifactorial nature of perioperative arrhythmogenesis, it is quite clear that an anaesthetic may be arrhythmogenic in one situation, and anti-arrhythmic in another.

Anaesthesia as an outcome determinant

From the above discussion, it is apparent that a number of factors may be theoretically important in delivering anaesthesia safely to a patient undergoing CABG surgery. However, the relative importance of each of these factors is less well understood. For example, we need to know how important close control of global haemodynamics and the preservation of myocardial oxygen balance actually is, and whether tachycardia or hypotension has been shown to adversely effect outcome, as opposed to simply being theoretically undesirable. The relevance of the quality of anaesthesia as an outcome determinant in cardiac surgery continues to be debated, but the data that have emerged have only answered a small part of the question.

There is no doubt that an anaesthetic mishap such as a wrong drug, incorrect drug dosage, or equipment failure can have a catastrophic effect on any surgical patient. However, apart from these considerations, there has hitherto been a belief that anaesthesia, although important to the care of the patient, has had no significant impact on outcome from CABG surgery. This may reflect the simplistic belief that, provided we do what we think is best, the anaesthetic management of the patient could not be significantly bettered, and therefore the outcome could not be improved. It certainly reflects the fact that until recently outcome studies have not been an important part of anaesthesia research.

The audit triad used to evaluate quality of patient care consists of *structure*, *process*, and *outcome*. In anaesthetic practice, structure would refer to the resources available to the anaesthetist to deliver care. This might include the availability of different monitoring systems or pain relief systems in the perioperative setting. Process refers to the use of those systems, for example whether pulse oximetry or patient-controlled analgesia (PCA) is available and used on every patient recovering from CABG surgery on the first postoperative day. The assumption of medical practice previously has been that, if structure and process are optimized, then outcome will invariably improve or at least not deteriorate. This is not necessarily true. The assumption that process and outcome are invariably linked may be quite fallacious. Early data from Cobb *et al.* showed that ligation of the internal mammary artery, a procedure used to produce a diversion of blood to the coronary arteries and supposedly associated with increased exercise tolerance and relief of angina, was in fact no more effective than a sham operation (86). The assumption that process developments and outcome are invariably beneficially linked is even more erroneous. The availability of oxygen and its use in high inspired concentrations to hypoxic neonates was eventually shown to be associated with eye and lung damage, and not with an improved outcome at all. These examples show that optimizing the structure and process may in fact be either be irrelevant to outcome or produce an adverse outcome, and therefore outcome studies are a crucially important part in the delivery of quality care.

Interest in outcome studies has been generated by the need for cost control in medicine, and cardiac surgery has been one of the areas under the closest scrutiny. The role of anaesthesia in this has also been examined, but other scientific considerations have also generated interest. The controversy surrounding the use of isoflurane anaesthesia in cardiac patients is partly responsible for the current interest that is being shown in outcome studies.

The literature regarding studies of isoflurane anaesthesia in patients with ischaemic heart disease is a good example of the need for outcome studies as a means of determining practice rather than relying on intermediate haemodynamic variables such as coronary blood flow and myocardial lactate extraction ratio.

Many outcome studies in cardiac anaesthesia and surgery refer to only one alternative outcome, life or death. In fact there is a wide variety of potential outcomes. Outcomes have been defined as those changes either favourable or unfavourable that occur in actual or potential health status after prior or concurrent care (87). In this context, health status may mean physiological parameters (haemodynamics, ECG abnormality, etc.), or broadened to include psychological concepts including patient satisfaction. For example, PCA may not reduce perioperative mortality but it may well improve patient satisfaction. That itself is an important outcome and one which anaesthetists should not disregard. Certainly the patients do not disregard it, and many hospitals advertise the availability of PCA for surgical patients in the knowledge that patients value it. It is therefore necessary to define each outcome, although highly objective outcomes such as survival are clearly more easy to define in a reproducible manner than subjective outcomes such as patient satisfaction. In fact many outcomes are surprisingly difficult to define. For example, perioperative infarction may be defined by ECG changes (Q wave, non Q wave), enzyme changes (M-CPK, troponin T), or functional image changes (radionuclide scanning, single photon emission computer tomography, etc.).

In each setting therefore, an outcome study needs to define its terms. What outcome is being measured and how it is being measured are important. When it is being measured is also important, particularly for anaesthetists. For example, perioperative infarction occurring at any time within the first 30 days following surgery may be of less relevance than perioperative infarction within the first 4 days.

The design of outcome studies is difficult, and particularly so in cardiac anaesthesia. CABG surgery has a variable mortality, but in low risk patients (i.e. Parsonnet score 0) the mortality is rarely over 2%. The impact on mortality of changing the main anaesthetic agent may be as little as 0.03%. This increase is certainly not trivial to the 3 in 10 000 extra patients who die as a result, and it would be reasonable to investigate further. However, the sample size needed would be simply enormous. For example, the largest prospective randomized study of anaesthetic outcome in non-cardiac patients failed to conclude on the advisability of different anaesthetic agents, simply because the incidence of perioperative myocardial infarction and death in an otherwise healthy population is so low. Although they studied 17 201 patients in order to detect a 50% reduction in death rate, with one anaesthetic agent with a statistical power of 95%, assuming an anaesthesia-related death rate of 0.03%, the authors estimated they would have to have studied more than 1 million patients (40). This is not realistic. Of course cardiac patients may be more vulnerable, and smaller numbers may be adequate. Multicentre trials may also be one way of generating greater numbers, and meta-analyses may have a role to play. However, variability between institutions may be a confounding factor, the Coronary Artery Surgery Study (CASS) noted a 21-fold variability in mortality between institutions (88). Single institution studies are more controllable, but they often take too long. The result is that changes in the patient population, cardiological management, and surgical and perfusion techniques may have taken place which invalidate the study as a controlled study of anaesthetic management. One study of the rate of myocardial reinfarction may well have suffered from this disadvantage as it took 9 years to complete (89). The undisputed advantage of the Texas Heart studies is that they were able to gather approximately 1000 patients undergoing CABG surgery in less than 1 year, thereby eliminating many of these confounding variables (24,32).

Finally, the CABG population is often assumed for study purposes to be a homogenous group with regard to cardiovascular and other disease, and yet we know they are not. All the relevant studies have identified that survival from CABG surgery reduces with increasing chronic health score (51–57), and yet few if any of the anaesthetic outcome studies match patients for equal chronic health scores. If this had been the case, it is possible that a clearer picture of the relationship between choice of anaesthetic and survival in CABG patients might have emerged, although it may still have been confounded by the effects of surgery. As has been previously stated, in the clinical situation anaesthesia and surgery are inevitably linked together, and the results of outcome studies are necessarily the results of the combination (90).

As a result of these difficulties, although less scientific than a properly controlled randomized prospective clinical trial, the use of observational data may be the only realistic way of linking process to outcome when the outcome itself is rare. However, despite all these problems it is clear that outcome studies in anaesthesia do have a role to play and that even now we can identify some anaesthetic factors that may be influential.

The anaesthetist

There is data to show that the experience of the surgeon and the number of procedures undertaken by an institution, and hence its familiarity with managing CABG patients, has an influence on outcome (53,91). There are now many countries where 'part-time' cardiac surgery by both individuals and institutions is actively discouraged.

The situation regarding anaesthesia is quite different. Training in anaesthesia includes training in all the areas of hospital practice which are within the anaesthetic domain, including intensive care and chronic pain relief as well as the more familiar surgical specialities. It is rare for a UK training programme to include more than 1 year of exposure to cardiothoracic anaesthesia, and frequently not only is the time spent much less than 1 year, but also it is not taken in one continuous period. The extent to which trained specialists practice cardiothoracic anaesthesia may also be relevant. The Association of Cardiothoracic Anaesthetists in the UK currently recommends that cardiothoracic anaesthetists should spend at least 50% of their clinical time involved in the care of cardiac surgery patients, including time spent in postoperative or intensive care. The relevant question is whether the anaesthetist who anaesthetizes one cardiac case per week can be expected to retain the intellectual and technical skills of those anaesthetists doing nothing but cardiothoracic anaesthesia.

Slogoff and Keats were the first to show that the identity of the anaesthetist may be an actual outcome determinant in CABG surgery (24). They found that one anaesthetist, who also was least active in cardiothoracic anaesthesia when compared to the rest of the cohort, had a preoperative infarction rate that was 11 times higher than the anaesthetist with the lowest incidence. They further showed that in their institution an increased incidence of perioperative infarction has been shown to correlate with increased mortality, a finding confirmed by others elsewhere. Since that time, Merry *et al.* have also shown that the identity of the anaesthetist may be an independent variable that affects outcome (92).

Needless to say, these studies have been given a mixed reception. The main point of them, and certainly of the Slogoff and Keats data, would appear to be that it is the totality of poor quality anaesthesia rather than failure to control one specific factor that is important. This is reflected in the fact that the infamous 'anaesthesiologist number 7' of their study also had the highest incidence of hypertension, tachycardia, and ischaemia, reflecting a failure to control haemodynamics adequately and an overall poor quality of anaesthesia. However, the most important consideration from these data is simply that it raises the question in a scientific manner. Beforehand, anaesthesia was often felt to be either largely irrelevant to a poor outcome or wholly responsible for it. The challenge for the future will be to try to further refine the concept of surrogate or intermediate outcomes which may identify poor quality anaesthesia before the patient is actually harmed. One important aspect now under study is the interrelationship between the surgeon and anaesthetist, and how the team is able to effectively differentiate their tasks while retaining a co-ordinated approach for the intraoperative management of the patient.

The anaesthetic

Any investigation regarding the safety of an anaesthetic drug or technique must take into account the clinical condition of the patient being anaesthetized. In 1943 Halford published data regarding the use of thiopentone for emergency anaesthesia for Pearl Harbour casualties (93). The results were widely regarded as catastrophic. However, other data appeared showing that thiopentone was a safe and effective anaesthetic in elective surgery patients (94). This demonstration of the obvious importance of the clinical condition of the patient saved thiopentone from being abandoned as an anaesthetic, and has influenced the speciality of anaesthesia ever since. As previously stated, there is a large body of evidence to show that patient factors have a powerful impact on many outcomes, including survival, in CABG patients. These patient factors may either be used as single entities or combined and given differential weighting, and the system can then be scored to produce a risk profile. The subject of risk stratification and the assessment of patient factors is dealt with in Chapter X.

Haemodynamic control

From the discussion earlier in this chapter, it is clear that close haemodynamic control forms a large part of the anaesthetic management of CABG patients. For this to be proven as an outcome-determining therapy, we should expect that those patients whose anaesthetic provides for close haemodynamic control should have a lower incidence of ischaemia, perioperative infarction, and death. In fact the studies so far reported give partial support to this theory. Slogoff and Keats showed that preoperative tachycardia did correlate with the development of ischaemia, and that perioperative ischaemia correlated with myocardial infarction (24). (Others have shown the correlation between perioperative myocardial infarction and death.) However, they also found that in a higher proportion of patients who had evidence of ischaemic episodes, no haemodynamic abnormality occurred at the time of the ischaemia. They suggested that these ischaemic episodes are different in aetiology to those seen in association with sympatho-adrenal activation, and might be related to alterations in coronary vasomotion which possibly may be related to other factors, including anaesthetics. However, they and others have also shown that continuation of beta-blockers reduces the incidence of perioperative ischaemia, presumably by minimizing sympathetic activation (47,95). The situation regarding the continuation of calcium channel blockers is more controversial. Studies have both suggested and refuted preoperative calcium channel blockade as effective anti-ischaemic therapy (48,49,96). It therefore appears that close haemodynamic control may help to minimize the incidence of ischaemia and infarction, but that there is a background incidence of ischaemia which is unresponsive to manipulation of haemodynamics.

Anaesthetic drugs

Following the isoflurane controversy, recent studies have tried to evaluate the effect of different anaesthetics on outcome in CABG patients. Comparisons of intravenous opioid, volatile, and combined techniques have failed to show a difference between the various anaesthetic techniques described (32,41). One further study suggested that isoflurane was associated with a higher incidence of perioperative infarction than enflurane. However, the two groups were incompletely controlled, even to the extent of the enflurane patients receiving significantly more nitroglycerin than the isoflurane group (97).

Further studies have been undertaken, specifically with the aim of identifying whether isoflurane anaesthesia may adversely affect outcome. Isoflurane was not more commonly associated with ischaemia or infarction, even in patients with steal-prone coronary anatomy, when compared to other volatile (32,98) or opioid-based techniques (99). The current consensus is that provided that other principles of safe anaesthesia are followed, the primary anaesthetic agent appears to have little influence on outcome in CABG surgery.

Intraoperative monitoring

Modern cardiac anaesthesia for cardiopulmonary bypass procedures uses a patient monitoring format which is well standardized. Intra-arterial and central venous cannulation, ECG monitoring, and a method of measuring core temperature have been recommended for routine use. Pulse oximetry and expired gas capnography have been included (100). Recently many countries have developed minimum monitoring standards that are recommended for every patient undergoing anaesthesia. In some countries these standards carry the force of law, but even in the remainder the medico-legal consequences of ignoring them make such practice inadvisable.

However, the dilemmas concerning monitoring in CABG surgery concern the use of sophisticated ECG monitoring, pulmonary artery catheter monitoring, and transoesophageal echocardiography.

The main benefit of sophisticated ECG monitoring in this setting is the accurate diagnosis of ischaemia. A number of newer monitoring systems have been developed which allow for on-line trend analysis of ST segment change, but there is no data yet on whether the use of these systems has permitted the more accurate diagnosis of ischaemia which, when appropriately treated, has affected outcome. However, data from London et al. have validated the use of multilead ECG monitoring as a more effective way of diagnosing ischaemic episodes (101). They found that monitoring standard lead II, V4 and V5 detected 98% of those episodes that were detected by a full 12-lead ECG. Single-lead monitoring with standard lead I detected no episodes at all.

The value of pulmonary artery catheters (PAC) continues to be closely questioned, and there is no doubt that there is a wide diversity of view regarding their value (102,103). There are studies that both support and refute the hypothesis that accurate clinical assessment is an acceptable alternative to pulmonary artery catheterization in patients with a range of conditions (89,104–106). Many studies have been carried out with the aim of validating the use of PAC in patients undergoing non-cardiac surgery, and groups have reported positively on the value of such monitoring (89,107,108). In patients undergoing non-cardiac surgery, perioperative pulmonary artery catheterization may be useful in revealing haemodynamic information that was not available either by clinical examination or by routine preoperative tests. In contrast, in patients undergoing cardiac surgery, preoperative cardiac catheterization will reveal data on cardiac index, ejection fraction, and left ventricular end diastolic pressure which may be more comprehensive than data from pulmonary artery catheterization.

There is no consensus view as to whether pulmonary artery catheterization improves outcome in patients undergoing CABG surgery, particularly in the low risk patients. Centres that have not used PAC monitoring as a routine have shown excellent surgical results, and despite many calls for randomized controlled trials, doubt has been cast about the practicality of such studies or their value (103,109). In fact the problem of correlating the use of PACs to outcome in CABG surgery highlights many of the problems of outcome studies. One would feel intuitively that more accurate haemodynamic monitoring should allow for earlier recognition of problems and prompt treatment, which should improve outcome.

However, the patient numbers in such a study would need to be very large, and some have questioned the ethics of continuing to withhold the use of a PAC in those patients who are haemodynamically unstable (106). It is salutary to remember that a PAC is a monitor and not a therapeutic procedure; if the use of a PAC is to affect outcome, the catheter must be properly sited, the data gathered correctly and interpreted, and a therapeutic decision made based on such data. Given that many workers have studied only the use of the PAC and not the therapeutic decisions based on the data gathered from their correct use, it is not surprising that many studies have failed to identify an improvement in outcome. However, for individual patients a PAC may be the most effective way of optimizing the patient's haemodynamic state, and the most appropriate task may be therefore to identify those patients in whom PAC monitoring is unnecessary, and those in whom it is advisable or mandatory. This view will vary, even between equally prestigious centres in the same country. 'Swan-Ganz catheters may be life-saving in Atlanta, but mostly are a nuisance in Houston' (90).

The use of intraoperative transoesophageal echocardiography has become widespread in recent years, and its value is well established. It can provide excellent data on aspects of ventricular function, including ventricular volumes and ejection fraction, segmental wall motion abnormalities, and hypo/akinesia, as well as data on valve function and intracardiac directional blood flow. Transoesophageal echo has been shown to identify ischaemic episodes faster and more sensitively than the ECG (110,111) or PAC (112), and persistent segmental wall motion abnormalities following surgery have been shown to be clearly associated with myocardial ischaemia and postoperative morbidity (113,114). The value of intraoperative echo in patients with concomitant valve disease is beyond doubt, but attention has been drawn to the fact that considerable training is essential for diagnosing lesions with reasonable accuracy (115). One drawback of transoesophageal echo as a monitor of intraoperative ischaemia is that it is often used only after induction of anaesthesia and endotracheal intubation, which is of course a time of high stress and with a high incidence of ischaemia. Despite the reduction in size of the current generation of transoesophageal probes, episodes of oesophageal trauma due to insertion of the probe have been reported (116).

Postoperative management

A more detailed account of postoperative management is provided in Chapter 7.

One aspect of patient management that is clearly in need of further outcome studies is the effect of changing the postoperative management of the patient. This may include the routine use of anti-ischaemic drugs including intravenous nitrates in order to prevent ischaemic episodes, and the use of vasodilators or inotropic agents or the newer inodilator drugs such as the phosphodiesterase inhibitors in order to improve cardiac output and prevent the development of a low output state. Many institutions have their own protocols for the routine use of vasoactive drugs following surgery, and such protocols are based on logical therapeutic sequences, but it is surprising how little data there are that address the question of whether routinely used treatments, as opposed to those that are specifically designed to correct a measured abnormality, carry any benefit.

One postoperative area under close scrutiny at the moment is the need for prolonged periods of intermittent positive pressure ventilation (IPPV) following routine CABG surgery. Following early reports (117–119), many centres are now content to reduce the period of postoperative ventilation to a few hours before the patient may be woken and extubated. Patients may then be discharged to a postoperative care area requiring less nursing than the traditional 1 : 1 nurse/patient ratio required for ventilator-dependent patients, thereby improving patient throughput and reducing unit costs. In this way, ever-spiralling health care costs and lengthening waiting lists can successfully be tackled. Despite increasing popularity, this method of postoperative management has left many questions unanswered concerning the ideal duration of postoperative IPPV. It is clearly unnecessary to ventilate many patients for prolonged periods, and indeed there may be hazards involved in so doing (increased use of sedative or paralyzing drugs, the hazard of disconnection from the ventilator or blockage of the endotracheal tube, etc.). Although there are some workers who believe that IPPV of whatever duration may be undesirable (120), most feel that the extubation criteria of awake, haemodynamically stable, with good gas exchange and minimal bleeding are still appropriate. Specific to CABG surgery, it has been shown that the incidence of post-revascularization ischaemic complications is minimal after 8 hours following revascularization, and that after this time there is little need to delay recovery and extubation (121). However, reducing the period of postoperative IPPV to 8 hours does not solve the problem of resource utilization, since many centres now look toward the idea of early discharge from the intensive therapy unit or other early postoperative care facility, as a prerequisite to reusing the same bed space in the same day. For this to be feasible, the early part of the patient's postoperative recovery, following which the patient can be transferred to a lower dependency facility, needs to be completed in about 4 hours. This has led to a reappraisal of many aspects of anaesthetic, perfusion, and surgical management. In particular, the use of long-acting drugs as premedicants and high doses of opioids during anaesthesia is best avoided in the low risk case scheduled for early extubation and discharge, and balanced opioid/volatile based techniques have been advocated as preferable (122). Large volumes of crystalloid solution in the bypass prime are best avoided as they may exacerbate the tendency to increase extravascular lung water and lead to poor gas exchange in the early postoperative period. In the critical early period following CABG surgery, there is clear data that gas exchange is worse in patients receiving one or two internal mammary grafts when compared to those patients who received saphenous vein grafts (123).

Another important aspect of postoperative management is the need for adequate early postoperative analgesia. This has been highlighted by Mangano (123) and it is questionable whether spontaneous respiration is compatible with adequate opioid analgesia in the early postoperative period. One way around the problem of opioid-induced respiratory depression is to use epidural analgesia, a technique which has been shown to provide effective analgesia and good haemodynamic stability (124). However, there are drawbacks to epidural analgesia, particularly in patients with abnormal coagulation.

Significant haemorrhage is a contraindication to early extubation, and a number of strategies have been adopted to minimize postoperative bleeding. The indications and dosage of aprotinin have been the subject of study (125–127), and although some workers advocate the routine use of aprotinin to reduce postoperative bleeding, there is no clear data to show that it improves outcome (i.e. facilitates early extubation) in this setting. This problem is clearly complicated by the fact that there are a number of causes of postoperative bleeding, including inadequate surgical haemostasis, and therefore no single agent or strategy is likely to be fully effective. Furthermore, there is no doubt that aprotinin has a variety of effects on coagulation and an incidence of adverse effects including anaphylaxis (128).

The effect of postoperative management on outcome is an important area of study, and it is complicated by the fact that we have few good indicators of imminent risk in those patients who appear to be doing well. It is not clear why a number of these patients suffer a setback in the postoperative period, particularly if haemodynamic parameters and the ECG are within normal limits. However, it is important to realize that the highest actual number of deaths (in contrast to the highest proportional mortality) still occur in the large group of patients who have a low preoperative risk score and would therefore be deemed to be acceptable candidates for early extubation and discharge (Fig. 6.4). Outcome studies in this and comparable situations are particularly important because, rather than expecting each individual patient to benefit from early extubation and discharge, we are intending that the patient should do as well as previously (or come to no harm) but for less cost. However, the statistical difficulties inherent in outcome studies, and in particular the problems of a large sample size, are very relevant to this question, and until a number of centres start to report well monitored series thereby allowing meta-analyses, the whole range of questions of cost-benefit analysis will not be adequately answered.

In conclusion, there are a number of anaesthetic factors that may affect patient outcome, in addition to the more widely understood criteria relating to the state of health of the patient before surgery and the nature and conduct of the surgery itself. The challenge for the future will be to further define the importance of these anaesthetic factors, bearing in mind that it is equally

Mortality

		≤9	10–12	≥13
Parsonnet score	≥35	3 1 died 33%	0	6 4 died 66%
	18–34	53 1 died 1.8%	29 4 died 13.7%	12 4 died 33%
	≤17	925 23 died 2.5%	62 5 died 8%	11 1 died 9%

UKACTA score

Fig. 6.4 Mortality data from 1101 adult patients undergoing cardiac surgical procedures. Patients are stratified according to two risk stratification scoring systems (Parsonnet and UKACTA). The lowest score (i.e. Parsonnet <17, UKACTA <9) supposedly represents the least risk. The proportional mortality is low (2.5%). However, of the 43 deaths, 23 (55%) occurred in this subgroup (adapted from reference 57).

important to identify those aspects of anaesthetic management that do significantly affect outcome, and to identify anaesthetic factors that, despite theoretical considerations, do not appear to have any significant impact on outcome.

References

1. Sabiston DC, Jr. The coronary circulation. *Johns Hopkins Med J* 1974;**134:**314–29.
2. Garrett HE, Dennis EW, DeBakey ME. Aorto-coronary bypass with saphenous vein graft: seven-year follow-up. *JAMA* 1973;**223:**792–4.
3. Favaloro RG. Saphenous vein graft in the surgical treatment of coronary artery disease. Operative technique. *J Thorac Cardiovasc Surg* 1969;**58:**178–85.
4. Johnson WD, Flemma RJ, Lepley D, Jr., Ellison EH. Extended treatment of severe coronary artery disease. A total surgical approach. *Ann Surg* 1969;**170:**460–70.
5. Keown KK. *Anesthesia for surgery of the heart*. Springfield, MO: Charles C Thomas, 1956.
6. Wynands JE, Sheridan CA, Kalkar K. Coronary artery disease and anesthesia. (Experience in 120 patients for revascularization of the heart). *Can Anaesth Soc J* 1967;**14:**382–98.
7. Lowenstein E, Hallowell P, Levine FH, Doggett WM, Austen WG, Laver MB. Cardiovascular response to large doses of intravenous morphine in man. *N Engl J Med* 1969;**281:**1389–93.
8. Lowenstein E. Morphine 'anesthesia' — a perspective. *Anesthesiology* 1971;**35:**563–5.
9. Lunn JK, Stanley TH, Eisele J, Webster L, Woodward A. High-dose fentanyl anesthesia for coronary artery surgery: Plasma fentanyl concentrations and influence of nitrous oxide on cardiovascular responses. *Anesth Analg* 1979;**58:**390–5.
10. deLange S, Boscoe MJ, Stanley TH, Pace N. Comparison of sufentanil-oxygen and fentanyl-oxygen for coronary artery surgery. *Anesthesiology* 1982;**56:**112–8.
11. Robbins GR, Wynands JE, Whalley DJ *et al*. Pharmacokinetics of alfentanil and clinical responses during cardiac surgery. *Can J Anaesth* 1990;**37:**52–7.

12. Bland JHL, Lowenstein E. Halothane-induced decrease in experimental myocardial ischemia in the non-failing canine heart. *Anesthesiology* 1976;**45**:287–93.

13. Ramsay JG, DeJesus JM, Wynands JE *et al*. Pure opiate vs opiate-volatile anesthesia for coronary bypass surgery. [Abstract] *Anesth Analg* 1989;**68**:S233.

14. Naunheim KS, Fiore AC, Wadley JJ *et al*. The changing profile of the patient undergoing coronary artery bypass surgery. *J Am Coll Cardiol* 1988;**11**:494–8.

15. Lytle BW, Cosgrove D, Loop FD. Future implications of current trends in bypass surgery. *Cardiovasc Clin* 1991;**21**:265–78.

16. Edwards FH, Clark RE, Schwartz M. Coronary artery bypass grafting: the Society of Thoracic Surgeons national database experience. *Ann Thorac Surg* 1994;**57**:12–19.

17. Little DM, Jr. Classical file. *Survey of Anesthesiology* 1981;**25**:270–8.

18. Traber DL, Wilson RD, Priano LL. The effect of alpha-adrenergic blockade on the cardiopulmonary response to ketamine. *Anesth Analg* 1971;**50**:737–42.

19. Kumar SM, Kothary SP, Zsigmond EK. Plasma free norepinephrine and epinephrine concentrations following diazepam-ketamine induction in patients undergoing cardiac surgery. *Acta Anaesth Scand* 1978;**22**:593–600.

20. Tyson GS, Sladen RN, Spainhour V, Savitt MA, Ferguson TB Jr, Wolfe WG. Blood conservation in cardiac surgery. Preliminary results with an institutional commitment. *Ann Surg* 1989;**209**:736–42.

21. Crystal GJ. Myocardial oxygen supply-demand relations during isovolemic hemodilution. *Adv Pharmacol* 1994;**31**:285–312.

22. Berne RM, Levy MN. Special circulations. In: Berne RM, Levy MN, eds, *Physiology*. St. Louis: CV Mosby, 1988, pp. 540–60.

23. Underwood SM, Davies SW, Feneck RO, Lunnon MW, Walesby RK. Comparison of isradipine with nitroprusside for control of blood pressure following myocardial revascularization: Effects on hemodynamics, cardiac metabolism, and coronary blood flow. *J Cardiothorac Vasc Anesth* 1991;**5**:348–56.

24. Slogoff S, Keats AS. Does perioperative myocardial ischaemia lead to postoperative myocardial infarction. *Anesthesiology* 1985;**62**:107–14.

25. Hickey RF, Sybert PE, Verrier ED, Cason BA. Effects of halothane, enflurane, and isoflurane on coronary blood flow autoregulation and coronary vascular reserve in the canine heart. *Anesthesiology* 1988;**68**:21–30.

26. Sahlman L, Henriksson B, Martner J, Ricksten S. Effects of halothane, enflurane, and isoflurane on coronary vascular tone, myocardial performance, and oxygen consumption during controlled changes in aortic and left atrial pressure. Studies on isolated working rat hearts *in vitro*. *Anesthesiology* 1988;**69**:1–10.

27. Hohner P, Nancarrow C, Backman C *et al*. Anesthesia for abdominal vascular surgery in patients with coronary artery disease (CAD). Part I: Isoflurane produces dose-dependent coronary vasodilatation. *Acta Anaesth Scand* 1994;**38**:780–92.

28. Buffington CW, Davis KB, Gillespie S, Pettinger M. The prevalence of steal-prone coronary anatomy in patients with coronary artery disease: an analysis of the Coronary Artery Surgery Study registry. *Anesthesiology* 1988;**69**:721–7.

29. Stevens WC, Cromwell TH, Halsey MJ, Eger EI, II, Shakespeare TF, Bahlman SH. The cardiovascular effects of a new inhalation anesthetic, Forane, in human volunteers at constant arterial carbon dioxide tension. *Anesthesiology* 1971;**35**:8–16.

30. Reiz S, Bålfors E, Sorensen MB, Ariola S, Friedman A, Truedsson H. Isoflurane — a powerful coronary vasodilator in patients with coronary artery disease. *Anesthesiology* 1983;**59**:91–7.

31. Moffitt EA, Barker RA, Glen JJ *et al.* Myocardial metabolism and hemodynamic responses with isoflurane anesthesia for coronary arterial surgery. *Anesth Analg* 1986;**65**:53–61.

32. Slogoff S, Keats AS, Dear WE *et al.* Steal-prone coronary anatomy and myocardial ischemia associated with four primary anesthetic agents in humans. *Anesth Analg* 1991;**72**:22–7.

33. Cason BA, Verrier ED, London MJ, Mangano DT, Hickey RF. Effects of isoflurane and halothane on coronary vascular resistance and collateral myocardial blood flow: Their capacity to induce coronary steal. *Anesthesiology* 1987;**67**;665–75.

34. Hartman JC, Kampine JP, Schmeling WT, Warltier DC. Volatile anesthetics and regional myocardial perfusion in chronically instrumented dogs: Halothane versus isoflurane in a single-vessel disease model with enhanced collateral development. *J Cardiothorac Anesth* 1990;**4**:588–603.

35. Buffington CW, Romson JL, Levine A, Duttlinger NC, Huang AH. Isoflurane induces coronary steal in a canine model of chronic coronary occlusion. *Anesthesiology* 1987;**66**:280–92.

36. Gewirtz H, Gross SL, Williams DO, Most AS. Contrasting effects of nifedipine and adenosine on regional myocardial flow distribution and metabolism distal to severe coronary arterial stenosis: Observations in sedated, closed-chest, domestic swine. *Circulation* 1984;**69**:1048–57.

37. Lillehaug SL, Tinker JH. Why do 'pure' vasodilators cause coronary steal when anesthetics don't (or seldom do). *Anesth Analg* 1991;**73**:681–2.

38. Merin RG, Lowenstein E, Gelman S. Is anesthesia beneficial for the ischemic heart? III. *Anesthesiology* 1986;**64**:137–40.

39. Moffitt EA, Sethna DH. The coronary circulation and myocardial oxygenation in coronary artery disease: Effects of anesthesia. *Anesth Analg* 1986;**65**:395–410.

40. Forrest JB, Cahalan MK, Redher K *et al.* Multicenter study of general anesthesia. II. Results. *Anesthesiology* 1990;**72**:262–8.

41. Tuman KJ, McCarthy RJ, Spiess BD, DaValle M, Dabir R, Ivankovich AD. Does choice of anesthetic agent significantly affect outcome after coronary artery surgery. *Anesthesiology* 1989;**70**:189–98.

42. Priebe H. Isoflurane and coronary hemodynamics. *Anesthesiology* 1989;**71**:960–76.

43. Moore PG, Kien ND, Boldy RM, Reitan JA. Comparative effects of nitric oxide inhibition on the coronary vasomotor responses to etomidate, propofol, and thiopental in anesthetized dogs. *Anesth Analg* 1994;**79**:439–46.

44. Nugent M. Anesthesia and myocardial ischemia. *Anesth Analg* 1992;75:1–3.

45. Marcus ML. Metabolic regulation of coronary blood flow. In: Marcus ML, ed. *The coronary circulation in health and disease*. New York: McGraw-Hill, 1983, pp. 65–92.

46. Thomson IR, Bergsrom RG, Rosenbloom M, Meatherall RC. Premedication and high-dose fentanyl anesthesia for myocardial revascularization: A comparison of lorazepam versus morphine scopolamine. *Anesthesiology* 1988;**68**:194–200.

47. Slogoff S, Keats AS, Ott E. Preoperative propranolol therapy and aortocoronary bypass operation. *JAMA* 1978;**240**:1487–90.

48. Slogoff S, Keats AS. Does chronic treatment with calcium entry blocking drugs reduce perioperative myocardial ischemia. *Anesthesiology* 1988;**68**:676–80.

49. Chung F, Horston PL, Cheng DCH *et al*. Calcium channel blockade does not offer adequate protection from perioperative myocardial ischemia. *Anesthesiology* 1988;**69**:343–7.

50. Thomson IR, Hudson RJ, Rosenbloom M, Meatherall RC. A randomized double-blind comparison of fentanyl and sufentanil anaesthesia for coronary artery surgery. *Can J Anaesth* 1987;**34**:227–32.

51. Killip T, Pasamani E, Davis K, the CASS Principal investigators and Their Associates. Coronary Artery Surgery Study (CASS): A randomized trial of coronary bypass surgery. Eight years follow-up and survival in patients with reduced ejection fraction. *Circulation* 1985;**72**(suppl V):102–9.

52. Parsonnet V, Dean D, Bernstein AD. A method of uniform stratification of risk for evaluating the results of surgery in acquired adult heart disease. *Circulation* 1989;**79**(suppl I):3–12.

53. O'Connor GT, Plume SK, Olmstead EM *et al*. A regional prospective study of in-hospital mortality associated with coronary artery bypass grafting. *JAMA* 1991;**266**:803–9.

54. Hannan EL, Kilburn H, O'Donnell JF, Lukacik G, Shields EP. Adult open heart surgery in New York State: An analysis of risk factors and hospital mortality rates. *JAMA* 1990;**264**:2768–74.

55. Grover FL, Hammermeister KE, Burchfiel C, the Cardiac Surgeons of the Department of Veterans Affairs. Initial report of the Veterans Administration preoperative risk assessment study for cardiac surgery. *Ann Thorac Surg* 1990;**50**:12–28.

56. Paiemont B, Pelletier C, Dyrda I *et al*. A simple classification of the risk in cardiac surgery. *Can Anaesth Soc J* 1983;**30**:61–8.

57. Duncan F, Feneck RO. Outcome predictors in cardiac surgery: A comparison of UKACTA data and Parsonnet risk stratification scoring systems. [Abstract] *Br J Anaesth* 1995;**74**:(suppl 2):A115.

58. Goldman L. Multifactorial index of cardiac risk in noncardiac surgical procedures: Ten year status report. *J Cardiothorac Anesth* 1987;**1**:237–44.

59. Pasternack PF, Imparato AM, Riles TS *et al*. The value of radionuclide angiography as a predictor of perioperative myocardial infarction in patients undergoing lower extremity revascularization procedures. [Abstract] *Circulation* 1984;**70**:II–163.

60. Van Trigt P, Christian CC, Fagraeus L *et al*. Myocardial depression by anesthetic agents (halothane, enflurane and nitrous oxide): Quantitation based on end-systolic pressure-dimension relations. *Am J Cardiol* 1984;**53**:243–7.

61. Housmans PR, Murat I. Comparative effects of halothane, enflurane, and isoflurane at equipotent anesthetic concentrations on isolated ventricular myocardium of the ferret. I. Contractility. *Anesthesiology* 1988;**69**:451–63.

62. Kemmotsu O, Hashimoto Y, Shimosato S. The effects of fluroxene and enflurane on contractile performance of isolated papillary muscles from failing hearts. *Anesthesiology* 1974;**40**:252–60.

63. Prys-Roberts C, Roberts JG, Foëx P, Clarke TNS, Bennett MJ, Ryder WA. Interaction of anesthesia, beta-receptor blockade, and blood loss in dogs with induced myocardial infarction. *Anesthesiology* 1976;**45**:326–39.

64. Lynch C, III. Differential depression of myocardial contractility by halothane and isoflurane *in vitro*. *Anesthesiology* 1986;**64**:620–31.

65. Tarnow J, Brückner JB, Eberlein HJ, Hess W, Patschke D. Haemodynamics and myocardial oxygen consumption during isoflurane (Forane) anaesthesia in geriatric patients. *Br J Anaesth* 1976;**48**:669–75.

66. Pagel PS, Kampine JP, Schmeling WT, Warltier DC. Influence of volatile anesthetics on myocardial contractility *in vivo*: Desflurane versus isoflurane. *Anesthesiology* 1991;74:900–7.

67. Kikura M, Ikeda K. Comparison of effects of sevoflurane/nitrous oxide and enflurane /nitrous oxide on myocardial contractility in humans. Load independent and non-invasive assessment with transesophageal echocardiography. *Anesthesiology* 1993;**79**:235–43.

68. Lawson D, Frazer MJ, Lynch C, III. Nitrous oxide effects on isolated myocardium: A re-examination *in vitro*. *Anesthesiology* 1990;**73**:930–43.

69. Pagel PS, Kampine JP, Schmeling WT, Warltier DC. Effects of nitrous oxide on myocardial contractility as evaluated by the preload recruitable stroke work relationship in chronically instrumented dogs. *Anesthesiology* 1990;**73**:1148–57.

70. Seltzer JL, Gerson JI, Allen FB. Comparison of the cardiovascular effects of bolus v. incremental administration of thiopentone. *Br J Anaesth* 1980;**52**:527–9.

71. McCammon RL, Hilgenberg JC, Stoelting RK. Hemodynamic effects of diazepam and diazepam-nitrous oxide in patients with coronary artery disease. *Anesth Analg* 1980;**59**:438–41.

72. Ruff R, Reves JG. Hemodynamic effects of a lorazepam-fentanyl anesthetic induction for coronary artery bypass surgery. *J Cardiothorac Anesth* 1990;**4**:314–17.

73. Schulte-Sasse U, Hess W, Tarnow J. Haemodynamic responses to induction of anaesthesia using midazolam in cardiac surgical patients. *Br J Anaesth* 1982;**54**:1053–7.

74. Kwar P, Carson IW, Clarke RSJ, Dundee JW, Lyons SM. Haemodynamic changes during induction of anesthesia with midazolam and diazepam (Valium) in patients undergoing coronary artery bypass surgery. *Anaesthesia* 1985;**40**:767–71.

75. Sebel PS, Lowden JD. Propofol: A new intravenous anesthetic. *Anesthesiology* 1989;**71**:260–77.

76. Merin RG. Propofol causes cardiovascular depression. *Anesthesiology* 1990;**72**:394–5.

77. Underwood SM, Davies SW, Feneck RO, Walesby RK. Anaesthesia for myocardial revas-cularization. A comparison of fentanyl/propofol with fentanyl/enflurane. *Anaesthesia* 1992;**47**:939–45.

78. White PF, Way WL, Trevor AJ. Ketamine — its pharmacology and therapeutic uses. *Anesthesiology* 1982;**56**:119–36.

79. Kaplan JA, Bland JW Jr, Dunbar RW. The perioperative management of pericardial tamponade. *South Med J* 1976;**69**:417–19.

80. Atlee JL, III. Causes for perioperative cardiac dysrhythmias. In: Atlee JL, III. ed. *Perioperative Cardiac Dysrhythmias*, 2nd edn, Chicago: Year Book Medical Publishers, 1990, pp. 187–273.

81. Hauswirth O, Schaer H. Effects of halothane on the sino-atrial node. *J Pharmacol Exp Ther* 1967;**158**:36–9.

82. Hauswirth O. Effects of halothane on single atrial, ventricular, and Purkinje fibers. *Circ Res* 1969;**24**:745–50.

83. Reisner LS, Lippman M. Ventricular arrhythmias after epinephrine injection in enflurane and in halothane anesthesia. *Anesth Analg* 1975;**54**:468–70.

84. Johnston RR, Eger EI, II. Wilson C. A comparative interaction of epinephrine with enflurane, isoflurane, and halothane in man. *Anesth Analg* 1976;**55**:709–12.

85. Atlee JL, III. Halothane: Cause or cure for arrhythmias. *Anesthesiology* 1987;**67**:617–18.

86. Cobb LA, Thomas GI, Bruce RA *et al.* Preliminary report of a double blind evaluation of ligation of the internal mammary arteries. [Abstract] *Circulation* 1958;**18**:704.

87. Donabedian A. The quality of care. How can it be assessed. *JAMA* 1988;**260**:1743–8.

88. Kennedy JW, Kaiser GC, Fischer LD *et al.* Clinical and angiographic predictors of operative mortality from the Collaborative Study in Coronary Artery Surgery (CASS). *Circulation* 1981;**63**:793–802.

89. Rao TLK, Jacobs KH, El-Etr AA. Reinfarction following anesthesia in patients with myocardial infarction. *Anesthesiology* 1983;**59**:499–505.

90. Keats AS. The Rovenstein Lecture, 1983: Cardiovascular anesthesia — perceptions and perspectives. *Anesthesiology* 1984;**60**:467–74.

91. Hannan EL, Kilburn H, Jr, Bernard H, O'Donnell JF, Lucacik G, Shields EP. Coronary artery bypass surgery: The relationship between inhospital mortality rate and surgical volume after controlling for clinical risk factors. *Med Care* 1991;**29**:1094–107.

92. Merry AF, Ramage MC, Whitlock RML *et al.* First-time coronary artery bypass grafting: the anaesthetist as a risk factor. *Br J Anaesth* 1992;**68**:6–12.

93. Halford FJ. A critique of intravenous anesthesia in war surgery. *Anesthesiology* 1943;**4**:67–9.

94. Organe G, Broad RJB. Pentothal with nitrous oxide and oxygen. *Lancet* 1938;**2**:1170–2.

95. Pontén J, Häggendal J, Milocco J, Waldenström A. Long-term metoprolol therapy and neuroleptanesthesia in coronary artery surgery: Withdrawal versus maintenance of β-adrenoceptor blockade. *Anesth Analg* 1983;**62**:380–90.

96. Gottlieb SO, Ouyang P, Aschuff SC *et al.* Acute nifedipine withdrawal: Consequences of preoperative and late cessation of therapy in patients with prior unstable angina. *J Am Coll Cardiol* 1984;**4**:382–8.

97. Inouke K, Reichelt W, El-Banayosy A *et al.* Does isoflurane lead to a higher incidence of myocardial infarction and perioperative death than enflurane in coronary artery surgery? A clinical study of 1178 patients. *Anesth Analg* 1990;**71**:469–74.

98. Pulley DD, Kirvassilis GV, Kelermenos N *et al.* Regional and global myocardial circulatory and metabolic effects of isoflurane and halothane in patients with steal-prone coronary anatomy. *Anesthesiology* 1991;**75**:756–66.

99. Leung JM, Goehner P, O'Kelly BF *et al.* Isoflurane anesthesia and myocardial ischemia: Comparative risk versus sufentanil anesthesia in patients undergoing coronary artery bypass surgery. *Anesthesiology* 1991;**74**:838–47.

100. Feneck RO. Standards of monitoring. *J Cardiothorac Vasc Anesth* 1994;**8**:379–81.

101. London MJ, Hollenberg M, Wong MG *et al.* Intraoperative myocardial ischemia: Localization by continuous 12-lead electrocardiography. *Anesthesiology* 1988;**69**:232–41.

102. Weintraub AC, Barash PG. Pro: A pulmonary artery catheter is indicated in all patients for coronary artery surgery. *J Cardiothorac Anesth* 1987;**1**:358.

103. Roizen MF, Berger DL, Gabel RA *et al.* Practice guidelines for pulmonary artery catheterization. *Anesthesiology* 1993;**78**:380–94.

104. Eisenberg PR, Jaffe AS, Schuster DP. Clinical evaluation compared to pulmonary artery catheterization in the hemodynamic assessment of critically ill patients. *Crit Care Med* 1984;**12**:549–53.

105. Bashein G, Johnson PW, Davis KB, Ivey TD. Elective coronary bypass surgery without pulmonary artery catheter monitoring. *Anesthesiology* 1985;**63**:451–4.

106. Tuman KJ, McCarthy RJ, Spiess BD *et al*. Effect of pulmonary artery catheterization on outcome in patients undergoing coronary artery surgery. *Anesthesiology* 1989;**70**:199–206.

107. Joyce WP, Provan JL, Ameli FM, McEwan P, Jelenich S, Jones DP. The role of central haemodynamic monitoring in abdominal aortic surgery: a prospective randomized study. *Eur J Vasc Surg* 1990;**4**:633–6.

108. Berlauk JF, Abrams JH, Gilmour IJ, O'Connor SR, Knighton DR, Cerra FB. Preoperative optimization of cardiovascular hemodynamics improves outcome in peripheral vascular surgery: a prospective, randomized clinical trial. *Ann Surg* 1991;**214**:289–99.

109. Swan HJC, Ganz W. Hemodynamic measurements in clinical practice: a decade in review. *J Am Coll Cardiol* 1983;**1**:103–13.

110. Smith JS, Cahalan MK, Benefiel DJ *et al*. Intraoperative detection of myocardial ischemia in high risk patients: electrocardiography versus two-dimensional transesophageal echocardiography. *Circulation* 1987;**72**:1015–21.

111. Wohlgelernter D, Jaffe cc, Cabin HS, Yeatman LA Jr, Cleman M. Silent ischemia during coronary occlusion produced by balloon inflation: relation to regional myocardial dysfunction. *J Am Coll Cardiol* 1987;**10**:491–8.

112. van Daele MERM, Sutherland GR, Mitchell MM *et al*. Do changes in pulmonary capillary wedge pressure adequately reflect myocardial ischemia during anesthesia. *Circulation* 1990;**81**:865–71.

113. Gewertz BL, Kremser PC, Zarins CK *et al*. Transesophageal echocardiographic monitoring of myocardial ischemia during vascular surgery. *J Vasc Surg* 1987;**5**:607–13.

114. Simon P, Mohl W, Neumann F, Owen A, Punzengruber C, Wolner E. Effects of coronary artery bypass grafting on global and regional myocardial function: Intraoperative echo assessment. *J Thorac Cardiovasc Surg* 1992;**104**:40–5.

115. Kaplan JA. Monitoring technology: advances and restraints. *J Cardiothorac Anesth* 1989;**3**:257.

116. Daniel WG, Erbel R, Kasper W *et al*. Safety of transesophageal echocardiography: a multicenter survey of 10 419 examinations. *Circulation* 1991;**83**:817–21.

117. Quasha AL, Loeber N, Feely TW, Ullyot DJ, Roizen MF. Postoperative respiratory care: A controlled trial of early and late extubation following coronary artery bypass grafting. *Anesthesiology* 1980;**52**:135–41.

118. Chong JL, Grebenik C, Sinclair M, Fisher A, Pillai R, Westaby S. The effect of a cardiac surgical recovery area on the timing of extubation. *J Cardiothorac Vasc Anesth* 1993;**7**:137–41.

119. Aps C, Hutter JA, Williams BT. Anaesthetic management and postoperative care of cardiac surgical patients in a general recovery ward. *Anaesthesia* 1986;**41**:533–7.

120. Jindani A, Aps C, Neville E *èt al*. Postoperative cardiac surgical care: An alternative approach. *Br Heart J* 1993;**69**:59–63.

121. Higgins TL. Pro: Early endotracheal extubation is preferable to late extubation in patients following coronary artery surgery. *J Cardiothorac Vasc Anesth* 1992;**6**:488–93.

122. Shapiro BA. Inhalation-based anesthetic techniques are the key to early extubation of the cardiac surgical patient. *J Cardiothorac Vasc Anesth* 1993;**7**:135–6.

123. Mangano DT, Siliciano D, Hollenberg M *et al*. Postoperative myocardial ischemia: therapeutic trials using intensive analgesia following surgery. *Anesthesiology* 1992;**76**:342–53.

124. Joachimsson PO, Nystrom SO, Tyden H. Early extubation after coronary artery surgery in efficiently rewarmed patients: A postoperative comparison of opioid anesthesia versus inhalational anesthesia and thoracic epidural analgesia. *J Cardiothorac Anesth* 1989;**3**:444–54.

125. Dietrich W, Spannagl M, Jochum M *et al.* Influence of high-dose aprotinin treatment on blood loss and coagulation patterns in patients undergoing myocardial revascularization. *Anesthesiology* 1990;**73**:1119–26.

126. Royston D. Aprotinin prevents bleeding and has effects on platelets and fibrinolysis. *J Cardiothorac Vasc Anesth* 1991;**6**:18–23.

127. Dietrich W, Dilthey G, Spannagl M, Jochum M, Braun SL, Richter JA. Influence of high-dose aprotinin on anticoagulation, heparin requirement, and celite- and kaolin-activated clotting time in heparin-pretreated patients undergoing open-heart surgery. A double-blind, placebo-controlled study. *Anesthesiology* 1995;**83**:679–89.

128. Bidstrup BP, Underwood SR, Sapsford RN. Effect of aprotinin (Trasylol) on aorta-coronary bypass graft patency. *J Thorac Cardiovasc Surg* 1993;**105**:147–52.

7 Perioperative care and recovery

Catherine R. Grebenik

Preoperative evaluation

Thorough preoperative assessment of the patient undergoing surgery for ischaemic heart disease is a vital part of management. It enables intercurrent diseases to be evaluated and treated, provides a guide for anaesthetic care, allows assessment of the likelihood of postoperative complications, and permits planning for the type of postoperative care required.

Every effort should be made to optimize the patient's condition before operation provided that this is consistent with the urgency of surgery. In patients with immediately life-threatening disease, or those with catastrophic circulatory collapse, there is little or no time for any preparation, although in appropriate circumstances intra-aortic balloon counter pulsation may help to support and stabilize the circulation. In less urgent cases, however, preoperative control of hypertension, cardiac failure, diabetes, and chronic obstructive airways disease will improve surgical outcome.

Common concurrent disorders

Hypertension

High blood pressure is common in patients with ischaemic heart disease. Thickening of arteriolar walls reduces the luminal diameter and increases systemic vascular resistance, with a reduction in circulating blood volume. Compensatory left ventricular hypertrophy limits diastolic compliance and left ventricular filling. There is an upward shift in the autoregulatory parameters of cerebral and renal blood flow. Blood pressure tends to be labile in untreated hypertensives; exaggerated falls in arterial pressure associated with induction of anaesthesia (1) can precipitate renal, cerebral, or myocardial ischaemia. Similarly, marked rises in pressure in response to noxious stimuli such as intubation or sternotomy may also be associated with myocardial ischaemia. If possible, patients with severe untreated hypertension (diastolic pressure greater than 110 mm Hg) should have their surgery delayed until adequate blood pressure control has been achieved. The institution of beta-blockade before induction of anaesthesia will reduce heart rate and blood pressure variability and the incidence of associated myocardial ischaemia.

Cerebrovascular disease

The presence of coexisting cerebrovascular disease should be considered in all patients with ischaemic heart disease, particularly where there is a history of stroke, transient ischaemic attacks, diabetes, peripheral vascular disease, or hypertension. Detecting carotid stenosis by the presence or absence of carotid bruits is unreliable; a bruit may be present with a lesion that is haemodynamically insignificant and, conversely, may be absent when the lumen of the vessel is almost obliterated. Routine preoperative screening with ultrasound in patients undergoing coronary artery surgery will detect significant carotid stenoses in up to 16% of patients, but the benefits of such screening are uncertain. Although the presence of carotid disease seems likely to be a risk factor for development of new neurological deficits after cardiopulmonary bypass, not all studies have shown a correlation with the occurrence of perioperative stroke. Recent data suggest that carotid endarterectomy is of value only in those patients who are both symptomatic and have a greater than 70% carotid stenosis. Unfortunately there is no consensus on the best management strategy for coexisting coronary and carotid arterial disease, and the decision must be made for each case individually. The risk of stroke after coronary artery surgery must be weighed against the risk of myocardial infarction during or after carotid endarterectomy. The options include staged operations, with either the coronary or the carotid surgery being performed first, or, as in some institutions, a simultaneous procedure with carotid endarterectomy performed either immediately before or during cardiopulmonary bypass (2).

Respiratory disease

Breathlessness and abnormalities of lung function are common in patients with cardiac disease, especially cigarette smokers. The role of pulmonary disease in contributing to mortality and morbidity after open heart surgery has not been clearly determined, but severe disease is a risk factor for postoperative respiratory failure. Patients with significant symptomatic lung disease should undergo preoperative lung function testing. As a minimum this should include arterial blood gas analysis, and spirometry to determine the ratio of forced expiratory volume in one second to forced vital capacity (FEV_1/FVC) and the response to bronchodilator drugs. Elective surgery should be delayed if there is evidence of chest infection, acute worsening of baseline disease, or inadequately treated bronchoconstriction.

Patients who are cigarette smokers should be urged to give up — even as short a period of abstinence from cigarettes as 24 hours will reduce carboxyhaemoglobin levels and thereby improve oxygen carriage. Paradoxically, however, it has been suggested that cessation of smoking for a period of less than 8 weeks preoperatively actually increases complications after surgery (3).

Diabetes

Diabetes mellitus commonly coexists with coronary artery disease (4). Diabetic patients have an increased incidence of previous myocardial infarction, hypertension, peripheral vascular disease, and impaired renal function. They therefore represent a high risk group, who should undergo elective surgery only when their diabetic status is well controlled. Postoperative morbidity is increased, with an increased likelihood of sternal wound infection, renal failure, and cardiovascular complications. Strict blood sugar control and avoidance of hyperglycaemia over the perioperative period may reduce the incidence of sternal wound infection.

When surgery is elective, preoperative management of diabetic patients is simpler if the operation is scheduled early in the day. Long-acting oral anti-diabetic medication should be stopped on the day before surgery, and long-acting insulin preparations changed to a short-acting type. Insulin dependent diabetics should receive their normal dose of short-acting insulin on the evening before surgery. No insulin should be given on the morning of operation unless the timing of surgery is such that the

Table 7.1 Management of diabetic patients

	Non insulin dependent	Insulin dependent
Day before surgery	Stop long acting anti-diabetic drugs	Change long acting insulin to short acting type
Morning surgery	No food, no insulin. Check blood glucose 2 hourly	No food, no insulin. Check blood glucose 2 hourly
Afternoon surgery	Breakfast. Check blood glucose 2 hourly. If blood glucose > 10 mmol/l start glucose/potassium insulin as below.	Breakfast. Give half usual morning dose of subcutaneous insulin. Check blood glucose 2 hourly. If blood glucose > 10 mmol/l start glucose/potassium/insulin as below.
Surgery delayed	Start intravenous infusion of 500 ml 10% glucose with 10 mmol KCl and 10 units of Actrapid insulin at 100 ml/hour. Check blood sugar 2 hourly.	Start intravenous infusion of 500 ml 10% glucose with 10 mmol KCl and 10 units of Actrapid insulin at 100 ml/hour. Check blood sugar 2 hourly. If blood glucose >10 mmol/l increase insulin to 15 units/500 ml 10% glucose.
Operative period	Continuous intravenous infusion of insulin starting at 2 units/hour. Check blood glucose hourly	Continuous intravenous infusion of insulin. Add up usual total daily dose of insulin and divide by 24 to get initial starting dose. Check blood glucose hourly
Early postoperative period	Continuous intravenous infusion of insulin. Check blood glucose 2 hourly	Continuous intravenous infusion of insulin. Check blood glucose 2 hourly
Later postoperative period	Return to oral anti-diabetic drugs when eating	Return to subcutaneous insulin regimen when eating. Check blood glucose at least twice daily

patient may eat breakfast. In this case, the patient may be given half their usual morning dose of short-acting subcutaneous insulin. The blood sugar level should be checked 2 hourly and treatment instigated if it falls outside the acceptable range of 5–10 mmol/L (90–180 mg/dL). Usually no further insulin will be required until the start of surgery. If surgery is delayed an infusion of 500 ml of 10% glucose with 10 mmol KCl and 10 units Actrapid insulin should be started at 100 ml/hour (modified Alberti regimen). If blood glucose remains greater than 10 mmol/L the insulin should be increased to 15 units/500 mL. Non-insulin dependent diabetics will almost always require insulin over the operative period but this can usually be delayed until the start of surgery. Both types of diabetics are best managed with a continuous intravenous infusion of short-acting insulin. This should be started during surgery and the blood glucose level checked every hour. Basal insulin requirement is about 2 units/hour so that the infusion can be started at this level and adjusted in response to blood sugar estimations. Table 7.1 summarizes the management of diabetic patients.

Renal failure

Elevated creatinine is a risk factor for postoperative renal failure and thereby for increased mortality. A plasma creatinine that exceeds the normal range implies that glomerular filtration has fallen to less than one third of normal. Patients who are totally dependent on dialysis represent a significant challenge with regard to fluid and electrolyte management and related medical problems. Uraemia is associated with disturbances of coagulation that may cause troublesome postoperative bleeding. Dialysis should be performed in the 24 hours prior to surgery to restore volume and electrolytes towards the normal range. Anginal symptoms are exacerbated by the anaemia that commonly accompanies chronic renal failure, and preoperative red cell transfusion may be indicated in patients with unstable angina and a low haematocrit (less than 30%).

Laboratory investigations

Most relevant laboratory investigations will have been performed as part of the routine investigation of ischaemic heart disease; they do not need to be repeated before surgery if the patient's condition is stable and the operation is scheduled within 6 weeks. Mandatory preoperative tests are full blood count, serum electrolytes and creatinine, routine urine test, chest radiograph, and electrocardiogram. The INR (international normalized ratio) should be checked if the patient is taking oral anticoagulants, and a coagulation profile performed if the clinical history suggests disordered haemostasis. Liver function tests and blood glucose are not necessary unless there is an appropriate indication.

Blood crossmatching

Blood usage during coronary artery surgery varies considerably between institutions (5). For routine elective surgery 2–4 units of packed red cells are normally crossmatched, although more is required for re-operations. Patients who are on anticoagulants or aspirin, or those who have received thrombolytic agents in the 36 hours preoperatively, may be expected to bleed excessively after cardiopulmonary bypass, and may require other blood products to treat the resultant coagulopathy.

Increasing concern about the safety and cost of homologous blood transfusion has led to considerable attention being paid to autologous predonation of blood before surgery (6,7). Studies have shown the practice to be safe in patients with coronary artery disease, and to reduce the need for homologous blood by 30–40%. Nevertheless, predonation is suitable only for patients of body weight greater than 50 kg with a haematocrit of greater than 35%, and who are undergoing elective surgery. The logistic difficulties of collecting several units of blood preoperatively and the expense of running a predonation programme mean that very few patients donate autologous blood, and its cost-effectiveness has been questioned (8). A multicentre study of transfusion practice in the US, where enthusiasm for predonation is greater than in the UK, showed that only 3.3% of patients donate autologous blood (9). Red cell substitutes, notably stroma-free haemoglobin solutions and perfluorocarbons, are currently undergoing clinical trials. Such solutions may provide a safe and cost-effective alternative to current transfusion practices.

Psychological preparation for surgery

Few surgical procedures invoke as much anxiety as operations on the heart. Greater knowledge and understanding of the procedure may help to allay anxiety in some patients. Written or videotaped information about the surgery, with a description of the likely course of events during recovery and convalescence, should be supplemented by discussion with medical and nursing staff. Informed co-operation is needed in the postoperative period and will be helped by an explanation of the need for postoperative oxygen and the use of patient-controlled analgesia, breathing exercises, and assisted coughing. Patients and their relatives should be aware of the potential risks of surgery.

Medication

Medical treatment of cardiovascular disease should be continued up until the time of surgery. In particular, discontinuation of anti-hypertensives and anti-anginals should be avoided to prevent rebound hypertension and ischaemia. Diuretics may be safely omitted on the day of operation; this will avoid discomfort and embarrassment for the patient once confined to bed. Practices vary regarding the use of digoxin; in some centres it is discontinued 36 hours preoperatively to avoid possible toxicity, others continue up to operation, since digoxin may reduce the incidence of supraventricular tachydysrhythmias in the postoperative period.

Ideally, drugs that affect platelet function should be discontinued prior to surgery to reduce the likelihood of bleeding after cardiopulmonary bypass. The list of drugs that affect platelet numbers or function is long, and includes penicillin and ampicillin, frusemide, propranolol, phenothiazines, tricyclic antidepressants, nitroglycerin, sodium nitroprusside, non-steroidal anti-inflammatory drugs, heparin, dipyridamole, and of course, aspirin. This last, which irreversibly acetylates platelet cyclo-oxygenase, should be stopped for 10 days prior to surgery to allow time for generation of new platelets with normal function. In patients with unstable angina, however, aspirin and/or intravenous heparin may be continued until the day of surgery if the risks of stopping them are deemed to be greater than the risks of post-bypass bleeding. Oral anticoagulants should be stopped 3 days preoperatively and the INR ratio checked on the day of surgery to ensure that it is less than 2.

Premedication prior to surgery is usually prescribed by the anaesthetist with the aim of producing mild to moderate sedation and reducing anxiety-provoked stress on the cardiovascular system. Some patients develop anginal pain during the crescendo of anxiety immediately preceding operation, and may require additional intravenous sedation and nitrates. Long-acting benzodiazepines such as diazepam and lorazepam are best avoided in patients for whom early extubation is planned, since they may cause prolonged postoperative drowsiness, especially in the elderly. Supplementary oxygen should be given from the time of premedication to avoid hypoxaemia due to respiratory depression.

Postoperative recovery

The early years of open heart surgery were characterized by lengthy operations on patients who frequently were suffering from advanced heart disease. By today's standards, the bypass technology was primitive and it is not surprising that these patients often suffered from what was known as 'pump lung' — the damaging effect on the lungs of the inflammatory response induced by extracorporeal circulation. This problem, together with the risks of bleeding and haemodynamic instability and the effects of hypothermic bypass, led to the routine use postoperatively of a period of intermittent positive pressure ventilation in an intensive care unit. The popularity of high dose narcotic anaesthesia for cardiac surgery and the consequent prolonged respiratory depression added to the need for postoperative respiratory support.

More recently, improvements and modifications in anaesthetic and surgical techniques and in the technology for extracorporeal circulation have reduced the need for conventional intensive care after cardiac surgery. As operative mortality has fallen over the years, numbers of operations have increased. Much elective coronary bypass surgery is now routine and standardized, with most patients being operated on before their health has been severely compromised. The vast majority of these patients can be expected to make a rapid and uneventful recovery, and it has been demonstrated that they can be managed safely without either admission to an intensive care unit or a prolonged period of postoperative mechanical ventilation (10,11).

There remain, however, some patients who are likely to require intensive monitoring, or extended ventilatory, circulatory or other support after open heart surgery. Such patients include:

- those with severe preoperative ventricular dysfunction (recent infarction, ejection fraction less than 30% with increased left ventricular end-diastolic pressure), especially those who require preoperative inotropic or mechanical ventricular support or who are undergoing emergency surgery
- those with severe lung disease (asthma, chronic obstructive airways disease)
- the massively obese
- those with other disorders affecting the conduct of anaesthesia or surgery (e.g. chronic renal failure or neuromuscular diseases)
- those in whom intraoperative problems have led to prolonged aortic cross-clamp and/or cardiopulmonary bypass times.
- those undergoing operative procedures involving periods of total circulatory arrest.

This group encompasses up to 8% of patients undergoing surgery and their postoperative management may be complex

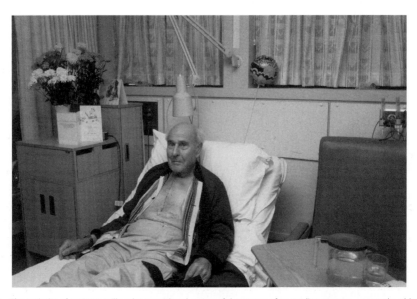

Fig. 7.1   The majority of patients will make a rapid and uneventful recovery after cardiac surgery — even the elderly.

On return from the operating theatre patients should be admitted to a recovery facility with the capacity to continue monitoring and support of vital functions. During the first 24–48 hours postoperatively a series of predictable physiological changes takes place with gradual recovery from the effects of surgery and cardiopulmonary bypass. The aim of postoperative care is to support and monitor the patient during this period, so that deviation from the normal pattern of recovery is detected and treated quickly and effectively, thus minimizing morbidity from complications.

Routine postoperative care

Patients who are not breathing spontaneously on return from the operating theatre are connected to a ventilator. Provided that gas exchange has been normal in the operating theatre, standard settings may be used initially, with a tidal volume of 10 mL/kg, respiratory rate of 12 breaths/minute and inspired oxygen of 40%. If the peripheral circulation is adequate, pulse oximetry demonstrates acceptable oxygenation. Ventilator settings should be adjusted according to subsequent blood gas analysis to produce normocarbia. Marked hypocarbia should be avoided, especially in the elderly, since it causes cerebral vasoconstriction and reduces cerebral blood flow. A heat and moisture exchanger in the breathing system will produce adequate humidification of inspired gas. Patients who are self-ventilating through an endotracheal tube should be sat upright and given humidified oxygen and air via a T-piece. The adequacy of ventilation should be checked clinically by observing the patient's colour and chest movement.

Monitoring and management of the cardiovascular system is continued in the recovery period as in the operating theatre. The electrocardiogram is reconnected and pressure transducers are connected and re-zeroed. The aim should be to ensure an adequate cardiac output with a favourable balance between myocardial oxygen supply and demand. The desirable range for mean arterial pressure in the early postoperative period lies between 65 and 90 mm Hg. Hypotension is likely to be accompanied by inadequate vital organ perfusion, but hypertension is equally undesirable as it may be associated with myocardial ischaemia and increased likelihood of bleeding. Adequacy of the circulation is demonstrated by well perfused peripheries, a urine output of more than 0.5 mL/kg per hour, normal acid-base balance, and a gradual rise towards normal in peripheral temperature.

Chest drainage tubes are connected to an underwater sealed drainage system with suction set at 20 cm H_2O; the volume collected being measured hourly or more frequently if bleeding is excessive. Blood loss is replaced as necessary with colloid to maintain the circulation, using packed red cells if the haematocrit is less than 25%. Patients undergoing cardiac surgery are routinely subjected to normovolaemic anaemia during surgery and acceptance of a lower transfusion 'trigger' of 22% has been shown to significantly reduce transfusion requirements without increase in morbidity (12). Acceptance of normovolaemic anaemia helps to reduce the need for blood transfusion at the cost of a compensatory increase in cardiac output to maintain oxygen delivery to the tissues. Although those with good left ventricular function may tolerate anaemia of this degree, the critical level of haemoglobin required to prevent regional myocardial ischaemia is likely to vary considerably between patients. Severe haemodilution may adversely affect oxygen delivery and increase myocardial work load excessively, especially in those with impaired left ventricular function. In general, patients with poor ventricular function or severely impaired respiratory mechanics should be transfused to maintain a haematocrit of at least 28% or possibly higher. The ideal haematocrit and the balance between risks and benefits of transfusion therefore varies from patient to patient, and there is enormous variation in transfusion practice between different cardiac centres.

Crystalloid input is restricted to 40–70 mL/hour of 5% glucose. Potassium chloride should be added to intravenous fluids to maintain a plasma potassium of 4.5–5.0 mmol/L. Up to 20 mmol of potassium can be added to each hour's fluids but frequent potassium estimations are needed as extracellular potassium levels can change rapidly. Plasma potassium levels fall with administration of insulin and catecholamines, both of which cause transfer of potassium ions into the intracellular space. Increases in plasma potassium may be related to large volumes of cardioplegic solutions or to transfusion of stored blood which is both acidotic and hyperkalaemic. Vital signs including urine output are charted hourly if the patient's condition is stable, or more frequently if there is haemodynamic instability. Rectal and peripheral temperatures are measured routinely. A hot air blanket or overhead radiant heater will speed re-warming in patients who are hypothermic on return from the operating theatre.

Soon after admission to the recovery unit, blood samples should be taken for arterial blood gas analysis, serum potassium, glucose, and haematocrit. The patient's conscious level should be briefly assessed and analgesia and sedation commenced as necessary. Prophylactic anti-emetics are prescribed routinely. A postoperative chest radiograph may be taken if there is an indication, such as a suspected pneumothorax or unexpected poor oxygenation, but otherwise radiography can safely be postponed until after removal of the chest drains. These can be removed once chest drainage is minimal (less than 20 mL/hour for three consecutive hours). If a left atrial line has been inserted at operation, this must be withdrawn before the chest drains, in case of haemorrhage from the line site.

There is a rapid step down in nursing dependency once a patient has been extubated. For the most efficient use of resources, those whose condition permits may be moved to a high dependency area after extubation and return from there to the ward on the first postoperative day.

Lung function after cardiopulmonary bypass

There is a consistent deterioration in lung function after cardiopulmonary bypass, with a decrease in lung volumes and carbon monoxide transfer capacity and an increase in right to left shunt and alveolar to arterial oxygen gradient. Oxygen consumption and carbon dioxide production increase in the early postoperative period and there is a change in the pattern of breathing, with a fall in tidal volume and a rise in respiratory rate and minute ventilation. The overall effect is to increase the work and oxygen cost of breathing. Pulmonary dysfunction is maximal around 24 hours postoperatively and there is usually a gradual return to normality over a period of days. The aetiology of these changes is unclear. They are similar, although greater in extent, to the changes seen after general anaesthesia for other types of surgery and may be due to a variety of factors including the mechanical effects of median sternotomy, atelectasis, phrenic nerve dysfunction, hydrostatic pulmonary oedema, and changes in endothelial function (13). Although mechanical ventilation will reduce the work of breathing, provided the patient is not 'fighting' the ventilator, there is no evidence to suggest that positive pressure ventilation has any effect in reducing the magnitude of pulmonary dysfunction or shortening its duration.

Postoperative ventilation

In the majority of patients the resumption of spontaneous breathing and subsequent extubation can follow the recovery of consciousness after surgery. Depending on the length of operation and anaesthetic management, this should take place within the first few hours after return from the operating theatre (14). In most cases postoperative ventilatory needs are dictated by the choice of anaesthetic technique rather than by than by the patient's pulmonary status. Although every patient should be considered individually, the normal criteria for discontinuing ventilation are:

- the patient is awake and responsive. If there is evidence of major neurological damage after surgery then ventilatory support may be continued for a longer period to avoid any degree of hypoxia and hypercarbia which might worsen the brain injury.
- the cardiovascular system is stable. This implies a reasonable cardiac output with adequate organ perfusion. A requirement for support with inotropic drugs or an intra-aortic balloon pump is not a contraindication to extubation provided that haemodynamics are either stable or improving.
- adequate gas exchange. The arterial P_{O_2} should be greater than 10 kPa with inspired oxygen concentration of 40% or less, and the P_{CO_2} near normal without excessive ventilation.
- normal core temperature. Shivering can increase oxygen consumption by up to 300%; patients who are hypothermic should be mechanically ventilated until core temperature is greater than 36°C.

Extubation can be performed when in addition to the above:

- breathing is clinically adequate with a respiratory rate of less than 30 breaths/minute
- oxygen saturation is above 90% with inspired oxygen concentration of 60% or less
- there is no excessive bleeding.

Unfavourable signs in the spontaneously breathing patient which may indicate a need for a further period of assisted ventilation include:

- tachypnoea (respiratory rate of more than 30–35 breaths/minute), agitation and sweating
- increasing acidosis (pH less than 7.25–7.30)
- a rise in either left or right atrial pressure
- tachycardia or dysrhythmias
- a fall in urine output.

A moderate elevation in arterial P_{CO_2} (up to 7.5 kPa) with mild respiratory acidosis is usually well tolerated and is not an indication for reventilation provided there is no hypoxia.

Although respiratory problems should not be considered in isolation, mechanical ventilation has therapeutic effects only in cases of severe congestive heart failure. In the dilated failing ventricle that is operating on the flat (depressed) portion of the cardiac function curve, a fall in venous return caused by positive pressure ventilation will reduce ventricular filling pressure and the associated decrease in wall stress may increase stroke volume. The failing ventricle may also benefit from the likely increase in arterial oxygen saturation and decrease in oxygen demand associated with ventilation. However, in patients whose ventricular or pulmonary function is not severely impaired the disadvantages of prolonged mechanical ventilation will usually outweigh any potential benefits. These adverse effects include:

- a reduction in venous return which is usually accompanied by a fall in cardiac output
- a consequent decrease in renal perfusion, and an increase in antidiuretic hormone (ADH)

- the effects of endotracheal intubation — cessation of mucus transport and impaired coughing which may predispose to atelectasis, and vocal cord ulceration and granuloma formation
- a greatly increased requirement for sedative drugs
- the potential for technical mishaps including ventilator disconnection.

Mechanical ventilation should therefore be seen as a method of supporting an intubated patient during illness, and its duration should not be unnecessarily prolonged in the postoperative period in the belief that overnight ventilation is somehow beneficial after cardiac surgery.

Postoperative analgesia

Pain is an inevitable result of surgical intervention and, together with anxiety and distress, is associated with adverse sympathetic nervous system effects of tachycardia and hypertension. Many of the biochemical components of the stress response, such as raised levels of catecholamines, the metabolic shift to a catabolic state, and immunosuppression are also closely linked to perioperative pain. Inadequate analgesia increases oxygen consumption and cardiac work, while inhibiting respiration by producing an acute restrictive type pulmonary defect, with a fall in tidal volumes, functional residual capacity, vital capacity, and forced expiratory volumes accompanied by an increase in respiratory rate. Good pain control is thus vital when early extubation is planned.

Preventing pain is more effective than attempting to abolish it after its onset. Persistence of the narcotics used during anaesthesia into the early postoperative period may therefore be beneficial, and the postoperative analgesic regimen should be started before the patient recovers full consciousness. Analgesia should not be withheld because of undue concern with maintaining normocarbia in the spontaneously breathing patient. Provided that there is no hypoxia, a state of mild hypercarbia (P_{CO_2} <7.5 kPa) is well tolerated. In some circumstances, improved analgesia may result in a fall in P_{CO_2} with a relaxation of pain-induced inhibition of breathing. The inevitable pain and discomfort of surgery is increased by factors such as movement, anxiety, fear, and fatigue; good nursing care can help the patient to relax and thus increase tolerance of the postoperative experience.

Currently the principal technique of intravenous opioid administration uses a continuous intravenous infusion after an initial loading dose. This avoids the peaks and troughs of plasma levels associated with intermittent bolus injections, but can be supplemented when necessary with small intravenous boluses. During the period of high-dependency care the infusion rate should be adjusted by the nursing staff to meet the needs of the individual patient. If extra bolus doses are required repeatedly the background infusion rate is increased. Similarly, excessive sleepiness or a respiratory rate of less than 8 breaths/minute is an indication to reduce the background infusion. The technique of on-demand or patient-controlled analgesia (PCA) requires a specialized infusion pump and the cooperation of the patient. Patients can anticipate painful experiences such as movement, physiotherapy, or coughing and administer additional drug, thus improving the quality of their pain control. Many patients are too sleepy to use the device effectively on the day of operation, but may be able to use it from the first postoperative day onwards. The major disadvantage of PCA is that it requires motivation and action by the patient and thus pain relief is not available when the patient is asleep or if he or she is confused. Also, since demand for analgesia is initiated by the presence of pain, analgesia is unlikely to be complete.

The addition of a non-steroidal anti-inflammatory drug such as diclofenac or ketorolac can frequently improve the quality of analgesia and has a 'morphine-sparing' effect. Diclofenac can be given intramuscularly but the injection is painful, and the most effective route is by suppository (50–100 mg, maximum of 150 mg/day). Ketorolac has the advantage of an intravenous formulation (initial dose 10 mg followed by 10–30 mg 4–6 hourly). Non-steroidal anti-inflammatory drugs should not be given to patients with impaired renal function because of their nephrotoxic effects and may precipitate an asthmatic attack in patients with that tendency. Other undesirable side effects include gastric ulceration and effects on platelet function.

Oral analgesia with paracetamol, dihydrocodeine, or non-steroidal anti-inflammatory drugs is usually sufficient to control pain by the second or third postoperative day. However, to achieve the best pain control these drugs should be given regularly by the clock rather than on demand.

Nausea and vomiting

Despite improvements in anaesthetic agents and techniques, postoperative nausea and vomiting is a common problem after cardiac surgery (15). The incidence depends on many variables including the size, age, and sex of the patient and the duration of surgery and postoperative ventilation. As well as being distressing and uncomfortable for the patient, retching and vomiting may be associated with vagally mediated bradycardias and hypotension. The addition of droperidol 5–10 mg to the opiate infusion is effective in reducing postoperative nausea and vomiting. Further anti-emetics may also be prescribed routinely, using either a centrally acting drug such as prochlorperazine (12.5 mg 6 hourly) or a dopaminergic antagonist such as metoclopramide (10 mg 6 hourly) which hastens gastric emptying.

Postoperative sedation

The residual effects of anaesthesia, together with the sedative effects of opiate analgesia, will usually produce sufficient sedation for a short period of postoperative ventilation. The routine administration of sedative drugs should be avoided as this is likely to prolong the duration of ventilator dependency. However, mechanically ventilated patients are subjected to a plethora of noxious stimuli and if positive pressure ventilation must be continued after recovery of consciousness then some degree of sedation is necessary to reduce the perception of and response to these stimuli. Cumulation of sedation can lead to confusion and respiratory depression, especially in elderly patients. A vicious circle may be created in which patients who have been sedated in order to tolerate ventilation are too sleepy to breath spontaneously, and therefore remain intubated for longer than necessary.

The ideal sedative drug would cause minimal cardiovascular depression, would not cumulate in patients with renal or hepatic impairment, and would have a pharmacokinetic profile that allowed a rapid return to full consciousness on ceasing drug administration, without residual respiratory depression. Such an agent does not, of course, exist. The choice of sedative agent lies between three groups of drugs, all of which have certain undesirable features.

Opioids produce sedation as a side effect of their analgesic action. Central depression of the cough reflex helps patients to tolerate the presence of an endotracheal tube, but prolonged respiratory depression may result from the administration of large doses, particularly in the presence of renal impairment. Nevertheless, infusions of opioids such as fentanyl, alfentanil, or morphine are frequently used to provide sedation, either alone or in combination with a benzodiazepine in which case the opiate requirement is significantly reduced.

Benzodiazepines are frequently used for long term sedation in patients in the intensive care unit. Midazolam has significant advantages over diazepam since it is shorter acting and water-soluble. Unfortunately there is considerable interpatient variability in response to midazolam; the half-life is unpredictable, and variations in protein binding effect clearance. Its action may be prolonged after cardiopulmonary bypass (16).

Propofol (a non-barbiturate intravenous anaesthetic agent) has a pharmacokinetic profile that allows rapid recovery (within about 10 minutes) after infusions of up to 72 hours duration. It produces excellent postoperative sedation after cardiac surgery (17). Unfortunately, however, it is not devoid of cardiovascular side effects and critically ill patients may be particularly sensitive to its cardiac depressant and vasodilator effects. It is also unlicensed for administration for longer than 3 days.

A perfect regime for sedation of mechanically ventilated patients does not exist. Propofol is probably the best choice for short periods of time, but when sedation must be continued for more than 12 hours, the least expensive narcotic with or without a benzodiazepine is as safe and effective as any other regime. In a stable mechanically ventilated patient intravenous morphine can provide excellent analgesia euphoria, and deep sedation with very little cardiovascular effect besides venodilatation. Paralysis with neuromuscular blocking drugs has no sedative or analgesic effect and should be used only when total control of the ventilatory pattern is necessary.

Control of blood glucose

Hyperglycaemia is common in the postoperative period, even in non-diabetic patients. The surgical stress and catecholamine release associated with the use of cardiopulmonary bypass increases gluconeogenesis and insulin requirements and produces a state of relative insulin resistance. Hence patients who are normally controlled with oral hypoglycaemic agents will usually require insulin over the acute operative period. Administration of catecholamines in sick patients after cardiopulmonary bypass can cause extreme insulin resistance, requiring very high doses (up to 20 units/hour) for control of blood sugar. Stabilization and improvement in cardiovascular status is usually associated with a decreased insulin requirement. The aim of diabetic management is to maintain a blood sugar level of between 5 and 10 mmol/L (90–180 mg/dL) in the early postoperative period, until the patient is eating and drinking normally and can return to his or her normal preoperative regimen. The simplest method of management is to use a continuous intravenous infusion of short-acting insulin which is titrated against regular measurements of blood sugar. Frequent estimations of both blood sugar and plasma potassium are needed, as both can change rapidly.

Postoperative complications

Hypertension

Postoperative hypertension is a common problem after coronary artery surgery and is related to neural reflexes, increased activity of the renin-angiotensin axis, and high levels of circulating catecholamines. Pain, anxiety, discomfort from a full bladder, hypoxia, hypercarbia, hypothermia, and struggling against mechanical ventilation may all contribute, and should be treated appropriately. Rebound hypertension may be expected after discontinuation of preoperative antihypertensive drugs, and oral medication should be restarted once the patient is able to swallow.

Nitroglycerin and sodium nitroprusside are the mainstays for the prevention or acute suppression of postoperative hypertension. Both drugs are vasodilators with different haemodynamic profiles but a similar cellular mode of action. Other agents which may be used include beta-blockers, calcium channel antagonists, and centrally acting α-agonists such as clonidine.

Nitroglycerin is a dilator of peripheral venous and coronary vascular beds but in sufficient dosage it also dilates arterioles and will counteract hypertension. When infused intravenously, nitroglycerin reduces both cardiac preload and afterload, reducing myocardial oxygen consumption and thereby having an anti-ischaemic effect. Nitroglycerin is also an effective dilator of the internal mammary artery and its routine use after mammary grafting may help to prevent spasm. However, its use as an anti-hypertensive may be limited by undesirable reflex tachycardia and by tachyphylaxis. At a cellular level it acts by penetrating the cell wall and forming nitric oxide. This activates guanylate cyclase, catalyzing the formation of cyclic guanosine monophosphate (c-GMP) which triggers the relaxation of vascular smooth muscle.

Sodium nitroprusside is also a vasodilator but has a greater effect on arteriolar resistance than nitroglycerin, and hence is a more effective antihypertensive agent. The haemodynamic effects are titratable but its dosage is limited by the production of toxic cyanide metabolites, the maximum infusion rate being 8 μg/kg per minute with a maximum 24 hour dose of 3.5 mg/kg.

Labetalol is a non-selective beta-blocker with additional weak α_1- adrenoreceptor antagonist activity. It is an effective antihypertensive agent that can be used either in bolus doses or by infusion, and has the advantage of suppressing reflex tachycardia.

Esmolol has the shortest duration of action of all currently known beta-blockers as it is metabolized within minutes by red cell esterases to inactive metabolites. It is a moderately selective β_1-blocker and is used primarily to reduce heart rate but it is an effective and easily titratable anti-hypertensive agent. However, because of its negative inotropic effects its use should be avoided in patients with severely impaired ventricular function.

Perioperative myocardial ischaemia

Revascularization is the obvious goal of coronary bypass surgery but many patients remain at risk of myocardial ischaemia or infarction since revascularization is frequently incomplete, either due to residual unbypassed vessels or to diffuse disease with poor distal runoff. The incidence of myocardial infarction after coronary bypass surgery is stated to be around 7% (18). Hypothermia appears to have deleterious effects on myocardial oxygenation; unintentional hypothermia (sublingual temperature less than 35°C) in postoperative vascular surgical patients has been shown to be associated with a relatively lower arterial P_{O_2} and myocardial ischaemia (19). Circulatory management should be directed at maintaining a favourable balance between myocardial oxygen supply and demand. If marked ischaemic changes are present after coronary artery surgery, particularly if there is haemodynamic compromise, then consideration should be given to revision of the grafts or intra-aortic balloon counter pulsation.

Recent data have indicated that patients undergoing coronary artery bypass surgery are especially vulnerable to myocardial ischaemia in the early period after revascularization. These ischaemic episodes appear to have greater severity than at other perioperative times, and it is suggested that there may be a relationship between post-bypass ischaemia and adverse outcome (20). This has led to the investigation of heavy sedative-analgesic regimes in the early postoperative period with the aim of blunting activation of the sympathetic nervous system and thus reducing myocardial ischaemia (21). In Mangano's study (21) the use of a continuous infusion of sufentanil reduced the incidence and severity of postoperative ischaemic episodes in comparison to intermittent intravenous morphine. However, on discontinuation of intensive analgesia the incidence of late postoperative ischaemia was similar in both groups of patients. Overall, there was no significant difference in adverse cardiac outcome between the two groups. This work obviously has major implications for postoperative care of patients after coronary artery surgery since the use of such analgesic regimes mandates postoperative ventilation for the first 24 hours.

The effects of early extubation on the incidence of postoperative myocardial ischaemia have yet to be determined. The only currently available information relating to early extubation is that of Cheng *et al.* (22), who found that the incidence of myocardial ischaemia appeared to decrease after extubation, whether this was performed early or late. This preliminary data thus suggests that early extubation certainly does not increase the risk of ischaemia or infarction when compared to late extubation, but much more work is needed to determine the exact relationship between perioperative stress, extubation time and myocardial ischaemia. Until the results of large outcome studies are reported, the use of heavy postoperative sedation regimes remains of unproved benefit.

Postoperative low cardiac output

Low cardiac output syndrome may be defined as a state in which the cardiac output is insufficient to meet the metabolic demands of the body. Postoperative loss of myocardial contractility leading to acute heart failure is usually the result of perioperative infarction or ischaemic stress and reperfusion injury provoked by the combination of aortic cross clamping and inadequate coronary perfusion. Some degree of ventricular dysfunction is almost invariable after surgery, with a gradual return to preoperative baselines in most patients within 24 hours (23). However, patients with pre-existing heart failure may develop more profound and prolonged ventricular dysfunction, the so-called 'stunned' myocardium. The combination of poor contractility, low coronary perfusion pressures, and increased filling pressures tends to produce a progressive downward spiral. This may be reversible if treatment is instituted to improve cardiac performance, reduce the workload of the heart, and maintain vital organ perfusion during the time required for myocardial recovery.

The therapy of postoperative cardiac failure requires the appropriate and simultaneous manipulation of heart rate, rhythm, contractility, and loading conditions to achieve an acceptable cardiac output whilst reducing myocardial oxygen demand. Each of these therapeutic modalities will be considered. The pharmacological strategy chosen must be based on the specific haemodynamic derangements that are involved and preferably on the measurement and monitoring of left heart filling pressures, cardiac output and vascular resistances. It may be necessary to insert a pulmonary artery catheter (PAC) to measure these variables. In many centres (particularly in the US) such monitoring is routine and forms part of the standard care of the cardiac surgical patient. There is, however, no conclusive evidence that the use of a PAC decreases mortality after cardiac surgery (24), and the data produced requires careful interpretation (25). Their routine use increases costs and also carries a risk of potentially fatal complications, even in skilled hands. Nevertheless, most clinicians find a PAC useful to direct treatment in a patient whose condition has deteriorated unexpectedly. A selective approach to their use may thus be both prudent and cost-effective.

Other abnormalities that may impair cardiac performance include hypoxia and hypercarbia, acidosis, and electrolyte imbalance. These factors should be treated appropriately.

Control of heart rate and rhythm

Establishing an atrioventricular conduction sequence at an appropriate rate is one of the most important initial therapeutic measures. The optimal heart rate may be as high as 100–110 beats/minute in the early postoperative period. However, the increase in cardiac output with tachycardia must be balanced against the associated rise in myocardial oxygen demand and decrease in diastolic time. Bradycardia is often a reflection of preoperative beta-blockade and calcium channel blockade and should be treated with atropine (0.6–1.8 mg intravenously), or isoprenaline (bolus of 2–20 μg or an infusion of 1–5 μg/min) or by pacing. Correctly timed atrial contraction may contribute up to 30% to ventricular filling. Patients with decreased left ventricular compliance require optimal loading conditions for a stiff, non-compliant ventricle so that rhythms other than sinus may seriously compromise cardiac output particularly when ventricular function is poor. Atrial or sequential atrioventricular pacing may be beneficial in such cases.

Avoidance of tachycardia is important since increased heart rate will aggravate ischaemia. Supraventricular tachycardias may be treated by electrical cardioversion, but recurrent dysrhythmias require pharmacological treatment. Amiodarone is an effective antiarrhythmic agent with a wide spectrum of activity against both supraventricular and ventricular dysrhythmias. It is probably the least negatively inotropic agent available and although oral administration is associated with multiple side effects, short-term intravenous administration is usually well tolerated. Its pharmacokinetic profile is such that it should be given as a loading dose of 5 mg/kg over 1 hour followed by an infusion of a further 12 mg/kg over the next 24 hours.

Ventricular loading

Maintenance of adequate filling pressures in both ventricles is a fundamental step in the management of low cardiac output. Hypovolaemia is frequently seen in the early postoperative period owing to excessive bleeding or diuresis, increased capillary permeability, and the effects of vasodilators or rapid rewarming. The optimal level of preload depends on baseline cardiac function and the nature of the cardiac lesion. In general if atrial pressures are low or normal (8–12 mm Hg), expansion of the circulating volume will usually produce an increase in cardiac output. If atrial pressures are elevated the response to a fluid challenge is less predictable and there is a danger of producing excessive ventricular dilatation, but the filling pressure needed for a chronically diseased heart may be considerably higher than that for a well-functioning ventricle. Where fluid infusion is needed to increase cardiac output, colloid solutions such as blood, albumin, hetastarch, or gelatine are preferable to crystalloids since a greater proportion of administered fluid will be retained in the circulation.

Although filling pressures are measured as a correlate of volume loading they are affected not only by the circulating volume but also by ventricular compliance, intrapericardial pressure, and intrathoracic pressure. Under most circumstances the pulmonary artery diastolic and wedge pressures accurately reflect left ventricular end diastolic pressure. This relationship does not hold true when high levels of positive end expiratory pressure are applied or when the heart rate is greater than 115 beats/minute (25).

Afterload reduction

Vasodilator therapy to reduce afterload and thereby decrease the impedance to left ventricular ejection may be markedly beneficial in the failing ventricle with elevated preload. Reduction in myocardial wall tension and improvement in diastolic ventricular compliance will reduce myocardial oxygen demand and is likely to increase stroke volume. A variety of vasodilator drugs is available to decrease ventricular loading. The most commonly used ones (nitroglycerin, isosorbide dinitrate, and nitroprusside) are nitric oxide based agents that produce varying degrees of both venodilation and arterial vasodilatation and thus affect both preload and afterload. Judicious fluid administration may be required to maintain an adequate circulating volume and prevent a fall in diastolic pressure which will reduce coronary perfusion. Vasodilators are frequently administered together with catecholamines in an attempt to attenuate the vasoconstrictor effects of the latter and avoid ventricular distension.

Inotropic drugs

Drug treatment to improve contractility with catecholamines or phosphodiesterase inhibitors is based on increasing the levels of cyclic AMP in the heart. Cyclic AMP is the important 'second messenger' that modulates phosphorylation of voltage-dependent calcium channels in the myocyte controlling calcium influx during depolarization. An increase in intracellular calcium binding increases the force of systolic contraction. Cyclic AMP also enhances diastolic relaxation of the heart by increasing the rate of resequestration of intracellular calcium during diastole.

The catecholamines used clinically include dopamine, dopexamine, dobutamine, adrenaline, noradrenaline, and isoprenaline which all affect heart rate, contractility, and vascular tone in differing degrees depending on their profile of receptor affinity (see Table 7.2). The response of the myocardium to inotropes varies with acute, chronic, or acute-on-chronic heart failure. Increased serum levels of catecholamines in patients with chronic heart failure lead to a reduction in β_1-receptor density thus reducing the effect of exogenous β-agonists.

Adverse effects of catecholamines include tachycardias and tachydysrhythmias, α-adrenergic mediated constriction of renal and splanchnic vascular beds, and β_2-mediated vasodilatation of muscle beds. All catecholamines will increase myocardial oxygen demand and this must be offset against the improvement in cardiac performance. The choice of first-line catecholamine depends on the underlying haemodynamics and desirability or otherwise of α-receptor stimulation, and on

Table 7.2 Starting doses of catecholamines

Drug	α-Receptors	β-Receptors	DA Receptors	Infusion dose (μg/kg per minute)
Dopamine	++	+++	++	2–20
Dopexamine	+	++	++	0.5–4
Dobutamine	+	++++		2–25
Adrenaline	+++	+++		0.03–0.5
Noradrenaline	++++	+++		0.03–0.5
Isoprenaline		++++		0.02–0.1

Key: +, mild activity; ++, moderate activity; +++, strong activity; ++++, very strong activity the personal preference of the clinician. Where appropriate, concomitant administration of vasodilators such as nitroglycerin or nitroprusside may be used to modify α-adrenergic mediated vasoconstriction.

Dopamine and dopexamine achieve much of their effects indirectly by releasing myocardial noradrenaline stores and reducing reuptake. Although maintaining coronary perfusion pressure, dopamine frequently causes tachycardia and increased diastolic ventricular filling pressure. Dopamine is widely quoted as having different effects depending on dosage; dopaminergic effects at low doses (> 2 μg/kg per minute), β effects at intermediate doses (2–5 μg/kg per minute), and α effects at high doses (> 10 μg/kg per minute), but in practice its effect is variable and there is considerable overlap of receptor stimulation. Both dopamine and dopexamine increase renal perfusion by stimulating renal dopaminergic receptors and are commonly used in low doses for this so-called 'renal protective effect' although scientific evidence to support this is lacking (26).

Dobutamine, a synthetic β-agonist, usually decreases diastolic filling pressures because of its vasodilator properties, but may cause unacceptable tachycardia.

Isoprenaline is a synthetic catecholamine with pure β-receptor activity, and is primarily used to treat right ventricular failure from pulmonary hypertension. A degree of tachycardia is often beneficial in this circumstance since the impedance to right ventricular ejection is diminished at higher heart rates.

Adrenaline is the most potent inotropic agent and bolus doses produce impressive cardiac stimulation. Despite what is quoted in older textbooks, adrenaline actually causes less tachycardia than equivalent inotropic doses of dopamine or dobutamine. Its combination of powerful α- and β-receptor stimulation and its low cost make it a common first choice of inotropic agent.

Noradrenaline maintains coronary perfusion without increasing heart rate, but its vasoconstrictor effects increase ventricular loading and may cause unacceptable ischaemia in other vital organs. Its primary indication is when hypotension is due to low systemic vascular resistance as for example in severe sepsis.

Phosphodiesterase inhibitors are a group of drugs that produce positive inotropic effects and vasodilatation by increasing intracellular cyclic AMP independently of the adrenergic receptor system. Because of their dual action they have been termed 'inodilators'.

Aminophylline is a non-specific phosphodiesterase inhibitor which tends to cause tachycardia and dysrhythmias.

Amrinone, milrinone, and enoximone are selective inhibitors of phosphodiesterase III. They improve contractility without significantly increasing heart rate and have beneficial effects on the diastolic relaxation and compliance of the left ventricle. They also cause relaxation of arteriolar and venous vascular smooth muscle and thus decrease both mean arterial and central venous pressures. This limits their usefulness as sole agents, but in combination with noradrenaline, adrenaline, or dopamine they may be effective when a plateau of effect has been reached with catecholamines (26). Despite their theoretical advantages, there is still controversy over the value of phosphodiesterase inhibitors and their place in the management of low cardiac output syndrome has yet to be fully established.

Mechanical support

Temporary mechanical ventricular support is a relatively safe and effective procedure in post-surgical low output states and is appropriate both in those in whom eventual ventricular recovery is expected and in those who require a 'bridge' to transplantation while awaiting a suitable donor organ. The aim is to diminish myocardial workload and oxygen consumption while increasing myocardial perfusion, thus encouraging recovery of 'stunned' myocardium. After technically satisfactory surgery a patient who remains in a low cardiac output state, despite conventional medical therapy, requires early mechanical support to avoid the sequelae of prolonged periods of inadequate tissue perfusion.

Postoperative bleeding

Excessive mediastinal bleeding is a serious complication of cardiac surgery and is associated with increased incidence of heart failure and mediastinal infection and increased mortality. Good surgical haemostasis at the end of cardiopulmonary bypass is the best prophylactic measure, but in the presence of a coagulopathy there may be diffuse bleeding from multiple surfaces that is impossible to deal with surgically. Strict control of arterial pressure is vital after operation, particularly where repair of high pressure structures is relatively fragile. Even brief episodes of hypertension may disrupt suture lines and arteriotomies, causing sudden heavy bleeding. The application of positive end expiratory pressure is a popular method of limiting bleeding after cardiac surgery. However, a randomized controlled trial failed to show any benefit from this manoeuvre (27) and it is likely to be deleterious in the hypovolaemic patient.

Postoperative bleeding sufficient to require reoperation occurs in 2–5% of patients after cardiac surgery. Active bleeding can be distinguished from the drainage of old blood by the colour and by comparison of the haematocrit of the drainage to that of the peripheral circulation; old blood is dark in colour and has a haematocrit less than that of the circulation. A continuing active loss of more than 5 mL/kg per hour is an indication for re-exploration of the chest, unless there are major abnormalities in coagulation. Rarely, sudden catastrophic bleeding necessitates immediate re-sternotomy in the recovery unit. This may be due to disruption of an anastomosis or cannulation site or by sutures tearing out of friable tissues. Recognition of excessive bleeding is more difficult when chest tube loss is minimal but drainage is impeded by clotted blood within chest tubes, or is occurring into extramediastinal structures not drained by the chest tubes, such as the pleural space. When continued blood loss is associated with significant abnormalities in coagulation, surgical exploration is indicated if bleeding persists despite attempted correction of haemostatic function.

Autotransfusion

Autologous transfusion is an area of uncertainty in cardiothoracic surgery, and practices vary widely between institutions. Postoperatively, shed mediastinal blood can be collected and reinfused, either directly or after washing and concentration in a cell-saver. Mediastinal blood undergoes extensive coagulation and clot lysis within the chest and is thereby incoagulable. It has a haematocrit of about 20%, low levels of platelets, extremely low levels of fibrinogen, antithrombin III, protein C, plasminogen, and factor VIII clotting activity and increased levels of fibrinogen degradation products and D-dimer protein. Shed mediastinal fluid supplies red cells without risk of viral transmission and autotransfusion of up to 700 mL of unwashed drainage appears to be safe (28). Unfortunately larger quantities may provoke derangement of haemostasis and cause further bleeding and thus may be counterproductive (29). Cell washing devices can be used to wash and pack shed mediastinal blood, thus eliminating many potentially deleterious substances that are associated with unwashed mediastinal blood and producing a product with a haematocrit of 55–80%. The disadvantages of such systems are the inherent time delay in producing red cells for reinfusion, and the cost in disposables and personnel required to operate them, particularly when only small quantities are salvaged.

Postoperative coagulopathy

Coagulation problems in cardiac surgical patients differ from those in other surgical specialities. Coagulation mechanisms are impaired by preoperative treatment with aspirin, non-steroidal anti-inflammatory drugs, and anticoagulants, and by the recent use of fibrinolytic drugs. Cardiopulmonary bypass with systemic heparinization and exposure of blood components to foreign surfaces and non-endothelial tissues produces further profound effects. Platelet numbers and function are reduced; there is dilution and consumption of clotting factors and production of fibrinolysins and other anticoagulant factors. Large doses of heparin given prior to perfusion are often reversed empirically with protamine, but in practice protamine deficiency (or excess) is an uncommon cause of serious postoperative haemorrhage.

Tests of haemostasis may be expected to be abnormal immediately postoperatively but should progressively return to normal with the passage of time. In the presence of bleeding a complete coagulation screen should be performed; this should include a platelet count, prothrombin time, and partial thromboplastin time or activated clotting time. Additional tests for the presence of accelerated fibrinolysis include fibrinogen level, level of fibrin degradation products, and euglobulin clot lysis time. Ideally, therapy should be aimed at correcting specific deficits in coagulation, but in practice, treatment is often empiric since there are frequently unavoidable delays in receiving the results of laboratory tests. Moreover, routine coagulation tests are unable to assess the major haemostatic disturbance resulting from cardiopulmonary bypass — the alteration of the interaction between the coagulation cascade and the platelet surface. The most likely cause of abnormal coagulation after cardiopulmonary bypass is a qualitative or quantitative decrease in platelets, and initial management should be directed to bring the platelet count to greater than $100\ 000/\mu l$. A unit of platelets for each 10 kg of body weight may be expected to raise the platelet count by 10 000 to 20 000. Fresh frozen plasma should be used to bring the prothrombin time to less than 1.5 times the control value. Red cell transfusion is needed to maintain haematocrit of greater than 25–30%. Cryoprecipitate may be required as a source of fibrinogen. Blood products should be warmed during infusion to avoid hypothermia which contributes to abnormal haemostasis.

Cardiac tamponade

Acute tamponade can be caused by the accumulation of a relatively small amount of blood or clot which limits cardiac filling. Its presence is suggested by low cardiac output in association with elevated and equalized right and left atrial pressures. Stroke volume is reduced but in mild tamponade sympathetic reflexes maintain cardiac output by an increase in heart rate and contractility. If bleeding continues, falling coronary blood flow is likely to precipitate ischaemia. The steep pressure–volume relationship that exists in acute tamponade means that haemodynamic collapse can occur rapidly.

The major differential diagnosis is from myocardial failure as a cause of low cardiac output, since the physical signs are similar, and indeed the two may coexist. Furthermore, both will respond, at least temporarily, to volume loading and inotropic support. Pulsus paradoxus (a fall in systolic blood pressure of more than 12 mm Hg with spontaneous inspiration) and electrical alternans (a regular variation in the height of the QRS complexes) are both classic signs of tamponade but are frequently absent. Other ECG changes that may occur are decreasing voltage complexes and T wave abnormalities. In the ventilated patient, tamponade may be suggested by a very marked respiratory variation in systemic arterial pressure. Chest radiography can be helpful — an acute increase in the size of the heart shadow is usually due to tamponade — but portable studies should not be compared with prior posterior–anterior films because the cardiac silhouette will always appear larger on the portable film. Echocardiography is frequently unhelpful in that there will always be some accumulation of blood around the heart in the immediate postoperative period and the echo density of clot is similar to that of muscle tissue. Thus, the diagnosis of tamponade must rest on a high index of clinical suspicion, and it may be necessary on occasions to reopen the chest in order to exclude a degree of tamponade as a cause of low cardiac output. Reopening the chest and removal of clot from around the heart usually produces a dramatic haemodynamic improvement.

Dysrhythmias

Dysrhythmias occur in between 10 and 70% of patients after coronary artery surgery, many of these being transient and self-limiting. The aetiology is multifactorial — intraoperative trauma, ischaemia, inadequate myocardial protection, electrolyte abnormalities, intrapericardial blood, beta-blocker and calcium antagonist withdrawal, and high catecholamine levels may all contribute. Abnormalities in serum potassium, in particular hypokalaemia, are a potent but easily treated cause.

Between 10 and 40% of patients undergoing coronary artery surgery will develop atrial flutter or fibrillation in the postoperative period, most commonly during the second and third postoperative days (30). Several risk factors have been identified including advanced age, pre-existing chronic airflow limitation, renal impairment, hypertension, postoperative withdrawal of beta-blockade, and the duration of cardioplegic arrest during surgery. These rhythm disturbances are seldom life-threatening but they cause considerable morbidity and will often prolong hospital stay. Studies of prophylaxis with a variety of drugs including digoxin, beta-blockers, verapamil, and magnesium suggest that the combination of beta-blockers and digoxin is more effective than either drug alone (31), although amiodarone may also have a useful effect (32). Atrial fibrillation is relatively benign in patients with good left ventricular function, but for those with impaired ventricular function the onset of fibrillation may precipitate haemodynamic deterioration due to loss of the atrial contribution to ventricular filling. Treatment is directed towards control of the ventricular rate and preferably reversion to sinus rhythm. The former can be managed with digoxin but the latter is probably best achieved by electrical cardioversion under light general anaesthesia.

Acute renal failure

Renal failure is uncommon in the routine patient although a transitory rise in creatinine may be seen postoperatively. Problems should be anticipated in those with pre-existing renal impairment, advanced cardiac failure or low cardiac output state, and the first manifestation is usually oliguria. The prevention of renal failure is of paramount importance as the established condition carries a high mortality after cardiac surgery — up to 70%, although the outcome depends on whether acute renal failure is associated with other organ failure (33). Low dose dopamine

(a)

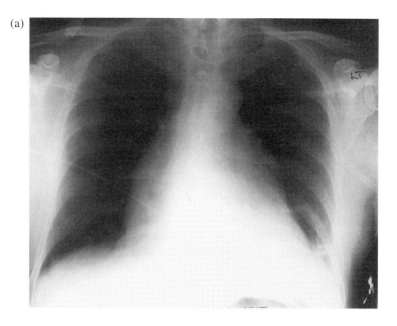

(b)

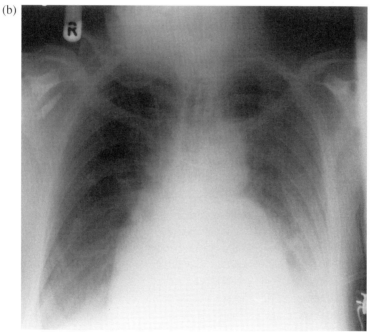

Fig. 7.2 A progressive increase in the size of the heart shadow on postoperative chest X-ray is a reliable, although far from invariable sign of tamponade. These two X-rays (a) and (b) taken two hours apart show acute widening of the mediastinum due to accumulation of blood and clot within the pericardium.

(2–4 μg/kg per minute) increases urine output and is widely used in an attempt to prevent acute renal failure in oliguric critically ill patients. The ability of dopamine to achieve this goal has never been scientifically demonstrated, but the maintenance of urine output may be useful in patients who are unresponsive to diuretics and may avoid the need for more invasive methods of fluid removal. Nevertheless the routine use of dopamine may not be innocuous, since it tends to increase heart rate, has vasoconstrictor effects and may hasten the onset of gut ischaemia in low output states. Controlled studies are needed to determine whether dopamine can prevent acute renal failure or is clinically beneficial.

The important features in prevention and treatment of renal dysfunction in the postoperative period include:

- the maintenance of adequate intravascular volume and state of hydration
- intraoperative and postoperative maintenance of a sufficient perfusion pressure and cardiac output
- avoidance of nephrotoxic drugs.

Loop diuretics cause renal vasodilatation and have been shown to preserve cortical blood flow during cardiopulmonary bypass. Their use in incipient renal failure may decrease the period of oliguria and anuria thus reducing the need for dialysis, but once again they have not been shown to influence survival.

Hyperkalaemia (>6.5 mmol/L) is a serious complication of renal shut-down and aggressive treatment is necessary to prevent serious dysrhythmias. An infusion of 50 mL of 50% glucose together with 10 units of soluble insulin given over 15 minutes will cause an intracellular shift of potassium. A similar effect is produced by an infusion of sodium bicarbonate (1–2 mmol/kg). Catecholamines are also effective at lowering extra cellular potassium levels and administration of a salbutamol nebulizer has been advocated as a method of treatment. Calcium chloride (10–20 mg/kg) will antagonize the cardiac effects of hyperkalaemia and should be given as a slow bolus if dysrhythmias are thought to be due to hyperkalaemia. These measures are all temporizing treatments and other manoeuvres to deplete potassium will be necessary. These include the administration of ion-exchange resins either orally or rectally and some form of dialysis or haemofiltration.

Stroke

Major central nervous system damage is a catastrophic event after cardiac surgery and carries a high mortality. Cerebral ischaemia may be due either to particulate or gas emboli or to global hypoperfusion. Fortunately overt stroke occurs in only 1–2% of patients but the incidence of subtle neuropsychological changes is much higher (34). Risk factors associated with an increased risk of stroke include advanced age, pre-existing cerebrovascular disease, prolonged perfusion times, and operations requiring intracardiac manipulations and total circulatory arrest. Of these, advanced age appears to be the most important (35).

Postoperative neurological deficits are treated along conventional lines. Primary cerebral damage is of course irreversible, but management should be directed towards prevention of secondary damage from further hypoxia or ischaemia. Maintenance of adequate arterial pressure and good oxygenation is vital. Mechanical ventilation should be continued in the early period after major cerebral injury to diminish the risks of hypoxia and hypercarbia and prevent the rise in venous pressure associated with laboured breathing. There is little or no evidence to support the use of steroids after acute brain injury, but cerebral oedema should be treated with osmotic or loop diuretics. Hyperthermia and convulsions should be treated aggressively, again to prevent secondary brain damage. Early CT scanning may occasionally detect surgically treatable lesions and may assist in assessing prognosis.

Post-cardiotomy psychosis is manifested by confusion, paranoia, or hallucinations and may be related to diffuse organic brain damage and cerebral dysfunction. Associated factors include advanced age, a prior history of psychological problems and alcoholism, sleep deprivation, hypoxia, and an unfamiliar and noisy environment. The condition usually resolves spontaneously over a matter of days but may pose a major problem for postoperative nursing care. Sedation tends to perpetuate confusion and should be avoided during the daytime unless it is necessary to prevent the patient from harming him- or herself by removing intravascular lines or monitoring equipment, in which case the most appropriate medication is haloperidol 5–10 mg parenterally.

Fever

Hyperthermia is not unusual in the early postoperative period and is treated with antipyretics such as paracetamol or aspirin. Fever beyond day 3 is not normal and should be investigated vigorously to locate the cause and permit appropriate treatment.

Late in-hospital care

The majority of patients will be fit to leave the critical care area within 24 hours of surgery. Indwelling lines and catheters should be removed as soon as the patient's condition permits, to avoid complications from sepsis. Daily survey should be performed to detect complications and review medication. Early detection and rapid treatment of complications helps to prevent the need for prolonged hospital stay. Daily haematocrit and electrolytes are unnecessary unless there is a clinical indication, but should be checked before discharge from hospital. Rehabilitation should start the morning after operation, with a carefully supervised progression of physical activity. Graded exercise including stair climbing is performed initially with the assistance of the physiotherapist. Early ambulation is beneficial in reducing the oedema of leg wounds, encouraging chest expansion, improving appetite and gastrointestinal function, and raising morale.

Postoperative stays after cardiac surgery have been gradually and progressively reduced. Whilst average stays in many hospitals 10 years ago were 10–12 days after coronary artery surgery, many centres now discharge patients after 5–7 days. More rapid discharge may be feasible in selected patients, but other factors including the level of family and home support and the distance from the hospital may affect whether or not a particular patient can be discharged. Elderly patients who live alone usually need a period of convalescence after surgery. A simple exercise test, as described by Krohn et al. (36) has been used as part of the criteria for early discharge.

Discharge criteria:

- successful completion of exercise test
- stable cardiac rhythm
- absence of temperature > 37.5°C
- adequate social/family support
- patient and family feel comfortable about going home
- no significant wound problems.

References

1. Prys-Roberts C. Anaesthesia and hypertension. *Br J Anaesth* 1984;**56**:711.
2. Perler BA, Burdick JF, Williams GM. The safety of carotid endarterectomy at the time of coronary bypass surgery: analysis of the results in a high risk patient population. *J Vasc Surg* 1985;**2**:558.
3. Warner MA, Offord KP, Warner ME, Lennon RL, Lonover MA, Janaaon-Schumacher U. Role of preoperative cessation of smoking and other factors in postoperative pulmonary complications: A blinded prospective study of coronary artery bypass patients. *Mayo Clin Proc* 1989;**64**:609–16.
4. Devineni R, McKenzie FN. Surgery for coronary artery disease in patients with diabetes mellitus. *Can J Surg* 1985;**28**:367.
5. Goodnough LT, Johnston MFM, Toy PTCY. The variability of transfusion practice in coronary artery bypass surgery. *JAMA* 1991;**265**:96–90.
6. Owings DV, Kruskall MS, Thurer BL, Donovan LM. Autologous blood donation prior to elective cardiac surgery: Safety and effect on subsequent blood use. *JAMA* 1989;**262**:1963–8.
7. Britton LW, Eastlund DT, Dziuban SW *et al.* Predonated autologous blood use in elective cardiac surgery. *Ann Thorac Surg* 1989;**47**:529–32.
8. Birkmeyer JD, AuBuchan JP, Littenberg B *et al.* Cost-effectiveness of preoperative autologous donation in coronary artery bypass grafting. *Ann Thorac Surg* 1994;**57**:161–9.
9. Goodnough LT, Johnston MFM, Shah T, Chernosky A. A two-institution study of transfusion practices in 78 consecutive adult elective open-heart procedures. *Am J Clin Pathol* 1989;**91**:468–72.
10. Aps C, Hutter JA, Williams BT. Anaesthetic management and postoperative care of cardiac surgical patients in a general recovery ward. *Anaesthesia* 1986;**41**:533–7.
11. Chong JL, Pillai R, Fisher A, Grebenik C, Sinclair M, Westaby S. Cardiac surgery: moving away from intensive care. *Br Heart J* 1992;**68**:430–3.
12. Cosgrove DM, Loop FD, Lytle BW. Determinants of blood utilization during myocardial revascularization. *Ann Thorac Surg* 1985;**40**:380–4.
13. MacNaughton PD, Braude S, Hunter DN, Denison DM, Evans TW. Changes in lung function and pulmonary capillary permeability after cardiopulmonary bypass. *Crit Care Med* 1992;**20**:1289–94.
14. Chong JL, Grebenik C, Sinclair M, Fisher A, Pillai R, Westaby S. The effect of a cardiac surgical recovery area on the timing of extubation. *J Cardiothoracic Vasc Anesth* 1993;**7**:1–5.
15. Grebenik CR, Allman C. Nausea and vomiting after cardiac surgery. *Br J Anaesth* 1996;**77**:356–9.
16. Mathews HML, Carson IW, Collier PS *et al.* Midazolam sedation following open heart surgery. *Br J Anaesth* 1987;**59**:557–60.
17. McMurray TJ, Collier PS, Carson IW, Lyons SM, Elliott P. Propofol sedation after open heart surgery. A clinical and pharmacokinetic study. *Anaesthesia* 1990;**45**:322–6.
18. Mangano DT. Multicenter outcome research. *J Cardiothorac Vasc Anesth* 1994;**8**:suppl 1:10–12.
19. Frank SM, Beattie C, Christopherson R *et al.* Unintentional hypothermia is associated with postoperative myocardial ischemia. *Anesthesiology* 1993;**78**:468–76.

20. Smith RC, Leung JM, Mangano DT. Postoperative myocardial ischemia in patients undergoing coronary artery bypass graft surgery. *Anesthesiology* 1991;**74**:464–73.

21. Mangano DT, Siliciano D, Hollenberg M *et al*. Postoperative myocardial ischemia. Therapeutic trials using intensive analgesia following surgery. *Anesthesiology* 1992;**76**:342–53.

22. Cheng DCH, Karski J, Peniston C *et al*. Safety of early extubation following coronary artery bypass graft (CABG) surgery: a prospective randomized controlled study of postop myocardial ischemia and infarction. *Anesthesiology* 1994;**81**:A81.

23. Breisblatt WM, Stein KL, Wolfe C *et al*. Acute myocardial dysfunction and recovery: A common occurrence after coronary bypass surgery. *J Am Coll Cardiol* 1990;**15**:1261–9.

24. Tuman KJ, McCarthy RJ, Spiess BD *et al*. Effect of pulmonary artery catheterization on outcome in patients undergoing coronary artery surgery. *Anesthesiology* 1989;**70**:199–206.

25. Tuman KJ, Carroll GC, Ivankovich AD. Pitfalls in interpretation of pulmonary artery catheter data. *J Cardiothorac Anesth* 1989;**3**:625–41.

26. Boldt J, Kling D, Moosdorf R, Hempelmann G. Enoximone treatment of impaired myocardial function during cardiac surgery: combined effects with epinephrine. *J Cardiothorac Anesth* 1990;**4**:462–8.

26. Duke GJ, Bersten AD. Dopamine and renal salvage in the critically ill patient. *Anaesth Intens Care* 1992;**20**:277–302.

27. Zurick AM, Urzua J, Ghattas M, Cosgrove DM, Estafnous FG, Greenstreet R. Failure of positive end-expiratory pressure to decrease postoperative bleeding after cardiac surgery. *Ann Thorac Surg* 1982;**34**:608–11.

28. Axford TC, Dearani JA, Ragno G *et al*. Safety and therapeutic effectiveness of reinfused shed blood after open heart surgery. *Ann Thorac Surg* 1994;**57**:615–22.

29. Schonberger JPAM, van Oeveren W, Bredee JJ, Everts PAM, de Haan J, Wildevuur CRH. Systemic blood activation during and after autotransfusion. *Ann Thorac Surg* 1994;**57**:1256–62.

30. Fuller JA, Adams GG, Buxton B. Atrial fibrillation after coronary bypass grafting. *J Cardiovasc Surg* 1989;**97**:821–5.

31. Kowey PR, Taylor JE, Rials SJ, Marinchak RA. Meta-analysis of the effectiveness of prophylactic drug therapy in preventing supraventricular arrhythmia early after coronary artery bypass grafting. *Am J Cardiol* 1992;**69**:963–5.

32. Butler J, Harriss DR, Sinclair M, Westaby S. Amiodarone prophylaxis for tachycardia after coronary artery surgery: a randomized, double blind, placebo controlled trial. *Br Heart J* 1993;**70**:56–60.

33. Zanardo G, Michielon P, Paccagnella A *et al*. Acute renal failure in the patient undergoing cardiac operation. *J Thorac Cardiovasc Surg* 1994;**107**:1489–95.

34. Shaw PJ, Bates D, Cartlidge NEF, Heaviside D, Julian DG, Shaw DA. Early neurological complications of coronary artery bypass surgery. *Br Med J* 1985;**291**:1384–7.

35. Tuman KJ, McCarthy RJ, Najafi H, Ivankovich AD. Differential effects of advanced age on neurologic and cardiac risks of coronary artery operations. *J Thorac Cardiovasc Surg* 1992;**104**:1510–17.

36. Krohn BG, Kay JH, Mendez MM, Zubiate P, Kay GL. Rapid sustained recovery after cardiac operations. *J Thorac Cardiovasc Surg* 1990;**100**:194–7.

8 Ventricular fibrillation with intermittent aortic cross clamping in coronary heart surgery

Ravi Pillai and J.E.C. Wright

Ventricular fibrillation induced either by electrical stimulation or by cooling is a long established technique used for surgery on the heart. Indeed, its use was widespread before the advent of a variety of solutions, both crystalloid and containing blood, that are currently used to arrest the heart and provide protection by hypothermia. The technique continues to be used in the setting of surgery for ischaemic heart disease by a small minority of surgeons in the world. The technique relies upon short periods of acute myocardial ischaemia, interrupted by normal coronary perfusion. Traditionally it is believed that as long as the periods of ischaemia are sufficiently short (6–12 minutes) complete myocardial recovery is obtained during the period of reperfusion. The practice of this technique has been supported more recently by the latterly observed myocardial protection effects of ischaemic preconditioning.

Ischaemic preconditioning

The theory of ischaemic preconditioning brings together the observation that if the myocardium is subjected to a short period of ischaemia, followed by reperfusion, it is protected from further periods of ischaemia subsequently and hence has the ability to recover full function. Furthermore, there is a great deal of evidence to suggest that the length of ischaemic time may be lengthened, with good recovery of myocardial function. Animal studies have demonstrated that short periods of ischaemia followed by reperfusion preserve high energy phosphates such as ATP and creatinine phosphate and reduce the rate at which such components are depleted during subsequent ischaemia. In addition, acidosis related to lactic acid production is also decreased. Functionally, myocardial recovery has been demonstrated as well as protection against arrhythmia. Although exact mechanism of ischaemic preconditioning is uncertain, it is possible that activation of adenosine receptors and protein kinase C may play a part. Studies in human hearts are limited by ethical considerations, but there is some evidence that the beneficial effect of this technique of performing coronary artery surgery is related to such preconditioning.

The technique of short periods of ischaemia by cross clamping the aorta with the heart fibrillating calls for an expeditious surgical technique, owing to the damaging effects of prolonged ischaemia at normotherma or moderate hypothermia, which may lead to irreversible myocardial dysfunction. The actual practice of the technique itself may vary and some aspects are discussed below. Apart from the theoretical advantages of this method there are several practical benefits.

Progressive revascularization

The majority of patients presenting for coronary artery surgery have multivessel coronary disease with tight proximal stenosis. In a significant proportion of these patients the myocardium may be chronically deprived of blood flow and the disease so severe that achieving myocardial protection using antegrade crystalloid or blood cardioplegia is not effective. Using the technique of distal coronary anastomoses with the heart fibrillating followed by completion of the proximal aortic anastomoses whilst the heart is reperfused, allows for each coronary artery to be bypassed and the corresponding area of myocardium to be revascularized progressively through the operation. This is particularly important in the setting of critical left coronary main stem stenosis and/or ostial stenosis of the left and right coronary arteries. preoperative planning of the sequence of anastomoses depending on severity of the vessel disease allows for effective protection and revascularization as one progresses through the operation.

In patients with no visible distal coronary vessels due to complete proximal occlusion, early revascularization and reperfusion of the myocardium is beneficial. This is particularly so in the subset of patients who have severely impaired left ventricular function with ejection fractions below 20%.

Assessment of graft patency

The completion of each graft by sequentially performing the proximal anastomoses following each distal end allows accurate assessment of graft patency. In addition to the observable flow within a graft, cardioversion following removal of the aortic cross clamp on completion of the distal anastomoses reverts the heart to sinus rhythm. If following completion of the graft the electrocardiogram (ECG) remains abnormal, then further inspection of the graft may be made in order to ascertain whether any technical problems have arisen with that particular graft. Abnormalities of the ECG and accurate assessment is difficult following other techniques which employ anastomoses of all the distal ends followed by aortic declamping and completion of proximal anastomoses. This approach should minimize the incidence of early perioperative infarction.

Reactive hyperaemia

Each period of ischaemic arrest causes the accumulation of metabolites in the myocardium. The coronary arteries, as with any other vessels, respond to such accumulations by dilating and ensuring a period of hyperaemic washout. Maximum dilation of the coronary artery allows for improved visualization and more accurate anastomoses. A minor consideration, but potentially an important one, is the increased ability to distinguish between the coronary arteries and veins, particularly in respect to identification of arteries that follow an intramuscular course. The retention of the normal colour of the myocardium allows for accurate dissection of deeply lying coronary arteries, by both palpation and visualization.

General considerations of technique

Ventricular fibrillation in modern day practice is induced by DC electrical stimulation, by using either an epicardial flat pad or a needle in close contact with the myocardium. At the time of

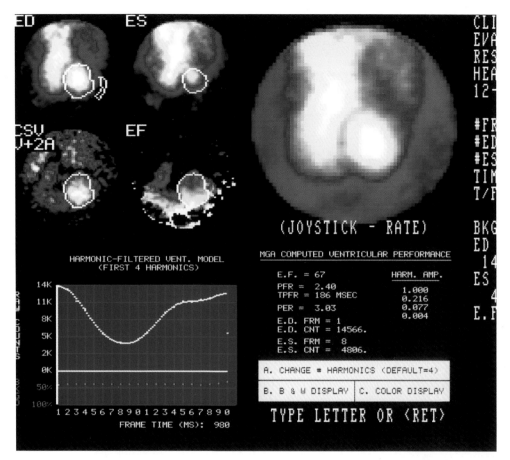

Plate 1 LAO image from an equilibrium radionuclide ventriculogram (see also Fig. 1.2, p. 12 for full caption).

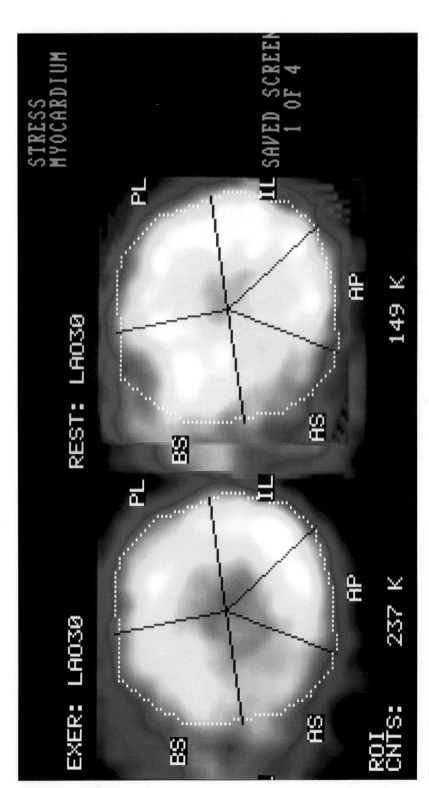

Plate 2 Thallium scan (see also Fig. 1.3, p. 14 for full caption).

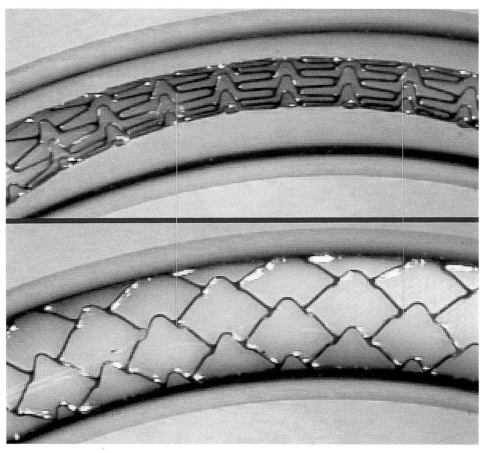

Plate 3 A coronary stent crimped on to a balloon (see also Fig. 2.2, p. 32 for full caption).

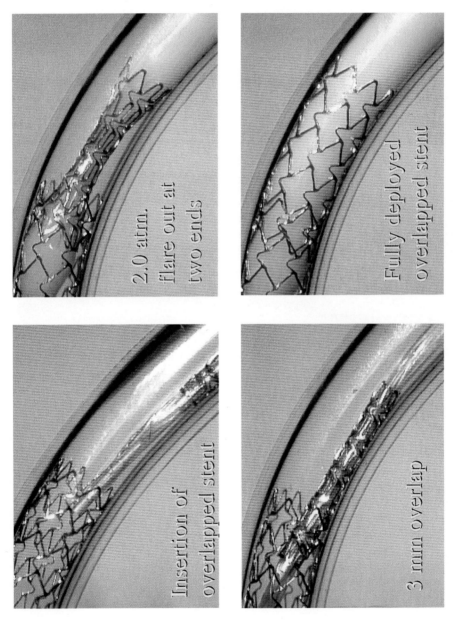

Plate 4 Techniques involved in sequential stenting of a long coronary stenosis (see also Fig. 2.3, p. 33 for full caption).

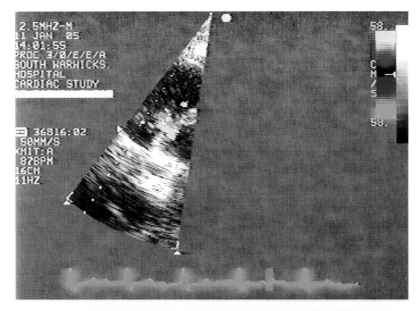

Plate 5 Doppler flow mapping demonstrating high velocity jet (see also Fig. 11.2, p. 196 for full caption).

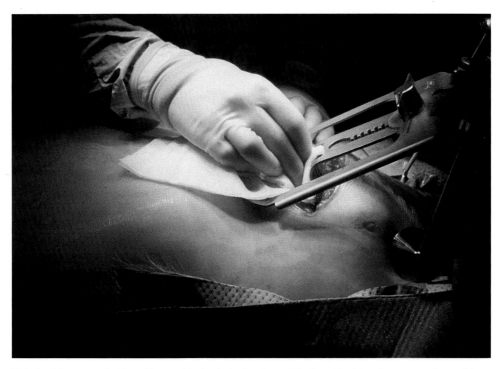

Plate 6 Submammary incision with a special retractor in place for mobilization of the internal mammary artery pedicle (see also Fig. 12.1, p. 219).

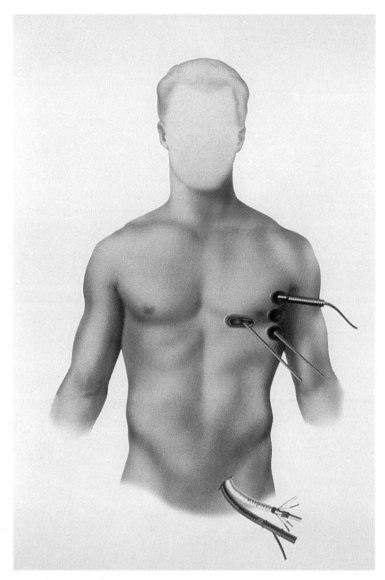

Plate 7 Location of ports in the third, fourth and fifth intercostal spaces in the mid-axillary line (see also Fig. 12.2, p. 220 for full caption).

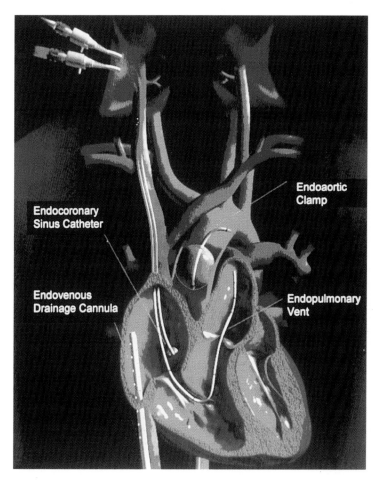

Plate 8 The Endovascular Cardiopulmonary Bypass System (see also Fig. 12.3, p. 221 for full caption).

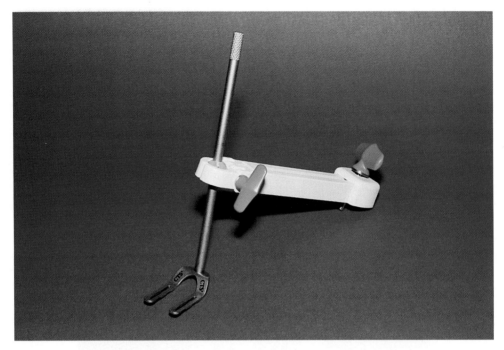

Plate 9 Coronary artery stabilizer (see also Fig. 12.4, p. 223 for full caption).

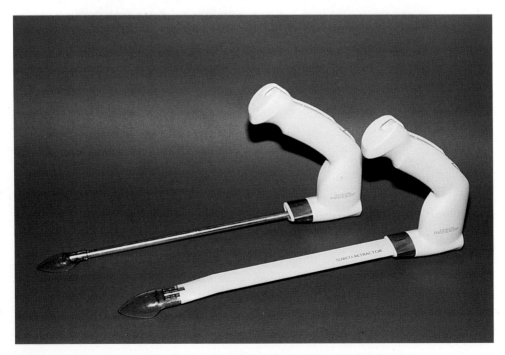

Plate 10 Dissectors for endoscopic saphenous vein harvest (see also Fig. 12.5, p. 225 for full caption).

aortic cross-clamping the heart is emptied and non-distended. This allows for minimum collateral flow and avoids flooding of the operating field. The manipulation of the venous drainage, particularly with the heart being held in a variety of positions, is an important aspect of preventing ventricular distension and irreversible subendocardial ischaemia. Some of the difficulties encountered in the past due to these factors have caused some surgeons to adopt modifications of the technique, such as continuous venting of the heart through the pulmonary artery, the superior pulmonary veins, or the left ventricular apex. Such manoeuvres add an unnecessary step to the operation and may indeed convert what is essentially a closed heart operation into an open one, with the subsequent need to de-air the heart to prevent air embolization. In addition to cardiac venting, active systemic cooling has also been a further modification. This has the disadvantage of making it difficult to cardiovert in between distal anastomoses while performing the proximal ones. As the circulating blood temperature falls below 32°C, spontaneous fibrillation of the heart usually occurs. Our preference is to maintain core temperature at normothermia or allow a degree of drift to about 34°C. In addition the maintenance of the serum potassium at 4–4.5 mmol/L ensures that persistent ventricular fibrillation is not due to an electroyle imbalance.

The removal of the electrical stimulant 2–3 minutes into the ischaemic period frequently spontaneously converts the rhythm to a slow ischaemic bradycardia. Although electrical activity is observed, there is very little mechanical response; this allows for an adequately still field. It may be argued that ischaemic asystole or bradycardia further reduces the myocardial oxygen demand and is therefore preferable to myocardial fibrillation. More often than not, following removal of the aortic cross clamp and in the absence of significant aortic regurgitation, the heart reverts to sinus rhythm with spontaneous restoration of normal rate and rhythm. Using this technique it is rare to see transient or temporary complete or partial heart block that is so often associated with the use of cardioplegia. The ability to wean patients off cardiopulmonary bypass in stable sinus rhythm reduces the need for pharmacological or electrical cardiac support.

Specific considerations

The major aspects in the successful utilization of this technique are multifactorial and they include:

- preparation of the coronary artery
- optimization of the conditions for acute ischaemia
- meticulous anastomotic technique
- adequate reperfusion

Preparation of the coronary artery for anastomoses

Suitable preparation of the coronary artery serves to minimize the period of myocardial ischaemia, as well as providing good exposure for anastomoses. It is our practice to sling the coronary artery on either side of the anastomotic site with two additional lateral sutures, holding the incised vessel open. We utilize 2/0 polypropylene sutures as slings that pass deep to the vessel through the myocardium. These sutures incorporate a substantial bulk of muscle between the suture and the coronary artery. The muscle buffer avoids damage to the vessel and prevents tearing. These sutures may be placed prior to ventricular fibrillation and aortic cross clamping when the distal right coronary artery, the left anterior descending artery, the diagonal of the anterior descending, or the intermediate vessels are being anastomosed. Although these sutures are placed with the heart beating, no attempt to fix their position is made at this juncture. To do so may lead to myocardial tears and haemorrhage. When vessels in the posterior or inferior aspects of the heart, such as the branches of the circumflex, the posterior descending artery, or the left ventricular branch of the dominant right coronary artery are being contemplated, it is more convenient to place such stay sutures after the induction of ventricular fibrillation with the aortic cross clamp in place. With the aorta cross clamped and the heart fibrillating and empty, the under-running polypropylene sutures are fixed to towelling at the edge of the wound, thereby displaying the vessel clearly with control of collateral blood flow. This allows for a dry field for anastomoses once the vessel is opened. In the case of the distal right coronary artery, polypropylene sutures are fixed along the left-hand side of the wound; for the left anterior descending and its branches and the intermediate vessel, the full sutures are fixed to the right of the wound. Such manoeuvres displace the vessels towards the middle of the pericardiotomy and also brings them forward, allowing for clearer visualization. The slight angulation that is caused contributes to the prevention of any blood flow into the operative field, obviating the need for any intraluminal device, clips, or continuous suction. The latter is well recognized as a possible cause of intimal injury at the time of graft anastomoses.

Optimization of the myocardial state

While the heart is fibrillating and the aorta is cross clamped it is essential that the ventricular chambers are maintained in an empty state. Any ventricular distension with subsequent subendocardial ischaemia may not be easily reversible; this is particularly the case in patients with pre-existing impaired ventricular function. In order to achieve this our preference is to drop the perfusion pressure momentarily and allow the heart to beat and empty itself with a reduced pump flow prior to placement of the aortic cross clamp and induction of ventricular fibrillation. Cross clamping the aorta with the perfusion pressure lowered also has the added advantage of avoiding damage to the aorta and causing an intimal tear. For the same reason it is our practice to vary the site of the aortic cross clamp if possible. Although it is easy to place the stay sutures for vessels in the front of the heart or the proximal right coronary artery with the heart beating, for vessels such as the branches of the circumflex system and the posterior descending artery it is more convenient to place the stay sutures while the heart is fibrillating and following aortic cross clamping. This again prevents undue distension of the heart. We routinely cannulate the right atrium with a Ross basket, which lies in the middle of the right atrial cavity. The utilization of the basket allows us to momentarily flick it into the right ventricle across the tricuspid valve in the event of the heart distending in spite of all the measure described above. Single venous cannulae now available which provide good drainage from the right atrium and the inferior vena cava are also suitable.

Meticulous anastomotic technique

The basis of achieving good anastomoses is dependent on adequate preparation, having delineated the site of anastomoses on the coronary artery and preparation of the conduit prior to aortic cross clamping. This approach maximizes the available anastomotic time during the period of ischaemia and provides the best operative field. This approach ensures that the major part of the cross clamp period is utilized for performing the distal anastomosis. Although it is accepted that 15 minutes is the maximum period allowable for normothermic myocardial ischaemia, it is important to ensure that the distal anastomoses is well performed with good proximal and distal blood flow.

Adequate perfusion

One of the great advantages of this technique is the ability to assess each coronary artery graft as it is performed. The visualization of blood flow in the coronary artery following removal of the aortic cross clamp, and the retrograde filling of venous or free arterial grafts, are important indicators of a good anastomosis. To reiterate what has been mentioned before, the restoration of the electrocardiogram to the preoperative state following completion of the proximal anastomosis in chronic stable angina is a useful indicator of graft patency and efficacy. The ability to assess each graft as well as the progressive revascularization of the heart makes the technique of coronary artery bypass grafting with ventricular fibrillation and intermittent cross clamping a challenging technique in managing the myocardium while carrying out coronary artery bypass grafting.

Acknowledgements

We wish to thank Dr Rhys Evans for his helpful review of this manuscript and advice. We thank Helen Blair and Alison Horner for their support in the preparation of the manuscript.

Further reading

Antunes MJ, Bernardo JE, Oliveira JM, Fernandes LE, Angrade CM. Coronary artery bypass surgery with intermittent aortic cross-clamping. *Eur J Cardiothorac Surg* 1992;**6**;189–94.

Bonchek LI, Burlingame MW. Coronary artery bypass without cardioplegia. *J Thorac Cardiovasc Surg* 1983;**88**:174–81.

Cohen M, Liu G, Downey J. Preconditioning causes improved wall motion as well as smaller infarcts after transient coronary occlusion in rabbits. *Circulation* 1991;**84**:341–9.

Cribier A, Korsatz L, Koning R *et al.* Improved myocardial ischaemic responses and enhanced collateral circulation with long repetitive coronary occlusion during angioplasty: a prospective study. *J Am Coll Cardiol* 1992;**20**:578–86.

Gross GL, Auchampach JA. Blockade of ATP-sensitive potassium channels prevents myocardial preconditioning in dogs. *Circ Res* 1992;**70**:223–33.

Jenkins DP, Steare SE, Yellon DM. Preconditioning the human myocardium; reent advances and aspiration for the development of a new means of cardioprotection in clinical practice. *Cardiovasc Drugs Ther (US)*; 1995;**9**(6):739–47.

Lasley RD, Mentzer RM Jr. Preconditioning and its potential role in myocardial protection during cardiac surgery. *J Card Surg (US)*; 1995;**10** (4 Pt 1):349–53.

Lui GS, Thornton J, Van Winkle DM, Stanley AWH, Olsson RA, Downey JM. Protection against infarction afforded by preconditioning is mediated by A_1 adenosine receptors in the rabbit heart. *Circulation* 1991;**84**:350–6.

Murry CE, Jennings RB, Reimar KA. Preconditioning with ischaemia: a delay of lethal cell injury in ischaemic myocardium. *Circulation* 1986;**74**:1124–36.

Murry CE, Richards VJ, Reimer KA, Jennings RB. Ischaemic preconditioning slow energy metabolism and delays ultrastructural damage during a sustained ischaemic episode. *Circ Res* 1990;**66**:913–31.

Perrault LP, Menasche P, Bel A *et al.* Ischaemic preconditioning in cardiac surgery: a word of caution. *J Thor Cardiovasc Surg (US)*;1996;**112(5)**:1378–86.

Speechly-Dick M, Mocanu M, Yellon D. Protein kinase C. Its role in ischaemic preconditioning in the rat. *Cir Res* 1994;**75**:586–90.

9 Technical aspects of coronary artery surgery

Ravi Pillai and J.E.C. Wright

Since the description of the use of saphenous vein for coronary artery bypass grafting by Favoloro in 1967 the procedure has been widely adopted across the world. Today it is the most common adult cardiac surgical operation. Its relative simplicity has led to the massive increase in the number of centres performing cardiac surgery in several countries. The fact that ischaemic heart disease is responsible for the largest number of deaths in most western countries has ensured that coronary artery surgery, as well as other interventional procedures for treating ischaemic heart disease, has occupied a position of importance alongside preventive measures as far as allocation of resources are concerned.

With the expansion of the number of centres, and the increasing number of cardiac surgeons performing the precedure, innumerable methods and techniques have been developed. Most techniques, however, require adherence to some basic principles in order to achieve the best results. Most surgeons acquire the skills required to perform coronary artery surgery during their training period in cardiac surgery. Individual surgical techniques may not only be confined to different methods of anastomosis but also to myocardial preservation, the use of cardiopulmonary bypass as well as using visual aids. It is common place now to use magnification in the form of 'operating telescopes' (loops) attached to spectacles, or indeed an operating microscope to perform distal coronary anastomosis on the heart. There are, however, a substantial number of cardiac surgeons who do not use such aids.

Cardiopulmonary bypass

The general aspects of cardiopulmonary bypass have been dealt with elsewhere, but for convenience some of the more specific points are repeated in this section. Following general anaesthesia and the placement of appropriate instrumentation for heamodynamic monitoring, the heart is approached through a median sternotomy. The surgical approach can vary very occasionally for grafts to the left-sided coronary vessels. As previously described this could be through a left thoracotomy, as well as more recent reports of limited thoracotomy within the context of minimally invasive techniques. The latter may develop in the future. Currently cardiopulmonary bypass is established with aortic and venous cannulation, the latter through the right atrium. In the setting of re-operations, cannulation of a femoral artery for arterial return may be initially performed in order not only to assist in safe re-sternotomy but also to maximize the amount of aortic wall available for proximal coronary graft anastomoses. Nevertheless, aortic cannulation for arterial

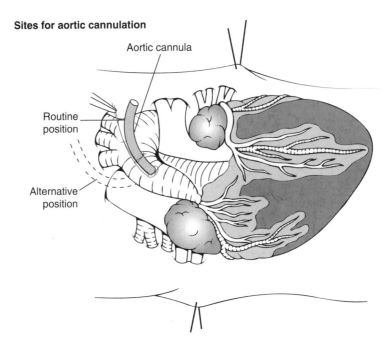

Sites for aortic cannulation

Aortic cannula

Routine position

Alternative position

Fig. 9.1 Sites for aortic cannulation.

return is the common practice. A more posterior or posterolateral insertion of the cannula into the aorta may be utilized in order to increase the amount of free anterior wall for proximal coronary graft anastomosis (Fig. 9.1).

Often patients with coronary artery disease have a varying degree of atheromatous plaque formation in the ascending aorta and arch. In view of this it is important to cannulate a clearly non-diseased part of the aorta if possible. Most commonly this is ascertained by palpation, which is adequate in most cases. The practice of routine transoesophageal echocardiography to delineate areas of plaque formation in the ascending aorta is utilized in certain practices. The length of the aortic arterial cannula may also be important. In general the arterial cannula should be short and lying freely in the aortic lumen, or long enough to pass down the arch of the aorta and lie in the mid part of the lumen. Intermediate lengths may either abut on the opposite aortic wall or may indeed lie in one of the head vessels. This may have the consequence of either disrupting plaques or, in rare cases, lifting the intimal layer. This could lead to dissection of the aorta or embolization of atheromatous plaques.

Venous return

Most practices use a two-stage cannula for obtaining venous return. Cannulation is achieved through the right atrial appendage. It is the authors' practice to utilize a metal basket lying in the right atrium such as the Ross venous basket. This method is particularly suited for the technique of intermittent cross clamping and fibrillation while coronary artery grafting is being carried out. The blunt end of the basket is ideal to be manipulated across the tricuspid valve into the right ventricle to decompress the heart in the event of ventricular distension. Separate venous cannulae may be employed passing from the right atrium into the superior and inferior venae cava in order to completely isolate the heart. This can be achieved more completely by snaring the superior and inferior vena cava along with the use of a left-sided vent. Complete isolation of the heart during bypass with hypothermia minimizes the collateral blood flow. Nowadays, however, it is not the authors' practice to routinely employ systemic hypothermia.

Myocardial protection

Intermittent cross clamping and fibrillation is the preferred technique of the authors for coronary artery surgery. A more detailed account of this technique is given in Chapter 8. Suffice to say here that the technique allows for progressive revascularization of the heart with the construction of sequential, distal, and proximal anastomosis. The technique also has the advantage of being able to identify specific problems with a particlar graft as well as allowing immediate revascularization of a territory of the heart that is at risk from acute ischaemia. This is useful in the setting of attempted resuscitation following cardiac arrest and emergency coronary artery surgery for unstable angina. It is our belief that it has important advantages in patients with poor ventricular function and those undergoing associated procedures such as left ventricular aneurysmectomy and repair of postinfarct ventricular septal defects. Visualization of the coronary arteries, particularly in re-operations or in the presence of pericarditis, is also facilitated.

Cardioplegia

A detailed account of this method of myocardial protection has been provided in Chapter 4. Briefly, the process of producing cardiac arrest by a combination of biochemical manipulation with or without hypothermia is achieved in three commonly utilized methods: antegrade, retrograde, or continuous cardioplegia.

Antegrade cardioplegia

Antegrade cardioplegia is most often delivered through the aortic root and may consist of a crystalloid cardioplegic solution or a cardioplegic solution made up in blood. Cardiac arrest is produced by a high concentration of potassium in the solution with other additives that bring about membrane stabilization. The most common technique involves the use of cold cardioplegic solution with infusions repeated at intervals of 20–40 minutes. More recently there has emerged a practice of infusing either warm blood cardioplegia from the outset or giving a short infusion of warm blood cardioplegia prior to reperfusion of the heart.

Retrograde cardioplegia

This technique utilizes essentially the same method of obtaining cardiac arrest but instead of the cardioplegic solution being infused through the aortic root the coronary sinus is cannulated by a specially manufactured catheter through the right atrium. This technique has the advantage of being able to perfuse all parts of the mycardium with a more even distribution of perfusate irrespective of the extent of coronary artery disease. Retrograde, venous perfusion is carried out at much lower perfusion pressures than aortic root perfusion. Proponents of this method point to the obvious advantages, particularly in re-operations for coronary artery disease in the setting of totally absent native vessels demonstrable on coronary angiography with or without patent coronary grafts.

Continuous cardioplegia

This technique is not commonly employed and consists of a continued slow infusion of cardio-plegic solution following initial cardiac arrest throughout the period of aortic cross clamping while the distal coronary anastomoses are performed. This continued infusion may be either ante-grade or retrograde, and is more often utilized with crystalloid cardioplegic solution.

The actual method of administering the cardioplegic solution varies enormously. In many prac-tices precise volumes are given at defined flow rates within pressure limits by being infused via a roller pump connected to the cardioplumonary circuit. Other methods included infusion into the aortic root utilizing infusion sets connected to a pressure bag. The relative merits of the different techniques remain unclear and it is likely that the lack of demonstrable differences in outcome following coronary surgery using the different techniques indicate little difference.

Coronary artery surgery without cardiopulmonary bypass

Grafting of single or multiple vessels without using cardioplumonary bypass has recently re-emerged as a technique in performing coronary artery surgery. Both the distal and proximal anas-tomoses are carried out with the heart beating with pharmacologically induced hypotension and bradycardia. These attempts are basically to eliminate the complications of cardiopulmonary bypass, both in relation to the often-discussed inflammatory response as well as other sequelae such as neuro psychological dysfunction. Given the techniques of modern day cardiopulmonary bypass, particularly with the advent of membrane oxygenators with improved anaesthetic and surgical techniques, the evidence that this particular method is superior in terms of long-term outcome and adequate revascularization remains debatable. Published series using this approach still remain small and include both operations with formal sternotomy, as well as more recently described minimally invasive techniques.

Manipulation of cardiopulmonary bypass

An often neglected aspect of open heart surgery is the use of the pump to vary the flow and per-fusion pressure while on cardiopulmonary bypass to facilitate the surgery. Much of what is described may seem obvious but is often overlooked. Tearing of the aorta or early dissection of the distal ascending aorta related to the site of cross clamping is a recognized complication. This is particularly true when there is significant aortic wall disease which is not always detectable either on angiography or by external inspection of the aorta at the time of surgery. Dropping the flow and thereby the aortic root pressure at the time of cross clamping enables one to clamp a soft non-rigid aorta safely. In addition this has the effect of emptying the heart, thereby preventing ventricular distension, and avoids forcing the heart to beat against a totally obstructed outflow. Prevention of ventricular distension is important, particularly in ventricles where function is impaired and is of importance whether one uses cardioplegia to arrest the heart or the technique of intermittent aortic cross clamping with fibrillation. An empty non-distended heart facilitates even distribution of cardioplegia and avoids tearing of the epicardial surface due to placement of stay sutures. On the other hand, patients with coronary artery disease are likely to have vascular disease involving other organs such as the brain and kidney as well as the gastrointestinal tract. In these circumstances long periods of low flows and hypoperfusion might result in an increased incidence of neurological sequelae or acute renal dysfunction in the postoperative period. The optimum management of cardiopulmonary bypass requires close co-operation between the surgical team and the perfusionists.

Perioperative technique

In common with all surgical approaches, coronary artery surgery requires meticulous planning and careful execution. Both these factors allow for an accurate anastomosis and expeditious surgery. Planning of surgery begins before the operation, taking into account the patient's general condition, age, symptoms, associated conditions, a careful judgement of diagnostic and angiographic findings, and a clear plan as to what is required in the treatment of the individual patient. A useful rule of thumb approach is that it is better to *stay* out of trouble than *get* out of it. This approach reinforces the concept of the need to have a preoperative plan, minimize surgical trauma, and observe the basic concepts of handling the heart, as well as cardiopulmonary bypass and expeditious surgical technique. The description below of anastomotic techniques, specifically describing both distal and proximal coronary artery anastomoses when applicable, sets out general principles which are universally applicable regardless of the conduit used. The conduits used require adequate preparation in terms of secure control of side branches of both arteries and veins. In preparing the saphenous vein, avoidance of a valve or attached fat at the site of anastomosis is essential. The distinction made between distal anastomosis and proximal anastomosis are only for the sake of clarity, since several of the points made in either section are relevant to both.

Frequently, either on viewing the angiogram or on inspection and palpation of the coronary artery it is clear that the length of the vessel is occupied by an atheromatous core. The vessel is likely to be totally occluded with no evidence of contrast flow. Under these circumstances, endarterectomy of the vessel following arteriotomy is carried out. This would be done through a limited or extensive arteriotomy. The atheromatous core is teased away from the media with longitudinal blunt dissection and counter-traction. A core of atheroma is then delivered through the arteriotomy. The dissection is carried out using spatulated instruments or rigid probes. Other techniques using jets of air or carbon dioxide have been previously described. The arterial wall left behind is usually much thinner and more friable. Vessels that have intermittent diffuse disease are less amenable to satisfactory endarterectomy.

Distal anastomoses

Several techniques for performing distal anastomosis have evolved over the last 25 years. Most are performed using 6/0, 7/0 or 8/0 polypropylene (Prolene) sutures, as continuous sutures which are interrupted at one, two, or four points, or as interrupted single sutures. Except in the absence of adequate conduit length it is prudent to use one conduit per coronary artery anastomosis. Although there is some theoretical advantage in having multiple anastomosis ('jump grafts') with improved runoff to produce long-term graft patency, there is little actual evidence of this. These general observations apart, there are important principles that allow for a good anastomotic technique, minimize the rate of perioperative infarction due to graft occlusion and enhance long-term graft patency. As part of planning, the vessel to be grafted is inspected and if possible an area free of disease chosen. Stay sutures are placed proximal and distal to the anastomotic point. Two further sutures placed laterally in the epicardial fat on either side of the anastomosis facilitate the anastomosis by keeping the arteriotomy open. The epicardium overlying the coronary artery is lightly incised with a scalpel and swept away. It must be noted that this process tends to weaken the wall of the artery and therefore should be limited to the length of the anastomosis only. Routine probing of coronary arteries either proximally or distally is unnecessary and may indeed damage the endothelium or raise atheromatous plaques. Clearly, if there is any doubt about the anastomosis itself gentle probing allows one to confirm patency. It is sensible in performing the anastomosis to pass the needle out from within the artery, thereby ensuring that the endothelium of the vessel or atheromatous plaques are not lifted. This is consistent with the general principles of vascular surgery. By ensuring that the anastomosis brings together the endothelium of the coronary artery with that of the conduit, one prevents the raising of flaps or leakage. If the coronary artery is diffusely diseased the use of a cutting needle prevents crumbling of the atheromatous plaque and indeed such a needle is easier to pass through the arterial wall. Most arteriotomies and anastomoses are 3–5 mm in length. By making the opening in the conduit, whether it be saphenous vein or an artery, slightly longer than the coronary arteriotomy, a cobra head effect is produced on completion of the anastomosis. Three techniques of anastomosis as practised by the authors are set out below. It is the author's preference to use different techniques for different vessels depending on the position of those vessels on the heart. The left anterior descending artery (LAD) and the diagonal branches (DLAD), as well as the right coronary artery (RCA) lie on the front of the heart, whereas branches of the circumflex vessels are approached with the heart lifted up exposing the posterior surface. The distal branches of the right coronary artery such as the posterior descending artery (PDA) and the left ventricular branch are on the inferior surface of the heart.

Left anterior descending artery and diagonal branches; right coronary artery

The **LAD, DLAD, and RCA** are easily accessible through a median sternotomy. Having determined the point of anastomosis and set-up as described previously the arteriotomy is performed and a clear bloodless field achieved. The anastomosis is performed using two 6/0 or 7/0 Prolene sutures anchoring the heel and the toe of the conduit (Fig. 9.2). The nearside suture line is carried out first, starting at the toe and placing two to three throws. Two or three more throws are placed from the heel towards the mid-line of the anastomosis. The sutures are tied at this point. Following this the far side suture line is performed, again starting at the toe for two or three throws and similarly completed at the midpoint of the anastomosis. Limiting the number of throws from the toe end to two or three ensures that retraction of the conduit and the epicardium on the opposite side provides good visualization of the heel end of the anastomosis. As with all anastomoses it is important that the sutures pass through the arterial wall only since inclusion of epicardial fat compromises the exposure.

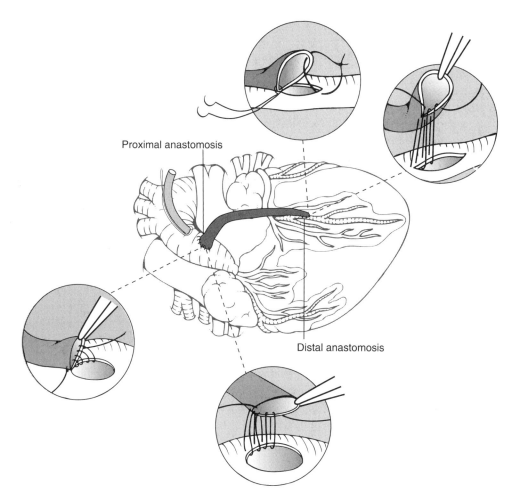

Proximal anastomosis

Distal anastomosis

Fig. 9.2 Principle of conduit construction.

Circumflex vessels

The circumflex vessels are approached with the apex of the heart lifted and held with the right edge of the sternotomy wound by the surgical assistant. Having set up, the authors' preference is to use one suture anchored at the heel with a continuous running suture, passing initially on the left hand side as seen by the operator all the way round the toe to the right-hand side towards the midpoint of the anastomosis (Fig. 9.2). The other end of the anastomosis suture is now completed by three or four throws towards the operator, passing outside in to the coronary artery. If the vessel is diffusely diseased then this one quarter of the anastomosis may also be performed placing the sutures inside out backhand. Releasing the stay sutures proximal to the arteriotomy or injecting cold saline while tying down the suture minimizes and avoids the 'pursestring effect'.

Posterior descending artery

Access to vessels on the diaphragmatic or inferior surface of the heart may be more difficult. In these circumstances the authors' preference is to use a two-suture technique whereby the first suture is placed at the heel of the anastomosis and the conduit tied down with not more than three throws. Three more throws are placed on either side, passing from the heel towards the midpoint of the arteriotomy. The second suture is now placed at the toe of the anastomosis and similarly tied down with three throws. The anastomosis is subsequently completed by running the sutures towards the midpoint and tying the suture from the heel.

In most instances, in order to preserve the principle of passing the needle from within the coronary artery, most nearside suture lines may be performed forehand while farside suture lines require a backhand technique.

Proximal anastomoses

The techniques described here pertain to venous grafts and free arterial grafts. Prior to performing the proximal anastomoses, the grafts are confirmed to be of adequate length (with the heart full), not twisted and reversed in the case of the saphenous vein. In most instances the proximal anastomosis is performed using a partially occlusive side-biting clamp, thereby ensuring that the heart is being reperfused at this period. Occasionally due to severe aortic wall disease the proximal anastomosis may be performed with the aortic cross clamp in place in order to avoid repeated clamping of the ascending aorta. Although this part of the aorta is the most common site for proximal anastomosis in certain circumstances the arch, or even the descending thoracic aorta, may be used. It is the authors' preference to use a small side-biting clamp for each of the proximal anastomoses. It is routine in most practices to use one large clamp to perform all the proximal anastomoses. Generally speaking grafts from left coronary arteries are anastomosed to the left side of the ascending aorta, and grafts from the right coronary and its branches to the right side. Depending on the position of the distal anastomosis right-sided grafts may be brought up to the ascending aorta either along the atrioventricular groove or around the right atrium. In some instances grafts to the distal circumflex vessels seem to lie better if anastomosed to the right side of the ascending aorta, having been brought through the transverse sinus.

As with the distal anastomosis, if possible a soft disease-free area of the aorta is identified for the proximal end of the graft. The defect created in the aorta may be square, circular, or triangular and achieved either with a pointed blade or an aortic punch. The authors' preference is for a circular defect created with a pointed knife, the size of the defect varying according to the conduit that is being utilized and its size. Occasionally on opening the aorta the endothelium is found to be heavily diseased and might indeed separate from the aortic wall. In these circumstances a meticulous technique is required whereby as the anastomosis is performed the separating layers are stitched together to prevent dissection at this point. The authors' preference is to anchor the heel of the conduit to the defect in the aorta in line with the tip of the left shoulder of the patient. Following this one limb of the suture is passed in a clockwise direction to 3 o'clock. The anastomosis is completed by running the other limb of the suture in an anticlockwise direction and tied at 3 o'clock. It is also common practice to perform this anastomosis using an open technique whereby the proximal end of the conduit is held away from the defect while a 5/0 or 6/0 Prolene suture is passed in a clockwise direction from 9 o'clock to 3 o'clock before parachuting the conduit down to the aortic defect. The anastomosis is then completed by passing the limb of the suture in an anticlockwise direction from 9 o'clock to 3 o'clock.

There may be a great degree of variability in the thickness of the aortic wall which might be important to consider when constructing the proximal anastomosis using free arterial grafts. If this wall thickness is found to be excessive, and therefore liable to distort the anastomosis, the defect in the aorta may be patched either using pericardium or vein in the first instance. Following this a defect is created in the middle of the patch and the proximal anastomosis performed.

On completion of each graft, residual air is removed by obliquely puncturing the conduit away from the proximal anastomosis with a 25 French gauge needle. At the same time simple palpation and 'distal' emptying of the conduit should confirm unrestricted flow into the coronary artery. As one approaches the end of the operation, the amount of cardiotomy suction required points to the degree of haemostasis. When the surgeon is satisfied that this is secure, the patient is weaned off cardiopulmonary bypass methodically with as low a filling pressure as possible. With the increasing age of the population being operated upon today, the minimization of bleeding and the maintenance of adequate perfusion pressures is a crucial in optimizing short- and long-term outcome.

Acknowledgements

We wish to thank Dr Rhys Evans for his helpful review of this manuscript and advice. We thank Helen Blair and Alison Horner for their support in the preparation of the manuscript.

Further reading

Alfieri O, Lorusso R. Developments in surgical techniques for coronary revascularization. *Curr Opin Cardiol* 1995;**10**(6);556–61.

Rashid A, Fabri BM, Jackson M *et al.* A prospective randomised study of continuous warm versus intermittent cold blood cardioplegia for coronary artery surgery: preliminary report. *Eur J Cardiothorac Surg* 1994;**8**(5);265–9.

Saatvedt K, Dragsund M, Bie-Larsen R, Nordstrand K. Video-assisted heart surgery — an alternative in the future? *Tidsskr Nor Laegeforen* 1996;**116**(25);3020–1.

10 Conduits for coronary artery surgery

S.M. Allen and R.S. Bonser

Relief of symptoms and long-term survival following coronary artery bypass grafting correlate to patency of the bypass conduit. Although early patency is determined by operative technique and the severity of pathological changes in the operated artery, the long-term patency depends upon the conduit used.

The ideal conduit will respond to physiological and anatomical requirements, will be available in sufficient quantities for complete revascularization, and will remain patent for the lifetime of the patient. No currently available conduit matches these ideals. An operation for myocardial revascularization therefore needs to be tailored to maximize the advantages and disadvantages of the available conduits within the constraints dictated by the patients age and risk factors, the urgency of treatment, and the experience and expertise of the surgeon.

Venous conduits

Long saphenous vein

Results

The long saphenous vein is expendable and available in sufficient length to reach the most distal coronary arteries. In 1968 Favoloro first reported the use of saphenous vein bypass grafts in occlusive coronary artery disease (1). Initially reserved for single vessels, the technique was soon applied to multiple vessels (2) and subsequently multiple sequential grafting was introduced (3). Comparative studies of saphenous vein and IMA grafts in the early 1970s suggested that the higher patency rates of IMA grafts was offset by lower flows (4,5) and the use of saphenous vein increased during this period.

Since then the patency rate of saphenous grafts has been the subject of many studies (6–17) that can be summarized as follows: In the early postoperative period 8–12% of grafts occlude and at 1 year between 12 and 20% of vein grafts are lost (9–10). Beyond the first year the occlusion rate decreases to 2% a year. At 5 years the cumulative percentage occlusion is 22–30% (12). Beyond 5 years the annual attrition rates doubles and up to 50% of grafts occlude within 10 years (6–17). Beyond 5 years 15–40% of patent grafts display irregularity, and by 10 years 50% of patent grafts have atheromatous changes with luminal compromise (9–10).

The outcome up to 20 years after operation has recently been reported (16) with graft patency of 81% at 0–5 years, 68% at 5–10 years, 60% at 10–15 years and 46% at 16–20 years.

Patients with graft stenoses, especially in grafts to the anterior descending artery, have a significantly worse prognosis than patients with comparable stenoses of native coronary arteries or with vein grafts with no stenoses (18).

Expanded use of long saphenous vein

Saphenous vein graft patency rates are lower for anastomoses to small coronary arteries or to arteries supplying scarred areas, because of reduced distal runoff. Superior patency has been postulated for sequential grafts because of the higher flow rates typically achieved. Several centres have reported satisfactory early (19–21) and late (22) patency with sequential saphenous vein grafts, with equivalent results to single grafts. The first side-to side anastomosis has the best patency and the terminal end-to-side anastomosis the worst. Patency of distal anastomoses is lower than that of single grafts to the same vessel (23). In a large series of patients with multiple endarterectomies accompanied by saphenous vein grafting in which the distal end of the vein served as a 10–15 cm onlay patch, early and late mortality was higher in patients with endarterectomy, but there was no significant difference in late graft patency between vein grafts to endarterectomized and non-endarterectomized vessels (24).

Causes of failure of long saphenous vein grafts

Early failure

Graft occlusion within 30 days is due to thrombosis, usually secondarily to technical error or vein damage during surgical preparation. Technical faults may be responsible for one-third of early graft occlusions (9) (Fig. 10.1). Endothelial injury leads to loss of endothelial integrity and impaired production of prostacyclin and endothelium-derived relaxing factor, which promotes platelet and leukocyte adhesion (13,14,25–27). Thrombosis is further favoured by poor flow resulting from distal coronary artery disease (28). Graft spasm can occur, but its frequency and importance is uncertain.

Fibrointimal hyperplasia

Grafts that remain patent may undergo uniform medial thickening followed by intimal thickening. The pathogenesis remains uncertain but is probably secondary to smooth muscle proliferation and migration (14,25,29). Intimal thickening may be further promoted by the laying down of increased amounts of extracellular matrix (14,25,29), derived possibly from organization of mural thrombos (13,27). However, intimal proliferation is not altered by endothelial regeneration, and is not apparently influenced by the initial degree of endothelial injury (29) or by anti-platelet treatment (28), and platelet-derived growth factor (PDGF) from vascular wall cells, rather than adherent platelets, may be the major causative factor in intimal hyperplasia (30). Thus it is likely that growth factor production is induced from the venous endothelium, smooth muscle layers, or monocytes that infiltrate in response to lipid accumulation (31). Intimal hyperplasia is present in 75% of grafts at 1 year (9) and is the leading cause of vein graft stenosis 6–24 months after operation.

Lower extremity veins are relatively inelastic when exposed to normal arterial pressure and changes may also represent intrinsic adaptation of the vein to the arterial circulation; experimental angiotensin-induced hypertension increases vein graft medial thickening and alters vasomotor function (32) and intimal hyperplasia impairs endothelium-dependent relaxation both in human and experimental vein grafts (33).

Increased wall tension is another stimulus for intimal hyperplasia. After a few weeks of implantation the average wall stress in the graft and the grafted artery are similar and the rate of smooth muscle proliferation slows (34).

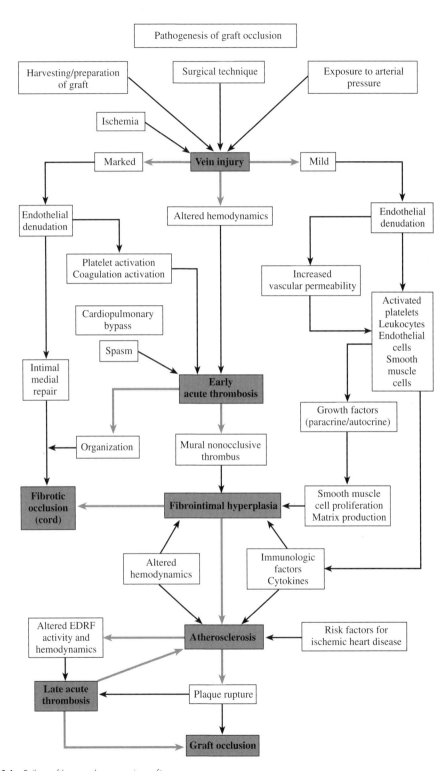

Fig. 10.1 Failure of long saphenous vein grafts.

Vein graft atherosclerosis

After the first year, lipid-laden atherosclerotic plaques appear (13,14,25).Vein graft atherosclerosis may occur in areas of existing intimal hyperplasia or as a separate process (35,36). Incorporation of lipids into the media of vein grafts is triggered by arterial implantation and distension during surgical preparation and exacerbated by hypercholesterolaemia (37). Most investigators believe that intimal hyperplasia provides a substrate for the development of atherosclerosis (25). Lipid deposition is followed by the appearance of cholesterol clefts, areas of calcification, ulceration, and thrombosis (14,25,38,39). By 6 years many grafts show histological evidence of advanced atherosclerotic changes (40). Rupture of the atheromatous plaque is an important factor leading to thrombotic occlusion of the graft. In a study of vein graft segments removed at reoperation late thrombosis was demonstrated in 69% of the residual grafts (41).

Measures to improve saphenous vein graft patency

Early patency

Patency in the early months can be improved by meticulous techniques of harvesting and anastomosis. Mechanical trauma and excessive distension of the vein during surgical preparation damage the endothelim, intima and media. Various techniques have been developed to avoid distending pressures of more than 300 mmHg (42–46). The nature and temperature of storage solutions and time of storage has less consistent damaging effects (42,43). Blood or crystalloid solutions that substitute all necessary electrolytes with additional albumin may preserve endothelial function of venous grafts better than saline solutions. Construction of the proximal anastomoses first may preserve endothelial cell integrity, function, and secretion of prostacyclin (47). Greater use of vein below the knee may avoid vein–artery size mismatch with reduced flow velocity, turbulence, and stasis.

Mid term patency

Because some degree of endothelial damage will inevitably occur despite meticulous technique, antithrombotic therapy is required. A recent meta-analysis provided conclusive evidence that antiplatelet treatment enhances the early patency of coronary vein grafts (48,49). Improved patency rates have been shown with aspirin alone, aspirin and dipyridamole, and sulphinpyrazone alone (50), but aspirin alone seems most effective. Preoperative aspirin is associated with increased bleeding complications and confers no additional benefit on early graft patency (51). However, administration of aspirin immediately or soon after surgery improves graft patency without increasing postoperative blood loss (52). The lowest dose of aspirin shown to have a consistent beneficial effect in clinical trials is probably 325 mg daily (49,53). Benefit of aspirin continued beyond 1 year is not established, although its continuation indefinitely has been recommended.

Oral anticoagulants are also effective in reducing early graft occlusion but require greater monitoring (54). Many surgeons limit their use to those patients who undergo endarterectomy (53,54).

Long-term patency

Late vein graft occlusion is unlikely to be influenced by antithrombotic therapies as these do not suppress smooth muscle proliferation. Agents not yet studied clinically that may have an antiproliferative effect on smooth muscle include cod liver oil (55), heparin (56,57), angiotensin-converting enzyme inhibitors (56,58), angiopeptin (59), and calcium channel blockers (60). Prevention of myointimal hyperplasia, however, is hampered by insufficient knowledge of its cellular and molecular basis. An organ culture model of human saphenous vein in which smooth muscle proliferation occurs reproducibly may overcome some limitations of isolated cell preparations (61). Preventive therapies are now being developed based on molecular biological concepts. Antibody to human PDGF reduced myointimal hyperplasia after balloon injury in rodent carotid arteries (62), and an antibody to basic fibroblast growth factor inhibited H-thymidine labelling, suggesting an effect on smooth muscle proliferation, after a similar injury (63). Other work is continuing on genetically manipulated cells (64) and genes (65).

The role of diet and reduction of serum lipids on the progression of graft atherosclerosis is unclear. In a dog model, fish oil (marine ω_3 fatty acids) reduced accelerated vein graft intimal thickening stimulated by diet-induced hypercholesterolaemia (66). There may be benefit from aggressive pharmacological reduction of low density lipoproteins (67,68).

Short saphenous vein

When long saphenous vein is not available the short saphenous vein may be used, with similar results.

Upper extremity vein

A cephalic vein length of at least 20 cm can usually be obtained, with shorter lengths of basilic vein. The calibre is generally smaller than that of the saphenous vein and the walls are often thin and friable. Patency rates have been considerably worse than those achieved with long saphenous vein (69,70).

Allogenic veins

Cryopreserved allogenic long saphenous vein

Clinical results of cryopreserved saphenous vein allografts used as coronary artery grafts have been disappointing (71–74). The degree of antigenicity of cryopreserved allograft veins is uncertain as there is little histological evidence of immune reaction after implantation. The freezing process destroys cellular elements in the vein, with only the collagen and elastic matrix remaining viable at implantation. Host cells repopulate the graft resulting in fibrosis. Work continues on the issues of long-term patency and possible immune rejection (75,76). Recent advances in cryopreservation techniques that preserve cellular viability and possibly decrease immunological responses to implantation have led to promising experimental results (77,78).

Fresh allogenic long saphenous vein

Clinical results using fresh allogenic long saphenous vein have been very poor (71,72). Experimental work suggests that fresh homologous vein grafts undergo a typical rejection reaction with histological changes noted within 5–10 days of implantation, and within 1 year the grafts are fibrotic and usually occluded.

Glutaraldehyde-fixed allogenic umbilical vein

Similar very poor clinical results have been achieved with glutaraldehyde-fixed umbilical vein (79) and there is also concern that these grafts may be predisposed to aneurysmal degenera-

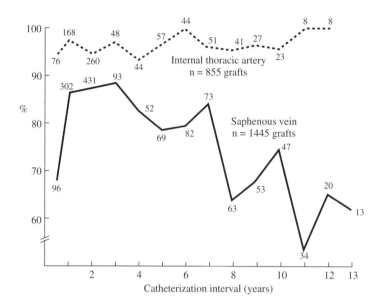

Fig. 10.2 IMA graft patency rates.

tion. The glutaraldehyde fixation probably abolishes antigenicity at the cost of a non-viable graft.

In summary, from present data the use of allogenic veins cannot be recommended.

Arterial conduits

The internal mammary artery

The single left internal mammary artery

Superior clinical results of internal mammary artery (IMA) grafts were first published in 1972 (80), but few surgeons adopted the technique until the mid-1980's when reports of IMA graft patency rates of over 90% up to 12 years following surgery (15,6,81) (Figure 10.2) coincided with the wider recognition of saphenous veins graft atherosclerosis (82,83). Along with increased graft patency it became clear that use of the IMA improved survival.

Large studies have since shown that one IMA to the anterior descending coronary artery significantly improves long-term survival in patients with both normal and poor left ventricular function compared with patients who have had venous grafts only (Figure 10.3). In addition, patients with an IMA graft have significantly less return of angina, few myocardial infarctions and reoperations, and overall improved event-free survival, with no increased mortality associated with its use (81,84–89). In the only randomized prospective study of IMA versus vein grafts to the left anterior descending artery (90), there was significantly higher survival and greater freedom from cardiac events in the IMA group.

With the extensive data available no doubt remains that the use of the single left IMA to the left anterior descending artery is associated with significantly improved long-term patency and survival when compared to saphenous vein. The patency advantage of the IMA when anastomosed to vessels other than the anterior descending is uncertain (91).

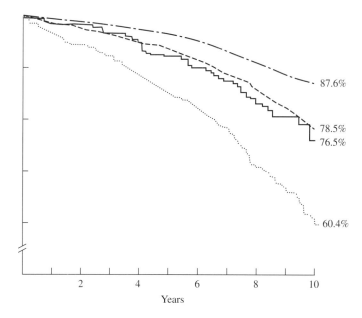

Years

Fig. 10.3 Effect of IMA grafts on long-term survival.

Extended use of the IMA

Given the favourable results with a single IMA graft it is logical to consider that additional arterial grafts may confer further benefit. Extended use of the IMA includes sequential, bilateral and 'free' aorto-coronary grafts.

The most common sequential combinations are the left IMA to the anterior descending and diagonal vessels or to two parallel circumflex branches. Early patency rates for sequential grafts to the left coronary system are about 95% (92–98). Sequential grafts to the right coronary system are less frequent because of constraints of length and angulation and patency rates are much lower (99,100). Skeletonizing the IMA may enable easier sequential grafting and provide greater length (101).

A different technique using the two terminal branches of the IMA to bypass either the left anterior descending and diagonal or two parallel circumflex branches in a Y-configuration has shown only 50% patency at 37 months (102).

The use of bilateral IMA grafting has been favoured by some surgeons, but no convincing survival benefit has yet been demonstrated (88,103–107). The use of bilateral IMA grafts raises the question of increased risk. In a comparison of patients matched for recognized risk factors (108), there was no difference in mortality between patients with vein grafts only, one IMA graft, or two IMA grafts, although those with two IMA grafts had a greater rate of sternal wound infections and greater transfusion requirements. In reoperations improved outcome following both single and bilateral IMA grafting has been reported (109,110).

The use of the IMA as a free graft from aorta to coronary gives additional graft length and enables the surgeon to avoid crossing the midline with the graft, which may jeopardize it at reoperation (111). Excellent early results with free IMA grafts have been reported (112,113) and 4 years patency rates of 84% have been achieved (111). These clinical results are backed up by a study in dogs (114) in which there was no difference in angiographic patency, vascular cell wall structure or perfusion of the vaso vasorum between *in-situ* and free grafts.

Another method of using the IMA is to divide it more proximally, for use retrogradely to enable distal vessels to be grafted. However, retrograde flow has shown to be only half antegrade flow (115).

Recently more ambitious methods of IMA grafting have been described. A Y-shaped graft can be created from a free segment of the distal left IMA (116) or right gastroepiploic artery (117) anastomosed end-to side to the *in situ* distal left IMA. Another technique is the extension of the right IMA end-to-end with a free inferior epigastric artery (118). The most ambitious use of the IMA is the circular left-IMA-right IMA graft that involves joining a free IMA end-to-end (119,120) or end-to-side (121) to the other *in situ* IMA as the sole conduit for multiple sequential anastomoses.

In summary, despite theoretical advantages the available evidence does not yet support the routine use of extended IMA grafting.

Biological properties of the IMA and other arterial conduits

There are a number of possible reasons why the IMA is such a durable conduit. It has a dense internal elastic lamina without gross deficiencies (122) and has relatively few smooth muscle cells in its thin-walled media (123). These two features are thought to be an important cause of the paucity of atheroma in the IMA, as migration of smooth muscle cells through fenestrations from the media to the intima, with proliferation across gaps in the internal elastic lamina, is a basic concept of atherogenesis. Media in the distal 10–20% of the IMA is more muscular with less elastic lamella in some individuals and it may be better not to use this distal portion of the IMA (124).

Histological studies have shown that the radial, ulnar, and gastroepiploic arteries have well-developed vasa vasorum that penetrate from the adventitia deep into the media. Experimental work (125,126) has shown that free arterial grafts are dependent on vasa vasorum for integrity and that the vasa vasorum cannot regenerate in time to prevent development of degenerative subintimal fibrous hyperplasia. The IMA, however, has a lack of vasa vasorum in the media and would appear to obtain the bulk of its nutrition through luminal substrates. This may help to explain the excellent patency rates when it is used as a free graft.

The low incidence of atherosclerosis is probably also related to protective vasoactive properties of the arterial wall. The IMA exhibits greater prostacyclin and nitric oxide production than saphenous vein (127,128). Endothelium-dependent relaxation is greater in the IMA than saphenous vein (129), and is apparently mediated by an endothelium-derived relaxing factor that is not prostacyclin. This factor may allow arterial grafts to autoregulate their flow. Enlargement of the IMA graft to increased demand has been shown on serial angiograms (130) and the growth potential of the IMA graft has been shown in children with Kawasaki disease (131).

Finally, injury to the endothelium is minimal because excessive handling is not required and its arterial wall is already accustomed to the high-pressure.

Reservations about the IMA

Although the IMA is generally regarded as the optimal conduit for coronary artery bypass grafting, praise for its qualities still exceeds its use (132). Many reservations about the use of the IMA have been expressed, some of which are valid and others not.

Flow rates

It has been contended that flows through IMA grafts are less than through vein grafts and may be inadequate for myocardial needs (133). However, adequate flow has been demonstrated through the IMA during operation (134), after operation by exercise stress test (135,136), or by actual measurement of coronary flow reserve by radionuclide techniques (137–140).

Operating time

Extra time is spent mobilizing the pedicle, although some time is saved as a proximal anastomosis is obviated. Techniques have been described to reduce the operative time (141,142).

Technical problems

The IMA is more difficult to handle than saphenous vein. Its wall is fragile and disruption of intima and media from adventitia can occur during suturing. Because of its smaller calibre it is more prone to stricture from deep sutures or purse-stringing of the anastomosis and the use of high magnification of ×8 to ×12 for these anastomoses has been recommended (106,143). The number of reports of successful treatment of such strictures by percutaneous balloon angioplasty (144–146) suggests that this is a genuine pitfall.

The IMA can be damaged during mobilization. Avulsion of branches or lacerations are immediately obvious, but more subtle damage, such as flow-limiting intimal dissections, can occur with excessive traction or too much diathermy current. There have been reports of disastrous consequences if this damage is not recognized (147,148) and the IMA should not be used if a major wall haematoma is identified. IMA anomalies may explain some injuries or poor IMA flow. Surgically significant abnormalities were observed in 118 out of 429 IMAs visualized by preoperative angiography (149). These consisted of common origin with another large collateral (11%), large-size collaterals of the IMA (9%), torturous IMA (5%), atypical course or origin (1%), atherosclerotic lesions (0.4%), and vasospasm (0.2%). An autopsy study showed 3.9% of patients had a total or near total occlusion of the subclavian artery and 3.1% had marked ostial stenosis of the IMA (123).

Insufficient IMA length can lead to tension on the anastomosis, leading to stricture or avulsion. Pedicled grafts are at risk of 360° torsion. If torsion or undue tension is recognized, the IMA should be converted to a free graft. A method of reducing tension on the graft is to suture a left flap of pericardium to the chest wall (150).

A particular danger of the free IMA grafts is stricture at the aortic anastomosis. If the aortic wall is thickened anastomosis to a vein patch may be necessary.

Bleeding

Mobilization of the IMA entails considerable dissection with division of the first six intercostal branches. Re-operations can be kept to a minimum by careful inspection of the pedicle and chest wall during and after mobilization. Bleeding has not been a significant problem in reported series, but a greater transfusion requirement in patients with bilateral IMA grafts compared to those with a single IMA graft or vein grafts alone has been reported (108).

Infection

Single IMA harvesting causes a significant decrease in sternal blood flow and bilateral IMA harvesting a further significant decrease, when compared to median sternotomy alone (151). A decrease in sternal blood supply would be expected to have an effect on sternal healing and wound infection has been reported to be higher in patients with bilateral IMA grafts (108,152–154). If infection occurs after bilateral IMA grafts spontaneous healing is rare, and closure with bilateral pectoralis major flaps or pedicled omentum is usually necessary (155). Careful use of diathermy and precise wound closure are the best preventive measures. It has been suggested that mobilizing the IMA without the surrounding tissue (skeletonized) may decrease the risk of infection in higher risk patients (101).

Spasm

Although some episodes of IMA graft 'spasm' may be strictures that prevent adequate flow reserve, true spasm has been documented angiographically (156,157). The use of intraluminal papaverine has been recommended to increase immediate IMA flow, facilitate construction of the anastomosis, and help distinguish low flow caused by technical errors from that caused by spasm (158). However, there is concern over possible detrimental effects to the intima and internal elastic lamina from this technique (159). Topical sodium nitroprusside may be more effective than topical papaverine in increasing IMA flow (160).

Nerve injury

Although upper extremity nerve injury has been reported in 10% of patients following cardiac surgery, the incidence does not seem to be influenced by IMA dissection (161). Excessive opening of the sternotomy retractor can lead to compression of the brachial plexus between the clavicle and the first rib, leading to paraesthesia in the ulnar or median distribution. The phrenic nerve lies obliquely behind the IMA at the level of the subclavian vein, and damage may occur from direct trauma during the proximal mobilization of the IMA. The incidence of an elevated left hemidiaphragm following coronary artery bypass grafting has been reported as 2.5% if no iced slush is used, 26% if topical iced slush is used, and 39% if the left internal mammary artery is also dissected (162).

Chest wall pain

Overzealous useof diathermy is probably the commonest cause of chest wall pain after IMA mobilization. Dissection of the IMA in a large pedicle with muscle and fascia can lead to inter-costal nerve injury. A higher prevalence of chest wall pain has been described in patients with IMA grafts (163).

Respiratory insufficiency

A significant increase in pleural effusions and left lower lobe atelectasis associated with mobil-ization of the IMA has been reported (164) but most centres have not experienced respiratory problems due to mobilization of the IMA or opening of the pleural space (143,165,166).

Re-operation

Re-operations on patients with one or more viable IMA graft are becoming more frequent and can be challenging. Over one-third of patent IMA grafts were injured during mobilization in one study (167), and an increased operative mortality (11%) has been reported (168). Dissection of the left ventricle after administration of cardioplegia helps to avoid damage to a patent left IMA graft. Operations where a patent right IMA crosses the midline cause particular concern and this can be avoided by using the right IMA as a free graft or routing it through the transverse sinus at the original operation (169). However, a previous IMA graft has been shown to have a lower risk of complication at reoperation than previous vein grafting alone (170). The hazard of embolization of vein graft atherosclerosis at reoperation is becoming widely recognized (171,172) and is responsible for much of the risk associated with reoperation.

Right gastroepiploic artery

The *in situ* right gastroepiploic artery rarely appears to be affected by atherosclerosis and may have all the advantageous features of the IMA graft. Experimental studies of endothelial function suggest it will have an excellent long-term patency (173), and *in vitro* responses to noradrenaline and serotonin are similar to those of the IMA (174). It does not differ from the IMA in size (175) and has a similar flow (176,177).

Two reports in1987 first described its successful use for coronary artery grafting (178,179). Larger series have subsequently been published (175–177,180–182) with a collective initial (3 months or less) patency rate of 96% for both *in situ* and free grafts and no increase in perioperative mortality (183). Adequate perfusion of myocardial territory supplied by gastroepiploic artery grafts under stress conditions has been demonstrated with thallium-201 scintigraphy (184). There are no long-term data available yet.

Drawbacks to the technique are the necessity for laparotomy, increased operating time, limited availability of the graft after previous gastric operations and the risk of graft damage in future laparotomies. Morbidity may be higher in patients who are obese and have hepatomegaly (182). Histological studies have suggested that the gastroepiploic artery may be more prone to intimal thickening than the IMA (122,185,186).

The use of the gastroepiploic artery as a free graft allows it to reach any coronary artery, can save time, avoids kinking of the pedicle across the diaphragm, avoids the consequences of coeliac artery disease and avoids trauma to the graft at subsequent laparotomy. However, spasm may be common in free gastroepiploic grafts (175,180,182). Its vasa vasorum are deep in the media, as is seen in veins and radial arteries but not with the IMA and there is no evidence that free gastroepiploic grafts behave similarly to free IMA grafts. Another drawback to its use as a free graft is the technically demanding proximal anastomosis that can be responsible for early graft failure (187).

Inferior epigastric artery

The inferior epigastric artery shows some analogies to the IMA in that it has a nearly intact internal elastic lamina and is thought to be largely nourished by diffusion of substrates as the vasa vasorum are confined to the adventitia. Although it has a more muscular media, it has a relatively low degree of intimal hyperplasia (188). It has an appropriate calibre (189) and can be harvested without entering the peritoneal cavity.

Since 1989 there have been reports of its use as a conduit for coronary artery grafting with mixed results (187,190–195). Superior results have been described where the artery was anastomosed to a vein or pericardial patch sutured to a large aortic orifice (190).Wound problems in obese and diabetic patients have been encountered (189). Greater follow-up is required to determine its reliability.

Radial artery

Use of the radial artery for coronary artery bypass grafting was prompted because of a number of potential advantages; the muscular wall is less friable than the IMA, the relatively superficial position facilitates harvesting, enough length for two grafts can usually be obtained, the lumen is regular throughout its length and compares well with the coronary artery lumen, and it seems to be rarely affected by atherosclerotic changes.

Encouraging early results were reported (196) but it soon became apparent that there were high rates of graft occlusion secondary to concentric intimal hyperplasia (197,198). These reports prompted abandonment of the radial artery for coronary artery bypass grafting, although it has recently enjoyed a resurgence of interest (199).

The cause of radial artery graft failure is unknown, but it may be due to the thickness of the media, the number of fenestrations in the internal elastic lamina, and injury to nutrient vessels and intima during preparation. It is interesting that the radial artery functions well when used by plastic surgeons as a free composite graft when both the venous and arterial blood supply are reconnected.

Splenic artery

As an autogenous, pedicled arterial graft it was hoped the splenic artery would have similar characteristics to the IMA graft (200,201). A number of problems are responsible for the failure of the splenic artery to become a popular conduit. Although initially efforts were made to avoid splenectomy, the remaining short gastric arteries proved inadequate to prevent splenic infarction in some cases. It is often large and tortuous with fibrous brands that require division to gain adequate length and prevent kinking. In addition, it is often diseased and in one autopsy series over a third had advanced atherosclerotic changes (202).

Lateral costal artery

The lateral costal artery arises from the IMA, subclavian, or superior intercostal arteries and occurs in up to 28% of patients. Since it most commonly arises from the IMA it may have the same favourable characteristics. Its use has been reported as a pedicled graft (203).

Free arterial heterografts

Bovine IMA grafts are treated with dialdehyde and sterilized with ethanol and propylene oxide. Patency up to 6 months of 85% has been reported (204) but other studies have shown an unacceptably high occlusion rate (205,206) and so far bovine grafts have proved to be a poor conduit for coronary artery grafting.

Synthetic conduits

Although large-bore vascular prostheses have been used with favourable results for more than three decades, results with smaller diameter grafts have been less successful. The initial results of coronary artery bypass grafts with expanded polytetrafluoroethylene (PTFE) grafts appeared promising (207–210), but long-term results have been poor (211) and do not justify the continued use these grafts for coronary artery surgery.

Attempts at seeding endothelium on to the surface of prosthetic vascular grafts have so far proved disappointing but if this technique can be refined if may prove to be beneficial (212).

Choice of conduit

Although saphenous vein is still extensively used for coronary artery bypass grafting it is clear that the IMA has superior patency and provides greater long-term survival. Most of the long-term data about IMA grafts relates to the left IMA to the left anterior descending artery. These show:

- no increase in operative mortality or morbidity
- patency over 90% up to 12 years
- significantly higher 10-year survival
- favourable effect on recurring angina, late myocardial infarction, reoperation and hospitalization from cardiac causes.
- potential to alter flow, with relief of ischaemia at peak myocardial demand.

Thus it can be firmly recommended that in stable conditions the left IMA should be used to revascularize the most important coronary artery, usually the left anterior descending. On the rare occasions that the anterior descending artery is not a very important vessel, the IMA should be used to graft another left-sided vessel.

To derive additional benefit from extended IMA grafting techniques and other conduits the operation must be accomplished with the same mortality, morbidity, and patency rates as achieved by using a single IMA graft with saphenous vein. Thus, recommendations for complex arterial grafts to vessels that do not carry the same prognostic implications as the left anterior descending cannot be made so firmly. Results of extended arterial grafting have come from centres with great expertise and experience. The technical learning curve for extended usage may initially cause suboptimal results. Most surgeons continue to use saphenous vein along with the left IMA.

As well as surgical bias and experience, the choice of conduit will also depend on the particular patient. Several patient factors may affect the choice of conduit.

- Complete revascularization with arterial grafts should be cnsidered wherever feasible in young patients under 40 years of age. Where both IMAs are not available the best alternative appear to be the gastroepiploic and inferior epigastric arteries, although the long-term results of these have not been determined. Use of the IMA in elderly patients is still controversial because the risk-benefit ratio has not yet been established (107,213). An uncontrolled trial in patients over 70 years did not allow firm conclusions but showed that IMA grafting can be safely performed in well-selected elderly patients (214). However, many surgeons would use vein grafts in patients over 75, particularly in women (215).
- In emergency patients in an unstable condition, for example following unsuccessful angioplasty, and those patients with poor left ventricular function, saphenous vein may be the safest choice of conduit; the operation is quicker and the risk of initial low flow through an IMA graft associated with low cardiac output is avoided.
- The IMA is the best conduit for patients with closed vein grafts, absent or unsuitable saphenous vein, or those who may need saphenous veins for lower limb arterial bypass.

- The presence of subclavian bruits should lead to angiographic investigtion before the IMA is used. Patients with previous mastectomy or chest wall irradiation may not have suitable IMAs. In these circumstances some surgeons would use saphenous vein only, although the successful use of the IMA in radiation-induced coronary artery disease has been described (216).

- The IMA is a particularly suitable conduit in **left main stem coronary disease** (217). An interesting alternative is a surgical left main stem angioplasty (218).

- The extended use of the IMA in **calcific aortic atheroma** can avoid proximal anastomoses onto a diseased aorta.

- In **Kawasaki's disease** the IMA has been shown to be superior in terms of the disappearance, improvement or reappearance of ischaemic changes in this condition (219).

- Endarterectomy of the coronary artery may lead to a long arteriotomy that can compromise use of the IMA. Options include a long onlay vein graft or anastomosing the IMA on to a vein patch (220).

- Patients with severe left ventricular hypertrophy and large coronary arteries may do better with a saphenous vein graft because of the initial flow requirements. The IMA is a particularly good conduit for patients with small coronary arteries (217).

- From the data on wound infection it is probably unwise to perform bilateral IMA grafts on diabetic patients, but use of a single IMA appears safe.

Summary

The standard conduits used for coronary bypass grafting are the saphenous vein and the IMA. The saphenous vein remains an important conduit for coronary revascularization as it is easy to procure and handle, can be used for many grafting patterns, and is large enough to provide an excess of blood flow for virtually any coronary artery. The IMA is a smaller vessel, more difficult to procure and handle, and less versatile. The patency rate of the IMA, however, is significantly better than that of saphenous vein. Expanded use of the IMA and the use of the gastroepiploic artery and inferior epigastric artery require further evaluation. The use of splenic artery, radial artery, cephalic and basilic vein, homologous fresh or cryopreserved saphenous vein, umbilical vein, free arterial heterografts, and synthetic conduits has proved disappointing.

The surgeon should consider all the advantages and disadvantages of each conduit and tailor an operation most suited to each individual patient.

References

1. Favoloro RG. Saphenous vein autograft replacement of severe segmental coronary artery occlusion. *Ann Thorac Surg* 1968;**5**:335–9.
2. Johnson WD, Flemma RJ, Lepley D Jr. Extended treatment of severe coronary artery disease. *Ann Surg* 1969;**170**;460–70.
3. Bartley TD, Bigelow JC, Page US. Aortocoronary bypass grafting with multiple sequential anastomoses to a single vein. *Arch Surg* 1972;**105**:915–17.
4. Grondin CM, Lesperance J, Bourassa MG, Campeau L. Coronary artery grafting with the saphenous vein or internal mammary artery. *Ann Thorac Surg* 1975;**20**:605–18.

5. Flemma RJ, Singh HM, Tector AJ, Lepley D Jr, Frazer BL. Comparative haemodynamic properties of vein and mammary artery in coronary bypass operation. *Ann Thorac Surg* 1975;**20**:619–35.
6. Lytle BW, Loop FD, Cosgrove DM, Ratliff NB, Easley K, Taylor PC. Long-term (5 to 12 years) serial studies of internal mammary artery and saphenous vein coronary bypass grafts. *J Thorac Cardiovasc Surg* 1985;**89**:248–58.
7. Grondin CM, Campeau L, Lesperance J, Enjalbert M, Bourasa MG. Comparison of late changes in internal mammary artery and saphenous vein grafts in two consecutive series of patients 10 years after operation. *Circulation* 1984;**70**(suppl I):213–21.
8. Szilagyi DE, Elliot JP, Hageman JH, Smith RF, Dallolmo CA. Biological fate of autogenous vein implants as arterial substitute. *Ann Surg* 1973;**178**:232–48.
9. Grondin CM, Lesperance J, Dourassa MG, Pasternac A, Campeau L, Grondin P. Serial angiographic evaluation in 60 consecutive patients with aortocoronary artery vein grafts 2 weeks, 1 year and 3 years after operation. *J Thorac Cardiovasc Surg* 1974;**67**:1–6.
10. Fitzgibbon GM, Leach AJ, Keon WJ, Burton JR, Kafka HP. Coronary bypass graft fate. Angiographic study of 1,179 vein grafts early, one year and five years after operation. *J Thorac Cardiovasc Surg* 1986;**91**:773–8.
11. Ulicny KS Jr, Flege JB Jr, Callard GM, Todd JC. Twenty-year follow-up of saphenous vein aortocoronary artery bypass grafting. *Ann Thorac Surg* 1992;**53**:258–62.
12. Grondin CM, Lesperance J, Solymoss BC *et al*. Atherosclerotic changes in coronary grafts six years after operation. *J Thorac Cardiovasc Surg* 1979;**77**:24–31.
13. Angelini GD, Newby AC. The future of saphenous vein as a coronary artery bypass conduit. *Eur Heart J* 1989;**10**:273–80.
14. Grondin CM. Later results of coronary artery grafting. Is there a flag on the field? *J Thorac Cardiovasc Surg* 1984;**87**:161–6.
15. Okies JE, Page US, Bigelow JC, Krause AH, Salomon NW. The left internal mammary artery: the graft choice. *Circulation* 1984;**70**(suppl I):213–221.
16. Lawrie GM, Morris JR GC, Earle N. Long term results of coronary bypass surgery: analysis of 1689 patients followed 15–20 years. *Ann Surg* 1991;**213**:377–87.
17. Fitzgibbon GM, Leach AJ, Kafka HP, Keon WJ. Coronary bypass graft fate: long-term angiographic study. *J Am Coll Cardiol* 1991;**17**:1075–80.
18. Lytle BW, Loop FD, Taylor PC *et al*. Vein graft disease: the clinical impact of stenoses in saphenous vein bypass grafts to coronary arteries. *J Thorac Cardiovasc Surg* 1992;**103**(5):831–40.
19. Bartley TD, Bigelow JC, Page US. Aortocoronary bypass grafting with multiple sequential anastomoses to a single vein graft. *Arch Surg* 1972;**105**:915–17.
20. Grondin CM, Limet R. Sequential anastomoses in coronary artery grafting. Technical aspects and early and late angiographic results. *Ann Thorac Surg* 1977;**23**:1–8.
21. Sewell WK, Sewell KV. Technique for the coronary snake graft operation. *Ann Thorac Surg* 1976;**22**:58–65.
22. Meeter K, Veldkamp R, Tijssen JGP, van Herweden L, Bos E. Clinical outcome of single versus sequential grafts in coronary bypass operations at 10 years' follow-up. *J Thorac Cardiovasc Surg* 1991:**101**:1076–81.
23. Campeau L, Enjalbert M, Lesperance J, Vasilic C, Grondin CM, Bourassa MG. Atherosclerosis and late closure of aortocoronary saphenous vein grafts: sequential

angiographic studies at 2 weeks, 1 year, 5 to 7 years and 10 to 12 years after surgery. *Circulation* 1983;**68**(suppl II):1–7.

24. Brenowitz JB, Kayser KL, Johnson WD. Results of coronary artery endarterectomy and reconstruction. *J Thorac Cardiovasc Surg* 1988;**95**:1–10.

25. Cox JL, Chiasson DA, Gotlieb AI. Stranger in a strange land: the pathogenesis of saphenous vein graft stenosis with emphasis on structural and functional differences between veins and arteries. *prog Cardiovasc Dis* 1991;**34**:45–68.

26. Amano J, Susuki A, Sunamori M, Tsudaka T, Numano F. Cytokines study of aortocoronary bypass vein grafts in place for less than six months. *Am J Cardiol* 1991;**67**:1234–6.

27. Angelini GD, Bryan AJ, Williams HMJ, Morgan R, Newby AC. Distension promotes platelet and leucocyte adhesion and reduces short term patency in pig arteriovenous bypass grafts. *J Thorac Cardiovasc Surg* 1990;**99**:433–9.

28. Fuster V, Cheseboro JH. Aortocoronary artery vein graft disease. Experimental and clinical approach for the understanding of the role of platelets and platelet inhibitors. *Circulation* 1985;**72**(suppl V):65–70.

29. Angelini GD, Bryan AJ, Williams HMJ, Soyombo AA, Williams S, Tovey J, Newby AC. Timecourse of medial and intimal thickening in pig arteriovenous bypass grafts: relationship to endothelial integrity and cholesterol accumulation. *J Thorac Cardiovasc Surg* 1992;**103**:1093–1103.

30. Yamaguchi M, Du W, Dieffenbach CW, Cruess DF, Sharefkin JB. Effect of aspirin, dipyridamole, and cyclic adenosine monphosphate on platelet-derived growth factor: A-chain mRNA levels in human saphenous vein endothelial cells and smooth muscle cells. *Surgery* 1991;**110**;377–84.

31. Newby AC. Intimal smooth muscle cell proliferation–underlying basis and possibilities for therapy. *Spectrum International* 1992;**32**:27–31.

32. O'Donohoe MK, Radic ZS, Schwartz LB, Mikat EM, McCann RL, Hagen PO. Systemic hypertension alters vasomotor function in experimental vein grafts. *J Vasc Surg* 1991;**14**:30–9.

33. Ku DD, Caulfield JB, Kirklin JK. Endothelium-dependent responses in long-term human coronary artery bypass grafts. *Circulation* 1991;**83**:402–11.

34. Zwolak RM, Adams MC, Clowes AW. Kinetics of vein graft hyperplasia: association with tangential stress. *J Vasc Surg* 1987;**5**:126–36.

35. Quist WC, Haudenschield CC, Lo Gerfo FW. Qualitative microscopy of implanted vein grafts: effects of graft integrity of morphologic fate. *J Thorac Cardiovasc Surg* 1992;**103**:671–7.

36. Ip JH. Fuster V, Badimon L. Syndromes of accelerated atherosclerosis: role of vascular injury and smooth muscle proliferation. *J Am Coll Cardiol* 1990;**15**:1667–87.

37. Boerboom LE, Olinger GO, Rodriguez ER, Ferrans VJ, Kissebah AH. Atherogenic effect of barotrauma on *in situ* saphenous vein grafts in monkeys. *J Thorac Cardiovasc Surg* 1991;**102**:448–53.

38. Lie JT, Lawrie GM, Morris GC. Aortocoronary bypass saphenous vein graft atherosclerosis: anatomic study of 99 vein grafts from normal and hyperlipidaemic patients up to 75 months postoperatively. *Am J Cardiol* 1977;**40**:906–14.

39. Fuchs JCA, Mitchener JS, Hagen PO. Postoperative changes in autologous vein grafts. *Ann Surg* 1978;**188**:1–15.

40. Shelton ME, Forman MB, Virmani R, Bajaj A, Stoney WS, Atkinson JB. A comparison of morphologic and angiographic findings in long-term internal mammary artery and saphenous vein bypass grafts. *J Am Coll Cardiol* 1988;**11**:297–307.

41. Solymoss BC, Nadeau P, Millette D, Campeau L. Late thrombosis of saphenous vein coronary bypass grafts related to risk factors. *Circulation* 1988;**78**(suppl I):140–3.

42. Bonchek LI. Prevention of endothelial damage during preparation of saphenous vein for bypass grafting. *J Thorac Cardiovasc Surg* 1980;**79**:911–15.

43. Adcock OT, Adcock GLD, Wheeler JR, Gregory RT, Snyder SO, Gayle RG. Optimal techniques for harvesting and preparation of reversed autogenous vein grafts for use as arterial substitutes. A review. *Surgery* 1984;**96**:886–94.

44. Angelini GD, Bryan AJ, Hunter S, Newby AC. A surgical technique that preserves human saphenous vein functional integrity. *Ann Thorac Surg* 1992;**53**:871–74.

45. Lo Grefo FW, Quist WC, Crawshow JM, Haudenschild CC. An improved technique for preservation of endothelial morphology in vein grafts. *Surgery* 1981;**90**:1015–24.

46. Gundry SR, James M, Ishihara T, Ferrans VJ. Optimal preparation technique for human saphenous vein grafts. *Surgery* 1980;**88**:758–94.

47. Angelini GD, Breckenridge IM, Williams HM, Newby AC. A surgical preparative technique for coronary bypass grafts of human saphenous vein which preserves medial and entholial functional integrity. *J Thorac Cardiovasc Surg* 1987;**94**:393–8.

48. Underwood MJ. The aspirin papers. *BMJ* 1994;**308**:71–2.

49. Antiplatelet Trialists collaboration. Collaborative overview of randomised trials of antiplatelet treatment II. Maintenance of vascular graft or arterial patency by antiplatelet therapy. *BMJ* 1994;**308**:159–68.

50. Goldman S, Copeland J, Moritz *et al.* Improvement in early saphenous vein graft patency after coronary artery bypass surgery with antiplatelet therapy: results of a Veterans Administration Cooperative Study. *Circulation* 1988;**77**(suppl VI):1324–32.

51. Goldman S, Copeland J, Moritz T *et al.* . Starting aspirin therapy after operation: effect on early graft patency. *Circulation* 1991;**84**:520–6.

52. Gavaghan TP, Mstag VG, Baron DW. Immediate postoperative aspirin improves vein graft patency early and later after coronary artery bypass graft surgery: a placebo controlled randomised trial. *Circulation* 1991;**83**:1526–33.

53. Israel DH, Adams PC, Stein B, Chesbro JH, Fuster J. Antithrombotic therapy in the coronary vein graft patient. *Clin Cardiol* 1991;**14**:283–95.

54. Golhlke H, Gohlke-Barwolf C, Sturzenhofecker P *et al.* Improved graft patency with oral anticoagulant therapy after aortocoronary bypass surgery: a prospective randomized study. *Circulation* 1981;**64**(suppl II):22–7.

55. Landymore RW, Kinley CE, Cooper JH, McCauley M, Sheridan B, Cameron C. Cod-liver oil in the prevention of intimal hyperplasia in autologous vein grafts used for arterial bypass *J Thorac Cardiovasc Surg* 1985;**89**:351–7.

56. Clowes AW, Clowes MN, Vergel SC *et al.* Heparin and cilazapril together inhibit injury-induced intimal hyperplasia. *Hypertension* 1991;**18**(suppl II):65–69.

57. Clowes AW. Regulation of smooth muscle cell function by heparin. *J Vasc Surg* 1992;**15**:911–13.

58. Roux SP, Clozel JP, Kuhn H. Cilazapril inhibits wall thickening of vein bypass grafts in the rat. *Hypertension* 1991;**18**(suppl):43–6.

59. Calcagno D, Conte JV, Howel MH, Foegh ML. Peptide inhibition of neointimal hyperplasia in vein grafts. *J Vasc Surg* 1991;**13**:475–9.

60. Guyotat IP, Guyotat J, Lievre M, Chignier E. Effect of nimodopine on subintimal hyperplasia of autologous vein bypass grafts in rats: a placebo controlled study. *Cardiovasc Pharmacol* 1991;**5**:778–85.

61. Angelini GD, Soyombo AA, Newby AC. Smooth muscle cell proliferation in response to injury in an organ culture of human saphenous vein. *Eur J Vasc Surg* 1991;**5**:5–12.

62. Ferns GA, Rainew EW, Sprugel KH, Motani AS, Reidy MA, Ross R. Inhibition of neointimal smooth muscle accumulation after angioplasty by an antibody to PDGF. *Science* 1991;**253**:1129–32.

63 Lindner V, Reidy MA. Proliferation of smooth muscle cells after vascular injury is inhibited by an antibody against basic fibroblast growth factor. *Proc Natl Acad Sci USA* 1991;**88**:3739–43.

64. Plautz G, Nable EG, Nabel GJ. Introduction of vascular smooth muscle cells and expression of recombinant genes *in vivo*. *Circulation* 1991;**83**:578–83.

65. Nabel EG, Plautz G, Nabel GJ. Site-specific gene expression *in vivo* by direct gene transfer into the arterial wall. *Science* 1990;**249**:1285–8.

66. Cahill PD, Sarris GE, Cooper AD *et al.* Inhibition of vein graft intimal thickening by eicosapentanoic acid: reduced thromboxane production without change in lipoprotein levels or low-density lipoprotein receptor density. *J Vasc Surg* 1988;**7**:108–18.

67. Blankenhorn DH, Nessim SA, Johnson RL, Sanmario ME, Azen SP, Cashin-Hemphill L. Beneficial effects of combined cholesterol-niacin therapy on coronary atherosclerosis and coronary venous bypass grafts. *JAMA* 1987;**257**:3233–40.

68. Cashin-Hemphill L, Mack WJ, Pogoda JM, Sammarco ME, Azen SP, Blackenhorn DH. Beneficial effects of colestipolniacin on coronary atherosclerosis: a 4 year follow-up. *JAMA* 1992;**264**:3013–17.

69. Prieto I, Basile F, Abdulnour E. Upper extremity vein graft for aortocoronary bypass. *Ann Thorac Surg* 1984;**47**;218–21.

70. Stoney WS, Alford WC JR, Burrus GR, Glassford DM Jr, Petracek MR, Thomas SF Jr. The fate of arm veins for aorto-coronary bypass grafts. *J Thorac Cardiovasc Surg* 1984;**88**:522–7.

71. Tice DA, Zerbino VR, Isom OW, Cunningham JN, Engelman RM. Coronary artery bypass with freeze-preserved saphenous vein allografts. *J Thorac Cardiovasc Surg* 1976;**71**:378–82.

72. Bical O, Bachet J, Laurian C, Camilleri JP, Goudot B, Menu P, Guilmet D. Aortocoronary bypass with homologous saphenous vein: long-term results. *Ann Thorac Surg* 1980;**30**:550–7.

73. Sellke FW, Stanford W, Rossi NP. Failure of cryopreserved saphenous vein allografts following coronary artery bypass surgery. *J Cardiovasc Surg (Torino)* 1991;**12**:820–3.

74. Laub GW, Muralidharan S, Clancy R *et al.* Cryopreserved allograft veins as alternative coronary artery bypass conduits: early phase results. *Ann Thorac Surg* 1992;**54**:826–31.

75. Deaton DW, Stephens JK, Karp RB *et al.* Evaluation of cryopreserved allograft venous conduits in dogs. *J Thorac Cardiovasc Surg* 1992;**103**:153–162.

76. Elmore JR, Gloviczki P, Brockbank KGM, Miller VM. Cryopreservation affects endothelial and smooth muscle function of canine autogenous saphenous vein grafts. *J Vasc Surg* 1991;**13**:584–92.

77. Brockbank EGM, Donovan TJ, Ruby ST, Carpenter JF, Hagen PO, Woodley MA. Functional analysis of cryopreserved veins: preliminary report. *J Vasc Surg* 1990;**11**:94–102.

78. Deaton DW, Stephens JK, Karp RB. Evaluation of cryopreserved allograft venous conduits in dogs. *J Thorac Cardiovasc Surg* 1992;**103**:153–62.

79. Silver GM, Katske GE, Stutzman FL, Wood NE. Umbilical vein for aortocoronary bypass. *Angiology* 1982;**33**:450–3.

80. Green GE. Internal mammary artery-coronary artery anastomosis; three year experience with 165 patients. *Ann Thorac Surg* 1972;**14**:260–71.

81. Loop FD, Lytle BW, Cosgrove DM *et al.* Influence of the internal mammary artery graft on 10 year survival and other cardiac events. *N Engl J Med* 1986;**314**:1–6.

82. Singh RN, Sosa J, Green GE. Long term fate of the internal mammary artery and saphenous vein grafts. *J Thorac Cardiovasc Surg* 1983;**86**:359–63.

83. Campeau L, Enjalbert M, Lesperance J *et al.* The relation of risk factors to the development of atherosclerosis in saphenous vein bypass grafts and the progression of disease in the native circulation. A study 10 years after aortocoronary bypass surgery. *N Engl J Med* 1984;**311**:1329–32.

84. Cameron AC, Kemp HG, Green GE. Bypass with the internal mammary artery graft: 15 year follow-up . *Circulation* 1986;**74**(suppl III):30–36.

85. Cameron A, Davis KB, Green GE, Myers WO, Pettinger M, Clinical implications of internal mammary artery bypass grafts: the Coronary Artery Surgery Study experience. *Circulation* 1988;**77**:815–19.

86. Ivert T, Huttunen K, Landou C, Bjork VO. Angiographic studies of internal mammary grafts 11 years after coronary artery bypass grafting. *J Thorac Cardiovasc Surg* 1988;**96**:1–12.

87. Johnson WD, Brenowitz JB, Kayser KL. Factors influencing long-term (10-year to 15-year survival after a successful coronary artery bypass operation). *Ann Thorac Surg* 1989;**48**:19–25.

88. Sergeant P, Lesaffre E, Flameng W, Suy R. Internal mammary artery: methods of use and their effect on survival after coronary artery bypass surgery. *Eur J Cardiothorac Surg* 1990;**4**:72–8.

89. Acinapura AJ, Rose DM, Cunningham JM, Jacobowitz IJ, Kramer MD, Zisbrod Z. Internal mammary bypass: effect on longevity and recurrent angina pectoris in 2900 patients. *Eur J Cardiothorac Surg* 1989;**3**:321–6.

90. Zeff RH, Kongtahworn C, Iannone LA *et al.* Internal mammary artery versus saphenous vein graft to the left anterior descending coronary artery: prospective randomised study with 10-year follow-up. *Ann Thorac Surg* 1988;**45**:533–6.

91. Huddleston CB, Stoney WS, Alford WC *et al.* Internal mammary artery grafts: technical factors influencing patency. *Ann Thorac Surg* 1986;**42**:543–9.

92. Rankin JS, Newman GE, Bashore TM *et al.* Clinical and angiographic assessment of complex mammary artery bypass grafting. *J Thorac Cardiovasc Surg* 1986;**92**:832–46.

93. Dion R, Verhelst R, Rousseau M, Chalant Ch-H. Sequential mammary grafting. *J Thorac Cardiovasc Surg* 1989;**98**:80–9.

94. Kabbani SS, Hanna ES, Bashour TT, Crew JR, Ellertson DG. Sequential internal-mammary coronary artery bypass. *J Thorac Cardiovasc Surg* 1983;**86**:697–702.

95. McBride LR, Barner HB. The left internal mammary as a sequential graft to the left anterior descending system. *J Thorac Cardiovasc Surg* 1983;**86**:703–5.

96. Oszulak TA, Schaff HV, Chesebro JH, Holmes DR. Initial experience with sequential internal mammary artery grafts to the left anterior descending and diagonal coronary arteries. *Mayo Clin Proc* 1986;**61**:3–8.

97. Boustany CW Jr, Flemeng W, Suy R. The sequential internal mammary artery graft. *J Cardiovasc Surg* 1988;**29**:596–600.

98. Van Sterkenberg SMM, Ernst SMPG, de la Riviere AB *et al.* Triple sequential grafts using the internal mammary artery: An angiographic and short-term follow-up study. *J Thorac Cardiovasc Surg* 1992;**104**:60–5.

99. Rivera R, Duran E, Ajuria M. Expanded use of the right and left internal mammary arteries for myocardial revascularization. *Thorac Cardiovasc Surg* 1988;**36**:194–7.

100. Accola KD, Jones EL, Craver JM, Weintraub WS, Guyton RD. Bilateral mammary artery grafting: avoidance of complications with extended use. *Ann Thorac Surg* 1993;**56**:867–71.

101. Cunningham JM, Gharavi MA, Fardin R, Meek RA. Considerations in the skeletonization technique of internal thoracic artery dissection. *Ann Thorac Surg* 1992;**54**:947–51.

102. Morin JE, Hedderich G, Poirier NL, Sampalis J, Symes JF. Coronary artery bypass using internal mammary artery branches. *Ann Thorac Surg* 1992;**54**:911–14.

103. Lytle BE, Cosgrove DM, Saltus GL, Taylor PC, Loop FD. Multivessel coronary revascularization without saphenous vein: Long-term results of bilateral internal mammary grafting. *Ann Thorac Surg* 1983;**36**:540–7.

104. Galbut DL, Traad EA, Dorman MY *et al.* Seventeen-year experience with bilateral internal mammary artery grafts. *Ann Thorac Surg* 1990;**49**:195–201.

105. Naunheim KS, Barner HB, Fiore AC. Update: results of internal thoracic artery grafting over 15 years: single versus double grafts. *Ann Thorac Surg* 1992;**53**:716–18.

106. Green GE, Cameron A, Goyal A, Wong SC, Schwanede J. Five-year follow-up of microsurgical multiple internal thoracic artery grafts. *Ann Thorac Surg* 1994;**58**:74–9.

107. Morris JJ, Smith R, Glower DD *et al.* Clinical evaluation of single versus multiple mammary artery bypass. *Circulation* 1990;**82**(suppl IV):214–23.

108. Cosgrove DM, Lytle BW, Loop FD *et al.* Does bilateral internal mammary artery grafting increase surgical risk? *J Thorac Cardiovasc Surg* 1988;**95**:850–6.

109. Galbut DL, Traad EA, Dorman MJ *et al.* Bilateral internal mammary artery grafts in reoperative and primary coronary bypass surgery. *Ann Thorac Surg* 1991;**52**:20–8.

110. Loop FD, Lytle BW, Cosgrove DM. Bilateral internal thoracic artery grafting in reoperations. *Ann Thorac Surg* 1991;**52**:3–4.

111. Loop FD, Lytle BW, Cosgrove DM, Golding LAR, Taylor PC, Stewart RW. Free (aorto-coronary) internal mammary artery graft: Late results. *J Thorac Cardiovasc Surg* 1986;**92**:827–31.

112. Barner HB. The internal mammary artery as a free graft. *J Thorac Cardiovasc Surg* 1973;**66**:219–21.

113. Schimert G, Vidne BA, Lee AB Jr. Free internal mammary artery graft: An improved surgical technique. *Ann Thorac Surg* 1975;**19**:474–7.

114. Daly RC, McCarthy PM, Orzulak TA, Schaff HV, Edwards WD. Histologic comparison of experimental coronary artery bypass grafts: similarity of *in situ* and free internal mammary artery grafts. *J Thorac Cardiovasc Surg* 1988;**96**:19–29.

115. Cohen AJ, Ameika JA, Briggs RA, Grishkin BA, Helsel RA. Retrograde flow in the internal mammary artery. *Ann Thorac Surg* 1988;**95**:1–10.

116. Slater AD, Gott JP, Gray LA. Extended use of bilateral internal mammary arteries for coronary artery disease. *Ann Thorac Surg* 1990;**49**:1014–15.

117. Koike R, Suma H, Takaiko O, Satoh H, Sawada Y, Takeuki A. Free arterial graft as internal mammary artery-Y complex. *Ann Thorac Surg* 1990;**49**:656–8.

118. Buche M, Schroeder E, Devaux P, Louagie YAG, Schoevardts J-C. Right internal mammary artery extended with an inferior epigastric artery for circumflex and right coronary bypass. *Ann Thorac Surg* 1992;**54**:381–3.

119. Gold JP, Shemin RJ, DiSesa VJ. Multiple-vessel revascularization with combined *in situ* and free sequential internal mammary arteries. *J Thorac Cardiovasc Surg* 1985;**90**:301–8.

120. Bakay C, Ak Cevin A, Suzer K *et al.* Combined internal mammary artery graft for coronary artery revascularization. *Ann Thorac Surg* 1990;**50**:553–6.

121. Tector AJ, Amundsen S, Schmal TM, Kress DC, Mohan P. Total revascularization with T-grafts. *Ann Thorac Surg* 1994;**57**:33–9.

122. Van Son JA, Smedts F, Vincent JG, Van Lier HJ, Kubat K. Comparative anatomic studies of various arterial conduits for myocardial revascularization. *J Thorac Cardiovasc Surg* 1990;**99**:703–7.

123. Sisto T. Atherosclerosis in internal mammary and related arteries. *Scand J Thorac Cardiovasc Surg* 1990;**24**:7–11.

124. Van Son JAM, Smedts F, de Wilde PCM *et al.* Histological study of the internal mammary artery with emphasis on its suitability as a coronary artery bypass graft. *Ann Thorac Surg* 1993;**55**:106–13.

125. Chiu C-J. Why do radial grafts for aortocoronary bypass fail? A reappraisal. *Ann Thorac Surg* 1976;**22**:520–3.

126. Conkle DM, Page DL, Curtis J, Foster JH, Bender HW. Subendothelial proliferation: A lesson observed in fresh arterial autografts. *Surg Forum* 1973;**24**:245–6.

127. Subramanian VA, Hernandez Y, Tack-Goldman K, Grabowski EF, Weksler BB. Prostacyclin production by internal mammary artery as a factor in coronary artery bypass grafts. *Surgery* 1986;**100**:376–83.

128. Chaikhouni A, Crawford FA, Kochel PJ, Olanoff LS, Halushka PV. Human internal mammary artery produces more prostacyclin than saphenous vein. *J Thorac Cardiovasc Surg* 1986;**92**:88–91.

129. Luscher TF, Diederich D, Siebenmann R *et al.* Difference between endothelium-dependent relaxation in arterial and in venous coronary bypass grafts. *N Engl J Med* 1988;**319**:462–7.

130. Singh RN, Beg RA, Kay EB. Physiological adaptability: The secret of success of the internal mammary artery grafts. *Ann Thorac Surg* 1986;**41**:247–50.

131. Kitamura S, Seki T, Kawachi K *et al.* Excellent patency and growth potential of internal mammary artery grafts in paediatric coronary artery bypass surgery: new evidence for a 'live' conduit. *Circulation* 1988;**78**(suppl I):129–39.

132. Lefrak EA. The internal mammary artery bypass graft: praise versus practice. *Tex Heart Inst J* 1987;**14**:139–43.

133. Kawasuji M, Tsujiguchi H, Tedoriya T, Taki J, Iwa T. Evaluation of postoperative flow capacity of the internal mammary graft. *J Thorac Cardiovasc Surg* 1989;**98**:73–9.

134. Canver CC, Dame NA. Ultrasonic assessment of internal thoracic artery graft flow in the revascularized heart. *Ann Thorac Surg* 1994;**58**:135–8.

135. Loop FD, Irarrazaval MJ, Bredee JJ, Siegel W, Taylor PC, Sheldon WC. Internal mammary artery graft for ischaemic heart disease: effect of revascularization on clinical status and survival. *Am J Cardiol* 1977;**39**:516–22.

136. Siegel W, Loop FD. Comparison of internal mammary artery and saphenous vein bypass grafts for myocardial revascularization. Exercise test and angiographic correlations. *Circulation* 1976;**54**:(suppl III): 1–3.

137. Green GE, Kemp H, Alam SE, Pierson RN Jr, Friedman MI, David I. Coronary bypass surgery. Five year follow-up of a consecutive series of 140 patients. *J Thorac Cardiovasc Surg* 1979;**77**:48–56.

138. Schmidt DH, Blau F, Hellman C, Grzeklak L, Johnson WD. Isoproterenol induced flow responses in mammary and vein bypass grafts. *J Thorac Cardiovasc Surg* 1980;**80**:319–26.

139. Johnson AM, Kron IL, Watson DD, Gibson RS, Nolan SP. Evaluation of postoperative flow reserve in internal mammary artery bypass grafts. *J Thorac Cardiovasc Surg* 1986;**92**:822–6.

140. Schvede K, Sigi S, Lee S. The effect of internal mammary artery grafting on the postoperative course. *J Cardiothorac Anesth* 1988;**95**:850–6.

141. Lee ME. Carbodissection of the internal thoracic artery pedicle. *Ann Thorac Surg* 1988;**46**:470–1.

142. Schachner A, Hauptman E, Deviri E, Ajuria M. A safe and rapid method for the mobilization of the internal mammary pedicle. *J Cardiovasc Surg* 1988;**29**:354–5.

143. Green GE. Use of internal thoracic artery for coronary artery grafting. *Circulation* 1989;**79**:(suppl I):30–3.

144. Crean PA, Mathieson PW, Rickards AF. Transluminal angioplasty of a stenosis of an internal mammary artery graft. *Br Heart J* 1986;**56**:473–5.

145. Steffenino G, Meier B, Finci L, von Segesser L, Velebit V. Percutaneous transluminal angioplasty of right and left internal mammary grafts. *Chest* 1986;**90**:849–51.

146. Singh S. Coronary angioplasty of internal mammary artery graft. *S Am J Med* 1987;**82**:361–2.

147. Sonmez B, Yorukoglu Y, Williams BT. Traction injury in the internal mammary artery: report of a case and review of the literature. *J Cardiovasc Surg (Torino)* 1990;**31**:592–4.

148. Dougenis D, Robinson MC, Brown AH. Acute dissection of the internal mammary artery: a fatal complication of coronary bypass grafting. *J Cardiovasc Surg (Torino)* 1990;**31**:592–4.

149. Bauer EP, Bino MC, Von Segesser LK, Laske A, Turina MI. Internal mammary artery anomalies. *Thorac Cardiovasc Surg* 1990;**38**:312–5.

150. Todd EP, Earle GF, Jaggers R, Sekela M. Pericardial flap to minimise mammary artery anastomotic tension. *Ann Thorac Surg* 1987;**44**:665–6.

151. Carrier M, Gregoire J, Tronc F, Cartier R, Leclerc Y, Pelletier L-C. Effects of internal mammary dissection on sternal vascularization. *Ann Thorac Surg* 1992;**53**:115–19.

152. Culliford AT, Cunningham JN Jr, Zeff RH. Sternal and costochondral infections following open heart surgery. *J Thorac Cardiovasc Surg* 1976;**52**:714–26.

153. Grossi EA, Esposito R, Harris LJ *et al.* Sternal wound infections and use of internal mammary artery grafts. *J Thorac Cardiovasc Surg* 1991;**102**:342–7.

154. Hazelrigg SR, Wellons HA Jr, Schneider JA, Kolm P. Wound complications after median sternotomy: relationship to internal mammary grafting. *J Thorac Cardiovasc Surg* 1989;**98**:1096–9.

155. Cohen M, Marshall MA, Silvermann VA, Levitsky S. Chest wall reconstruction for infected median sternotomy wounds. *Contemp Surg* 1988;**32**:13–20.

156. Kong B, Kopelman H, Segal BL, Iskandrian AS. Angiographic demonstration of spasm in a left internal mammary artery used as a bypass to the left anterior descending coronary artery. *Am J Cardiol* 1988;**61**:1363.

157. Sarabu MR, McClung JA, Fass A, Reed GE. Early postoperative spasm in left internal mammary artery bypass grafts.*Ann Thorac Surg* 1987:**44**:199–200.

158. Mills NL, Bribgaze WL. Preparation of the internal mammary artery graft. *J Thorac Cardiovasc Surg* 1989;**98**:73–9.

159. Van Son JAM, Tavilla G, Noyez L. Detrimental sequelae on the wall of the internal mammary artery caused by hydrostatic dilatation with diluted papaverine solution. *J Thorac Cardiovasc Surg* 1992;**104**:972–6.

160. Cooper GJ, Wilkinson GAL, Angelini GD. Overcoming perioperative spasm of the internal mammary artery: which is the best vasodilator? *J Thorac Cardiovasc Surg* 1992;**104**:465–8.

161. Roy RC, Stafford MA, Charlton JE. Nerve injury and musculoskeletal complaints after cardiac surgery: influence of internal mammary artery dissection and left arm position. *Anesth Analg* 1988;**67**:277–9.

162. Curtis JJ, Nawarawong W, Walls JT *et al.* Elevated hemidiaphragm after cardiac operations: incidence, prognosis, and relationship to the use of topical ice slush. *Ann Thorac Surg* 1989;**48**:764–8.

163. Eng J, Wells FC. Morbidity following coronary artery revascularization with the internal mammary artery. *Int J Cardiol* 1991;**30**:55–9.

164. Hurlbut D, Myers ML, Lefcoe M, Goldbach M. Pleuropulmonary morbidity: internal thoracic artery versus saphenous vein graft. *Ann Thorac Surg* 1990;**50**:959–64.

165. Loop FD, Lytle BW, Cosgrove DM. New arteries for old. *Circulation* 1989;**79**(suppl I): 40–5.

166. Wiener-Kronish JP. Postoperative pleural and pulmonary abnormalities in patients undergoing coronary artery bypass grafts. *Chest* 1992;**102**:1313 -14.

167. Ivert TSA, Ekestrom S, Peterffy A, Welti R. Coronary artery reoperations. *Scand J Cardiothorac Surg* 1988;**22**:111–18.

168. Joyce FS, McCarthy PM, Taylor PC, Cosgrove DM, Lytle BW. Cardiac reoperation in patients with bilateral internal thoracic grafts. *Ann Thorac Surg* 1994;**58**:80–5.

169. Ranstrom J, Lund O, Cadavid E, Oxelbark S, Thuren JB, Menze AC. Right internal thoracic artery for myocardial revascularization: early results and indications. *Ann Thorac Surg* 1993;**55**:1485–91.

170. Coltharp WH, Decker MD, Lea JW IV *et al.* Internal mammary artery graft at reoperation: risks, benefits, and methods of preservation. *Ann Thorac Surg* 1991;**52**:225–9.

171. Saloman NW, Page US, Bigelow JC, Krause AH, Okies E, Metzdorff MT. Reoperative coronary surgery. Comparative analysis of 6591 patients undergoing primary bypass and 508 patients undergoing reoperative coronary artery bypass. *J Thorac Cardiovasc Surg* 1990;**100**:250–60.

172. Grundy SR, Razzouk AJ, Vigesaa RE, Wang N, Bailey LL. Optimal delivery of cardioplegic solution for 'redo' operations. *J Thorac Cardiovasc Surg* 1992;**103**:896–901.

173. O'Neil GS, Chester AH, Allen SP *et al.* Endothelial function of human gastroepiploic artery: implications for its use as a bypass graft. *J Thorac Cardiovasc Surg* 1991;**102**:561–5.

174. Ochiai M, Ohno M, Taguchi *et al.* Responses of human gastroepiploic arteries to vasoactive substances: Comparison with responses of internal mammary arteries and saphenous veins. *J Thorac Cardiovasc Surg* 1992;**104**:453–8.

175. Mills NL, Everson CT. Right gastroepiploic artery: a third arterial conduit for coronary artery bypass. *Ann Thorac Surg* 1989;**47**:706–11.

176. Suma H, Takeuchi A, Hirota Y. Myocardial revascularization with combined arterial grafts utilizing the internal mammary and gastroepiploic arteries. *Ann Thorac Surg* 1989;**47**:712–15.

177. Verkalla K, Jarvinen A, Keto P, Virtanen K, Lehtola A, Pellinen T. Right gastroepiploic artery as a coronary bypass graft. *Ann Thorac Surg* 1989;**47**:716–19.

178. Pym J, Brown PM, Charrette EJP, Parker JO, West RO. Gastroepiploic-coronary anastomoses — a viable alternative coronary artery bypass graft. *J Thorac Cardiovasc Surg* 1987;**94**:256–9.

179. Suma H, Fukumoto H, Takeuchi A. Coronary artery bypass grafting by utilizing *in situ* right gastroepiploic artery: Basic study and clinical application. *Ann Thorac Surg* 1987;**44**:394–7.

180. Beretta L, Lemma M, Vanelli P *et al.* Gastroepiploic free graft for coronary bypass. *Eur J Cardiothorac Surg* 1990;**4**:323–8.

181. Suma H, Wanibuchi Y, Terada Y, Fukuda S, Takayama T, Funita S. The right gastroepiploic artery graft; clinical and angiographic midterm results in 200 patients. *J Thorac Cardiovasc Surg* 1993;**105**:615–23.

182. Gallo I, Saenz A, Alonso C *et al. In situ* right gastroepiploic artery: a conduit for coronary revascularization. *Eur J Cardiothorac Surg* 1991;**5**:110–11.

183. Suma H, Wanibuchi Y, Furuta S, Takeuchi A. Does use of the gastroepiploic artery increase surgical risk? *J Thorac Cardiovasc Surg* 1991;**101**:121–5.

184. Kusukawa J, Hirota Y, Kawamura K *et al.* Efficacy of coronary artery bypass surgery with gastroepiploic artery. *Circulation* 1989;**80**(suppl I):135–40.

185. Tavilla G, van Son JAM, Verhagen AF, Smedts F. Retrogastric versus antegastric routing and histology of the right gastroepiploic artery. *Ann Thorac Surg* 1992:

186. Suma H, Takanashi R. Arteriosclerosis of the gastroepiploic and internal thoracic arteries. *Ann Thorac Surg* 1990;**50**:413–16.

187. Fundaro P, Di Biasi P, Santoli C. Technical progress in coronary surgery. *Curr Opin Cardiology* 1991;**6**:892–7.

188. Schwartz DS, Factor SM, Schwartz JD. Histological evaluation of the inferior epigastric artery in patients with known atherosclerosis. *Eur J Cardiothorac Surg* 1992;**6**:438–41.

189. Milgator E, Pearl JM, Laks H *et al.* The inferior epigastric arteries as coronary bypass conduits. *J Thorac Cardiovasc Surg* 1992;**103**:463–5.

190. Puig LB, Ciongolli W, Cividanes VL *et al.* Inferior epigastric artery as a free graft for myocardial revascularization. *J Thorac Cardiovasc Surg* 1990;**99**:251–5.

191. Vincent JG, Van Som AM, Skotnicki SH. Inferior epigastric artery as a conduit in myocardial revascularization: the alternative free graft. *Ann Thorac Surg* 1990;**49**:323–5.

192. Buche M, Schoevaerdts J-C, Louagie Y *et al.* Use of the inferior epigastric artery for coronary bypass. *J Thorac Cardiovasc Surg* 1992;**103**:665–70.

193. Mills NL, Everson CT. Technique for use of the inferior epigastric as a coronary bypass graft. *Ann Thorac Surg* 1991;**51**:208–14.

194. Milgater E, Laks H, Drinkwater DC, Buckberg GD. The inferior epigastric arteries: additional arterial conduits for aorto-coronary bypass operations? *J Thorac Cardiovasc Surg* 1991;**101**:746–8.

195. Mills NL, Everson CT, Hockmuth DR. Free arterial grafts. *Curr Opin Cardiol* 1991;**6**:898–903.

196. Carpentier A, Guermonprez JL, Deloche A , Frechette C, DuBost C. The aorta-to-coronary radial artery bypass graft. *Ann Thorac Surg* 1973;**16**:111–21.

197. Curtis JJ, Stoney WS, Alford WC Jr, Burrus GR, Thomas CS Jr. Intimal hyperplasia — A cause of radial artery aorto-coronary bypass graft failure. *Ann Thorac Surg* 1975;**20**:628–35.

198. Fisk RL, Brooks CH, Callaghan JC, Dvorkin J. Experience with the radial artery graft for coronary artery bypass. *Ann Thorac Surg* 1976;**21**:513–18.

199. Acar C, Jebara V, Portoghese M. Experience with the radial artery for coronary artery bypass grafting. *Ann Thorac Surg* 1992;**54**:652–60.

200. Edwards WS, Lewis CE, Blakelley WR, Napolitano L. Coronary artery bypass grafts with internal mammary and splenic artery grafts. *Ann Thorac Surg* 1973;**15**:35–40.

201. Mueller CF, Lewis CE, Edwards WS. The angiographic appearance of splenic-to-coronary artery anastomosis. *Radiology* 1973;**106**:513–16.

202. Larsen A, Johanson A, Anderson D. Gastric arteriosclerosis in elderly people. *Scand J Gastroenterol* 1969;**4**:387–9.

203. Hartman AR, Mawulawde KI, Dervan JP, Anagnostopoulos CE. Myocardial revascularization with the lateral costal artery.*Ann Thorac Surg* 1990;**49**:816–18.

204. Suma H Oku T, Sato H, Koike R, Sawade Y, Takeuchi A. The bioflow graft for coronary artery bypass: preliminary report. *Tex Heart Inst J* 1990;**17**:103–5.

205. Donzeau-Gouge P, Touati G, Vouhe PR *et al.* Pontages coronaires par artere mammaire interne de boeuf. *Arch Mal Coeur* 1990;**83**:1811–15.

206. Mitchell IM, Essop AR, Scott PJ *et al.* Bovine internal mammary artery as a conduit for coronary revascularization: Long-term results. *Ann Thorac Surg* 1993;**55**:120–2.

207. Molina JE, Carr M, Yarnoz MD. Coronary bypass with Goretex graft. *J Thorac Cardiovasc Surg* 1978;**75**:769–71.

208. Yokoyama T, Gharavi MA, Lee Y-C, Edmiston WA, Kay JH. Aorta-coronary artery revascularization with an expanded polytetrafluoroethylene vascular graft: a preliminary report. *J Thorac Cardiovasc Surg* 1978;**76**:552–5.

209. Islam MN, Zikria EA, Sullivan ME *et al.* Aortocoronary Goretex graft: 18-month patency.*Ann Thorac Surg* 1981;**31**:569–73.

210. Sapsford RN, Oakley GD, Talbot S. Early and late patency of expanded polytetrafluoroethylene vascular grafts in aorta-coronary bypass. *J Thorac Cardiovasc Surg* 1981;**81**:860–4.

211. Chard RB, Johnson DC, Nunn GR, Cartmill TB. Aortocoronary bypass grafting with polytetrafluoroethylene conduits. *J Thorac Cardiovasc Surg* 1987;**94**:132–4.

212. Zilla P. Endothelialization of vascular grafts. *Curr Opin Cardiol* 1991;**6**:877–86.

213. Wareing TH, Saffitz JE, Kouchoukos NT. Use of single internal mammary grafts in older patients. *Circulation* 1990;**82**:224–8.

214. Azariades M, Fessler CL, Floten HS, Starr A. Five-year results of coronary bypass grafting for patients older than 70 years: role of internal mammary artery. *Ann Thorac Surg* 1990;**50**:940–5.

215. Jones EL, Lattouf O, Lutz JF, King SB III. Important anatomical and physiological considerations in performance of complex mammary-coronary artery operations. *Ann Thorac Surg* 1987;**43**:469–76.

216. Van Son JAM, Noyez L, van Asten NJC. Use of internal mammary artery in myocardial revascularization after mediastinal irradiation. *J Thorac Cardiovasc Surg* 1992;**104**: 1539–44.

217. Vijayanagar R, Bognolo D, Eckstein P *et al.* Safety and efficacy of internal mammary artery grafts for left main coronary artery disease. *J Thorac Cardiovasc Surg* 1987;**28**:576–80.

218. Dion R, Verheslt R, Matta A *et al.* Surgical angioplasty of the left main coronary artery. *J Thorac Cardiovasc Surg* 1990;**99**:241.

219. Ohara K, Yagihara T, Kishimoto H *et al.* Follow-up study of coronary artery bypass grafting after Kawasaki disease: early and late postoperative evaluation. *Nippon Kyobu Geka Gakkai Zasshi* 1989;**37**:103–9.

220. Fundaro P, Di Biasi P, Santoli C. Coronary endarterectomy combined with vein patch reconstruction and internal mammary grafting: experience with 18 patients. *Tex Heart Inst J* 1987;**14**:389–3.

11 Surgery for complication of ischaemic heart disease

G.M.K. Tsang and R.S. Bonser

Ischaemic heart disease is the most common cause of death in developed countries. Acute myocardial infarction (AMI) causes approximately 150 000 deaths per year in the UK and 500 000 deaths per year in the US. More than 60% of deaths associated with AMI occur within 1 hour of the event and are attributed to arrhythmias, mostly ventricular fibrillation. The in-hospital mortality for AMI is 10–15%. Most deaths are attributable to myocardial failure, a subset of which are secondary to mechanical complications.

Complications in ischaemic heart disease that may require surgical intervention include unstable angina, in particular following AMI, failure of percutaneous transluminal coronary angioplasty (PTCA), postinfarction ventricular septal defects, ischaemic mitral regurgitation, left aneurysms, and left ventricular free wall rupture.

Coronary artery bypass grafting in AMI and unstable angina

Clinically it has been convincingly shown that early reperfusion following AMI results in smaller infarction, better residual left ventricular function and survival (1–9). Reperfusion may be achieved by thrombolysis, PTCA, or coronary artery bypass grafting (CABG).

Currently thrombolysis may be achieved with either streptokinase, recombinant tissue type plasminogen activator (rt-PA) or anisoylated plasminogen streptokinase complex (APSAC). Agress (1952) showed that it was possible to achieve intracoronary thrombolysis with streptokinase under experimental conditions (10). Subsequent large clinical trials in patients with AMI with intravenous streptokinase have shown recanalization in 50% of patients (11), with subsequent improvement in short- and long-term survival confirmed by the European Cooperative study, the Thrombolysis in Myocardial infarction (TIMI) and the Gruppo Italia no per lo Studio della Streptochinasi nell' Infarto Miocardico GISSJ trials (7–9,12). The low specificity of streptokinase for thrombus-bound plasminogen have led to the introduction of rt-PA. Higher recanalization and lower complications have been shown when rt-PA is compared with streptokinase, but so far no convincing survival advantage has been shown (13,14). APSAC, which has more favourable pharmacokinetics, has not been shown to increase thrombolysis rate compared to intracoronary streptokinase (15,16). The drawback of thrombolysis therapy is a rethrombosis rate of 5–29% (17,18) presenting as persistent or post-infarction unstable angina. Reocclusion with threatened myocardium may require intervention either with emergency PTCA or CABG.

Table 11.1 Operative mortality for large series of early CABG following acute myocardial infarction

Series	Date	Number of patients	Mortality (%)
DeWood et al. (23)	1979	169	1.2
DeWood et al. (24)	1983	701	4.4
Phillips et al. (25)	1986	261	5.7
Naunheim et al. (26)	1988	313	4.7
Floten et al. (27)	1989	832	4.7
Applebaum et al. (28)	1991	406	6.7
Lichtenstein et al. (29)	1991	115	6.1
Sintek et al. (30)	1994	530	1.7

Primary PTCA is at least as effective as thrombolysis in achieving revascularization in patients with AMI. Recanalization rates of 85–95% have been shown with a lower re-occlusion rate than for thrombolysis (19–20). However, primary PTCA may not be logistically possible for the majority of patients with AMI. Therefore, PTCA is usually reserved for dilating re-occlusions or residual stenosis with success rates of greater than 75% for suitable lesions. Although mortality with secondary PTCA is low, very early or immediate PTCA for residual stenosis has not been beneficial and is associated with higher morbidity and mortality (18,21,22).

CABG may be used as primary treatment for AMI or following failed thrombolysis or angioplasty. Primary CABG has been shown to achieve revascularization with 7% overall mortality (Table 11.1) (23–30). Some smaller studies have reported mortality equivalent to elective CABG (30–32). Mortality is, however, strongly determined by preoperative factors such as age, residual left ventricular function, and in particular the presence of cardiogenic shock and perhaps the time interval from AMI to revascularization. Mortality rates as high as 65% and 43% have been reported in patients with cardiogenic shock and left ventricular ejection fraction of less than 30% respectively (24–27,33,34). Experimental revascularization following acute ischaemia has suggested that this should be performed within 6 hours for effective rescue of ischaemia myocardium (35). However, clinical studies have shown that revascularization may still be beneficial beyond this, suggesting that developed collateral circulation may help prolong ischaemic myocardium viability (8). The efficacy and relatively safety of performing of CABG within a short time interval between AMI and CABG appears inconclusive. Earlier studies have suggested that very early revascularization may be associated with a lower operative morality (7). Revascularization within 6 hours by primary CABG is probably not realistic for most patients, but it appears early CABG is associated with improvements in ejection fraction (23,31,33) although conclusive data to support whether this is translated to improved long-term survival are lacking. However, there are also suggestions that operative mortality is inversely proportional to the time interval between AMI and CABG (27,30) but statistical significance is not achieved and multiple regression analysis has shown other factors to be more important. Generally it appears that clinically stable patients may undergo CABG with a very acceptable risk.

For similar logistical reasons primary CABG is not available to the majority of patients with AMI. There is also very little data to differentiate the use of secondary PTCA or CABG for suitable residual lesions following initial thrombolysis. Currently emergency CABG is mostly indicated when, following thrombolysis, residual ischaemia persists and the coronary artery anatomy is not suitable for angioplasty or following failed PTCA. CABG following recent thrombolysis has been associated with increased perioperative blood loss. However, large studies have demonstrated that reoperation for haemorrhage is not higher in thrombolysed patients although most cases were operated on more than 24 hours following thrombolysis (36). The general consensus is that with CABG within 24 hours of thrombolysis, clotting screen including fibrinogen degradation products and fibrinogen levels should be assayed and appropriate replacement undertaken. The prophylactic used of antifibrinolytic products may also be indicated.

Coronary artery bypass grafting for failed elective percutaneous transluminal coronary angioplasty

Since it was first reported by Gruntzig in 1978 (37), percutaneous transluminal coronary angioplasty (PTCA) has become an accepted form of treatment for coronary artery disease. Technical advances have meant that there is an increasing number of patients who are suitable for PTCA with high success and low complication rates (38,39). It currently accounts for more than 50% of revascularization procedures (40). Nevertheless PTCA is not free of complications and 1–6% of patients will require emergency coronary artery bypass grafting (CABG) for acute ischaemia due to failed PTCA (41).

PTCA increases vessel lumen by 'cracking' and outward displacement of the associated atheromatous plaque. Local intimal dissection at the dilatation site can be seen radiographically. This does not usually interfere with antegrade blood flow but acute myocardial ischaemia caused by extensive dissection (Figure 11.1a–c) or thrombosis requires emergency revascularization procedures. A second PTCA may be successful at recanalization in over 50% of cases (42). Arterial stenting has been promising in associated dissections and intracoronary thrombolysis may be used in acute thrombosis. However, ultimate emergency CABG may be required with the best

Table 11.2 Results of emergency coronary artery bypass grafting in patients with failed percutaneous transluminal coronary angioplasty. Percentage figure in parenthesis.

Series	Total number	Emergency CABG	Q Wave infarction	Mortality (% in brackets)
Atkins and Black (43)	125	11 (8.8)	1 (9.1)	0
Cowley *et al.* (44)	3079	202 (6.6)	52 (25.7)	13 (6.4)
Golding *et al.* (45)	1831	81 (4.4)	37 (46)	2 (2.5)
Killen *et al.* (46)	3000	115 (3.8)	50 (43.5)	13 (11.3)
Pelletier *et al.* (47)	265	35 (13.2)	3 (8.6)	0
Reul *et al.* (48)	518	70 (13.5)	8 (11.4)	4 (5.7)
Roberts *et al.* (49)	175	14 (8)	3 (21)	0
Talley *et al.* (50)	NA	202	54 (27)	5 (2.5)
Klepzig *et al.* (51)	2850	100 (3.5)	29 (29)	12 (12)
Kinoshita *et al.* (52)	1315	9 (0.7)	2 (25)	1 (11)
Buffet *et al.* (53)	2576	100 (3.9)	57 (57)	19 (19)

NA, not available.

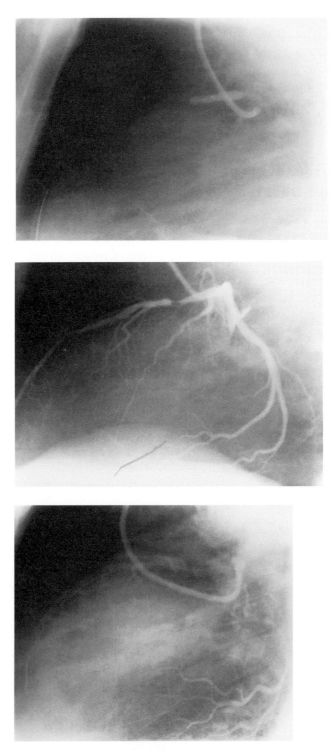

Fig. 11.1 Coronary angiogram showing critical proximal LAD stenosis (a), treated with balloon angioplasty (b) and subsequent dissection at site of dilatation with loss of distal perfusion (c).

chance of limiting injury being associated with a short ischaemic to reperfusion time. In patients requiring emergency CABG, use of a guide wire or perfusion catheter may be helpful in maintaining target vessel patience. Intra-aortic balloon pump support has been strongly advocated. Table 11.2 illustrates the in-hospital mortality of several series (43–53) of patients undergoing emergency CABG following failure of PTCA. Results are highly variable and difficult to compare, but in this collective series the referral rate for emergency surgery is approximately 5% with adverse outcome in terms of myocardial infarction and operative mortality being 40% and 8% respectively. Referral rates for emergency CABG have steadily declined since the 14% reported by Gruentzig in 1979 (38,54), owing to improved patient selection and technical ability. However, it may be expected to rise again as patients with more complicated and severe disease are selected for PTCA. The strongest predictive factor of poor outcome is cardiogenic shock and haemodynamic instability, although a 62% survival following salvage CABG has been achieved in patients with refractory cardiac arrest during cardiac catheterization procedures (55). Failure to dilate a target stenosis with primary PTCA or re-stenosis after successful dilatation requires further dilatations or elective CABG.

Given that arterial conduits have higher long-term patency rates, the choice of conduit for CABG following failed PTCA — particularly to the left anterior descending artery — is controversial. Studies employing extensive use of the internal mammary artery have yielded acceptable results, but perioperative myocardial infarction is higher than in groups using venous conduit (56). Patients who are stable and who would normally warrant the use of an arterial conduit are probably best served with an IMA graft. However, in unstable patients dissection of the IMA, even after the establishment of cardiopulmonary bypass, may unnecessary prolong myocardial ischaemia and potential early postoperative hypoperfusion with IMA grafts may add to the higher rate of perioperative myocardial infarction encountered. There is as yet no conclusive evidence that, in the failed PTCA situation, CABG using saphenous vein as to IMA as a conduit results in a lower long-term patency rate. During CABG for failed PTCA, other graftable vessels with significant stenotic disease should be grafted.

Postinfarction ventricular septal defects

Postinfarction ventricular septal defects (VSDs) complicate approximately 1–2% of cases of acute myocardial infarction (57–59). Development of a postinfarction VSD usually occurs within 2 weeks of an acute myocardial infarction. Anatomically, 60% of postinfarction VSDs are anteriorly or apically sites as a result of infarction located in the left anterior descending artery territory, with the remaining 40% sited in the posterior part of the septum owing to acute occlusion of the posterior descending artery (60). Involvement of the subvalvular apparatus in postinfarction posterior VSDs may cause severe mitral regurgitation which in addition to right ventricular dysfunction and increased technical difficulty of a posterior repair may contribute to their higher mortality when compared to anteriorly sited VSDs (61–63). Factors that have been associated with postinfarction VSDs include hypertension, left ventricular hypertrophy, female sex, and advanced age. Only a small percentage of these patients have sustained a previous myocardial infarction or had previous chronic symptomatic ischaemic heart disease. Thus, it is believed that VSDs occur following abrupt closure of a single vessel unsupported by a developed collateral circulation (64–67).

Diagnostically, postinfarction VSD is suspected when a pansystolic murmur, best audible at the left sternal edge, and an associated thrill develops shortly after an acute myocardial infarction.

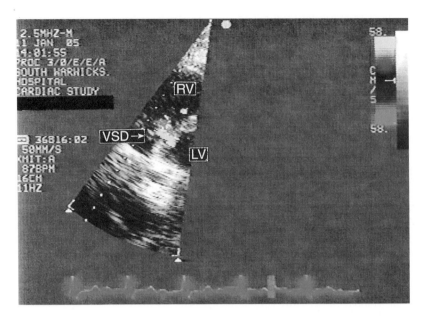

Fig. 11.2 Colour Doppler flow mapping demonstrating high velocity jet from the left ventricle (LV) to a dilated right ventricle (RV) through the VSD. See also colour plate section (Plate 5).

The haemodynamic status of the patient is variable depending on the size of the left to right shunt and associated left and right ventricular function. Differentiation with postinfarction mitral valve regurgitation may be difficult with the added difficulty that mitral regurgitation may occur in association with posterior VSDs. Changes in the appropriate ECG leads may point to the site of the VSD, but inferior infarction in association with an anterior VSD can occur because of a prominent LAD supplying part of the inferior septum (62). Echocardiography with colour flow Doppler is the investigation of choice in confirming the presence of a VSD, defining its anatomical position and quantifying the left to right shunt (Fig. 11.2) (68–70). Verification of the shunt may be obtained by Swan–Ganz catheterization with a step-up in blood oxygen saturation from the right atrium to the pulmonary artery seen. The size of the shunt may then be calculated.

Controversy exists as to whether concommittent coronary angiography and bypass grafting for significant stenosis should be performed (71–73). Single-vessel disease is more common in anterior postinfarction VSDs, whereas multiple-vessel disease is more common with posteriorly sited VSDs. Overall, grafting the vessel supplying the infarcted territory offers no benefit and generally concommitant CABG offers no advantage in early survival (62,66,67,71,72). However, it has recently been shown that it offers an advantage in late survival particularly in the group with multiple-vessel disease (72). This has led some to selectively investigate with coronary angiography those who have had an inferior infarction (66). However, the relationships between the infarcted territory, site of VSD, and coexisting coronary artery disease are not absolute. So, if the patient is haemodynamically stable, coronary angiography should probably be performed to delineate any significant coronary artery stenosis which should be bypassed at the time of surgery. Coronary angiography is a relatively safe procedure and with the diagnostic accuracy of two-dimensional echocardiography with colour mapping a left ventricular angiogram is probably not necessary, particularly in patients with a degree of heart failure. In haemodynamically unstable patients, time-consuming investigations should be avoided and surgery undertaken at the earliest opportu-

Table 11.3 Table illustrating recent 30 day mortality following operation for postinfarction ventricular septal defects

Series	Number of patients	30 day mortality (%)
Daggett *et al.* (62)	55	33
Jones *et al.* (78)	60	38
Teo *et al.* (80)	21	57
Komeda *et al.* (76)	31	10
Skillington *et al.* (66)	101	21
Deville *et al.* (79)	62	38
Loisance *et al.* (77)	66	45
Muehrcke *et al.* (72)	75	24
Parry *et al.* (67)	81	47
Lemery *et al.* (75)	52	55

nity. Interim support with either intra-aortic balloon pump support or percutaneous cardiopulmonary bypass has been advocated.

Due to the fact that postinfarction VSDs are now commonly regarded as surgical emergencies, their natural history can only be estimated from series published before surgical repair was common. These limited studies report a 30 day mortality rate of 80% (73–74). Nevertheless the high mortality rate of conservative therapy appears to be substantiated by recent studies that include a conservative therapy group, but of course these consist of highly selected patients and long-term survival with conservative therapy has been reported (67,75). Therefore mortality figures from conservative therapy may not reflect possible survival in the present era. There have been many retrospective series concerning surgical treatment of post-infarction VSDs, but many are small in number with results accumulated over a long period. Tables 11.3 and 11.4 (62,66,67,72,75–80) show the early and late survival rates respectively of a selection of recently published series with 20 or more patients studied. Operative mortality is generally high, but appears to be highly variable between centres. The total number of patients operated on this

Table 11.4 Long-term survival of patients following surgery for postinfarction ventricular septal defect

Series	Survival (%)		
	1 year	5 year	10 year
Jones *et al.* (78)	38	10	NA
Komeda *et al.* (76)	NA	83	NA
Skillington *et al.* (66)	76	70	40
Deville *et al.* (79)	57	44	30
Loisance *et al.* (77)	55	35	15
Muehrcke *et al.* (72)	NA	46	14
Lemery *et al.* (75)	NA	19	8

NA, not available.

selected group was 604 with a median of 3 cases per year (range 2–8). Mean 30 day mortality was 37% (range 10–57%). The 30 day mortality figures were better than that reported by Hill (59) in an earlier group analysis, but again these are highly selected comparisons. Nevertheless, within a number of reported series, the longitudinal data does suggest that for a number of reasons, mortality — although still high — is improving. Long-term survival data is limited. Within the series analysed the men 5 and 10 year survival is 44% (range 10–83%) and 21% (range 8–40%) respectively. Again there appears to be great inter-institution variation. The quality of life in survivors appear to be good, with over 80% of survivors being in NYHA classification I or II (81).

There are no randomized trials comparing conservative to surgical treatment, or early to delayed surgical treatment in post-infarction VSD. In fact currently it may be argued that such trials would be unethical. Therefore many of the conclusions on treatment are by necessity drawn from historical retrospective comparisons, spanning many years. Nevertheless the general consensus of opinion is that medical treatment, even with inotropic support and left ventricular off-loading with IABP, is associated with a high mortality (67,72–74) with Lemery showing that it is uniformly fatal, as is the delay in surgical treatment later than 48 hours in this group of patients. Therefore it is advocated that patients presenting or developing shock after conservative treatment should undergo emergency repair which offers a chance of survival. Stable patients may be treated conservatively but cardiovascular decompensation may be very rapid and a relatively elective would be changed to an emergency procedure. Therefore some have advocated emergency surgery for all. However, surgical series have consistently demonstrated better survival in the group of patients undergoing a delayed procedure after the development of the VSD whether as deliberate policy or due to late presentation. This may be due to self selection and the fact that the organized infarcted muscle offers better operating conditions. Survival figures following early surgery have been impressive in some series but these are difficult to compare because of the variation in the definition of early surgery. The terms 'early' and 'late' operation have been used inconsistently. Within the series shown in Table 3 early operation can be surgery within 48 hours or 1 week of developing a VSD after myocardial infarction, with some series having merely pointed to the mean difference in delay in operation between the survivors and non-survivors (77,79). In previous publications early surgery has meant operation up to 3 weeks following the development of the VSD (82). Parry and others have pointed out that very early surgery is associated with a very high mortality (67,76,83) and mortalities of 90% have been shown in patients when concomitant clinical shock is present (67,83). Therefore the additional number of patients salvaged by early surgery may not be high and the possibility arises that stable patients may have a better chance of survival if surgery is delayed. The improvement in survival in patients who survive to have a delayed operation has prompted some to use prolonged IABP support (84,85) or percutaneous catheter closure of the defect to achieve haemodynamic stability and hence delayed operation (86). The effect of his approach on operative mortality has not been fully evaluated. Although there are no randomized trials comparing early to delayed treatment for post-infarction VSDs, most units will now advocate repair at the earliest opportunity on the theoretical basis that despite persistent high operative mortality, the absolute number of patients salvaged is higher. It remains difficult to decide which patients, if any, should be denied surgery and which patients will be advantaged by a delayed approach.

The first successful surgical repair of a post-infarction VSD was performed by Cooley in 1957 (87). Since then intraoperative management, myocardial protection, and operative technique have improved and this may account for improvements in survival. Generally centres have reported improvement in survival over the last two decades. Operative techniques have been described in detail (88). Essentially, cardiopulmonary bypass may be instituted with bicaval drainage and snares with blood returning into the ascending aorta. The heart may be vented via the right superior pulmonary vein or pulmonary trunk. Systemic hypothermia and myocardial protection with intermittent cold antegrade crystalloid cardioplegia or intermittent aortic cross clamping and ventricular fibrillation may be used. The main principle of the operation is to close off the defect and preserve ventricular function. This may be achieved in various ways. Amputation of the apex and direct closure may be possible with apically sited VSDs, but except for the smallest anterior and posterior VSDs a patch repair using either synthetic material such as dacron, which may be lined with autologous pericardium, or biological material such as bovine pericardium is used. The ventriculotomy is made over the infarcted area of the left ventricle, although access can be gained through the right atrium (89) or ventricle (87). Daggett has advocated extensive debridement of the infarcted area, but others prefer to avoid this in an attempt to preserve left ventricular function but sutures must be placed to healthy myocardium. The use of biological glues has been advocated to improve tissue condition (90). With anterior VSDs the ventriculomy may be close primarily but the use of a patch closure of the posterior ventriculotomy have been advocated to preserve ventricular geometry and function (91).

Analysis of several series has shown that operative mortality is dependent on left and right ventricular function, the presence of cardiogenic shock, the site of the VSD, and the timing of surgical intervention. Right ventricular dysfunction may be exacerbated by right ventricular infarction in association with the large left to right shunt. In addition this is likely to be associated with posterior VSDs and mitral incompetence. Large degrees of right and left ventricular dysfunction are often associated with cardiogenic shock and multisystem failure which are the strongest preoperative predictive factors of short- and long-term outcome. Other factors such as the presence of diabetes mellitus, age, and the preoperative use of IABP have not been consistently shown to be correlated to survival.

Ischaemic mitral regurgitation

Ischaemic mitral regurgitation (MR) is a spectrum and may be classified into sudden onset MR caused by papillary muscle rupture or dysfunction associated with acute myocardial infarction, or MR in the presence of ischaemic heart disease with no primary leaflet or chordal pathology. It accounts for 6–10% of mitral valve disease requiring surgery (92–93) and should be distinguished from the two most common causes, degenerative and rheumatic mitral insufficiency, which can occur concomitantly with coronary artery disease.

Some degree of MR is common after myocardial infarction. In some studies approximately 50% of patients have been detected to have some degree of MR within 24 hours after myocardial infarction (94–95). Physical examination is generally a unreliable method of detecting MR as the characteristic murmur can be present only in a minority of patients. In a consecutive series of 849 patients admitted to the Multicentre Investigation of the Limitation of Infarct Size (MILIS), Barzilai (96) found that a mitral regurgitant murmur was present in 9% of admission with a further 11% developing the murmur between days 1 and 11. Lehmann (97) in the Thrombolysis in Myocardial Infarction (TIMI) trial reported that the murmur was audible in only 4% of the 13% of patients who was shown to have MR at left ventriculography. Echocardiography, in particular transoesophageal echocardiography, may be able to demonstrate the underlying mechanism for the MR (98).

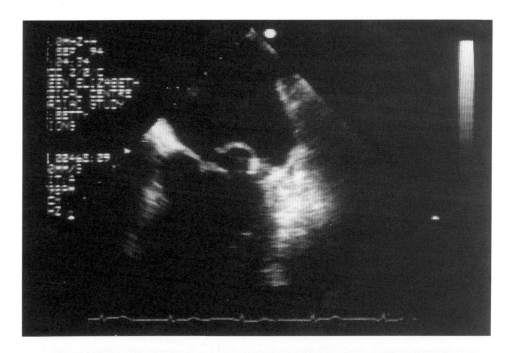

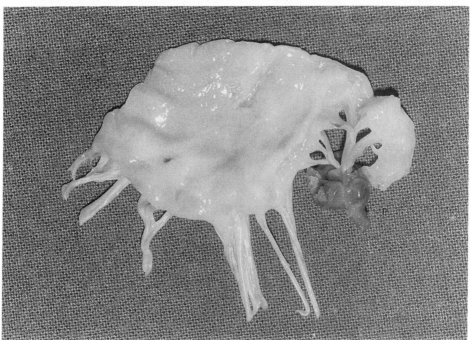

Fig. 11.3 (a) Echocardiogram: apical two-chamber view showing prolapsing posterior leaflet. (b) Excised valve leaflet seen in (a). P, papillary muscle.

Severe acute MR occurs in approximately 3% of patients after myocardial infarction (96,97,99). Without abnormalities in the valve leaflets MR may be caused by annular dilatation secondary to left ventricular dilatation as a consequence of left ventricular failure or dysfunction of the subvalvular apparatus. Dysfunction of the subvalvular apparatus may be caused by infarction and complete rupture of the papillary muscle (Fig. 11.3a,b) or, more commonly, the muscle insertion of one or more of the chordal attachments will tear causing moderate to severe mitral regurgitation. Alternatively, the papillary muscle may become intermittently ischaemic and fail to tighten the chordae during systole, or an infarcted but intact papillary muscle may undergo fibrosis, shorten, and distort the valve during systole leading to regurgitation. In all cases, there is loss of coaptation of the leaflets.

Severe mitral incompetence requiring prompt surgical intervention after myocardial infarction is usually due to rupture of a papillary muscle. Papillary muscle rupture commonly occurs in the first week after inferior myocardial infarction and has been associated with the lack of collateral circulation. The extent of left ventricular damage is less than that required to produce the clinical presentation of cardiogenic shock (99) that is often seen. Usually left ventricular function is relatively well preserved and the sudden severe MR causes high pressures in a normal sized and relatively low compliant left atrium with large V waves detectable in the pulmonary arterial wedge tracing, although this is not a universal finding. The sudden rise in pulmonary venous pressures leads to pulmonary oedema. Results from conservative therapy, despite pharmacological preload and afterload reduction and intra-aortic balloon support, are poor, with an 80% mortality from cardiogenic shock within 2 weeks (100–102). Therefore these patients require emergency surgical intervention. In stable patients cardiac catheterization is performed to define the anatomy of coronary artery disease as concomitant CABG has been shown to improve short- and long-term survival (103). The results of surgical intervention in acute MR following myocardial infarction are relatively poor. Table 11.5 (92,104–111) shows that the overall reported numbers are small and in this collective series of 134 patients the early mortality is 28%. However, the highest mortality appears to have occurred in patients who have a long delay between the development of shock and surgery. Mishimura managed to achieve zero mortality in a small group of patients operated on early following cardiovascular decompensation. These data suggest, although not conclusively, that early surgery before the onset of multisystem failure in this group of patients may be beneficial to survival. Survival for MR secondary to left ventricular dysfunction is less than for subvalvular apparatus dysfunction,

Table 11.5 Operative mortality for early mitral valve surgery for ischaemic mitral regurgitation

Series	Year	Number of patients	Mortality (%)
Tepe and Edmunds (104)	1985	11	50
Andrade et al. (105)	1987	13	39
David and Ho (106)	1986	15	20
Nishimura et al. (107)	1986	7	0
Yadav et al. (108)	1985	9	33
Rankin et al. (109)	1988	30	50
Defraign et al. (110)	1990	13	15
Loisance et al. (111)	1990	26	31
Hendren et al. (92)	1991	11	9

reflecting the fact that left ventricular function is a strong determinator of outcome. Operative techniques for mitral valve replacement for MR post myocardial infarction is essentially the same as for standard elective mitral valve replacement, but the left atrium and ventricle cavity are likely to be small. This may make access difficult and an alternative incision such as a transeptal or Dubost incision may be used. In addition a small ventricular cavity may make accommodation of a strutted or caged prosthesis difficult, and a low profile mechanical prosthesis is preferable.

Ischaemic mitral regurgitation which is not secondary to ischaemic papillary muscle or chordal rupture is more common. In this group of patients it is often difficult to judge whether concomitant valve and bypass surgery is necessary. It has been shown that successful vascularization often reduces the degree of MR (112–114) and therefore a simultaneous mitral valve procedure with an expected higher mortality is not necessary. Conversely, bypass surgery alone in the presence of significant MR results in higher mortality than when MR is absent. In the presence of severe MR, concomitant mitral valve surgery reduces operative mortality. Chronic severe ischaemic MR is therefore probably best served by a valve and bypass operation whereas a bypass operation alone is adequate for mild to moderate ischaemic MR. Both groups would achieve good symptomatic relief. The greatest difficulty occurs when the MR is moderate to severe. The necessity for a valve procedure is not well established. Some have used symptom severity in terms of NYHA and angina classification, together with objective measurements such as left atrial size, left ventricular end systolic volume, and pulmonary artery pressures measurements as guides to the necessity for valve replacement, but generally patients with predominantly anginal symptoms are best served with revascularization alone and expect some residual exertional dyspnoea which may incidentally improve, due to improve left ventricular function from a revascularized ventricle, than to undergo a concomitant valve procedure which have at least double the expected operative morality. Table 11.6 (92,109,115–121) shows the results of a collective series of concomitant mitral valve and bypass surgery for ischaemic MR. The overall mortality is 23% in a total of 514 patients. Figures between institutions are very variable, but it appears that in groups that perform a high proportion of mitral valve repairs the overall mortality are lower, with Kay and Hendren showing mortality figures of less than 10%. These figures are only matched by David who performed chordal preservation mitral valve replacement and suggests that the improvement in residual left ventricular function contributes to improvements in early and late survival. The true mortality for elective CABG and mitral valve procedure in chronic ischaemic mitral regurgitation is probably less because incorporated in some of these figures are patients operated on under emergency conditions for acute severe mitral regurgitation. Hendren has shown that over 75% of ischaemic MR including those that present as an emergency may be suitable for repair and the current trend towards repair may result in a reduction of mortality for ischaemic mitral regurgitation in the future.

Long-term survival following combined bypass and mitral valve surgery for ischaemic mitral regurgitation is approximately 48% at 5 years for the studies in Table 11.6 that have reached adequate follow up. Outcome following ischaemic mitral surgery has been shown to be dependent on several factors at presentation. These consistently included age, NYHA classification, left ventricular function, and severity of mitral regurgitation. Overall long-term survival for ischaemic mitral regurgitation with bypass surgery with or without a valve procedure is 75% at 5 years, but for patients with concomitant valve surgery for severe MR survival may be as poor as 33% (115–116). This appears to be irrespective of whether a repair or replacement is performed. Overall early and late survival following surgery for ischaemic mitral regurgitation is poor with a higher mortality than if these two factors are merely additive.

Table 11.6 Operative mortality for patients undergoing mitral valve surgery for mitral regurgitation

Series	Year	Number of patients	Early mortality (%)	Late survival (%) (years follow up)
Kay *et al.* (115)	1980	61	8	55
Pinson *et al.* (116)	1984	37	38	44
Czer *et al.* (117)	1984	107	20	40
McGovern *et al.* (118)	1985	23	22	NA
Connolly *et al.* (119)	1986	16	19	85
David and Ho (106)	1986	51	8	75 (4)
Rankin *et al.* (109)	1988	55	42	NA
Hendren *et al.* (92)	1991	65	9	63 (3)
Vidal *et al.* (120)	1991	39	36	55
Czers *et al.* (121)	1992	60	15	72 (1)

Ventricular aneurysms

Transmural myocardial infarction is the most common cause of left ventricular (LV) aneurysms. The reported incidence has been between 10% and 30%, with 85% sited anteriorly (122). False aneurysms as a consequence of a limited myocardial rupture are more common following an inferior myocardial infarction.

Diagnosis of an LV aneurysm may be difficult because of the heterogeneity in criteria used to define the presence of an aneurysm. Morphologically an LV aneurysm is a well delineated transmural thin-walled scar, virtually devoid of muscle, with loss of trabeculae on the inner surface. Angiographically this would correspond to an area of systolic akinesis, hypokinesis, or dyskinesis (Fig. 11.4a,b). The formation of an LV aneurysm usually takes several weeks following myocardial infarction. Clinically, following myocardial infarction the majority of patients present with angina alone or in combination with exertional dyspnoea secondary to congestive heart failure (123–125). Ventricular arrhythmias and systemic embolic symptoms account for less than 20% of presentation in most major series. Associated intraventricular thrombus occurs in up to 50% of LV aneurysms but yet only a small proportion of patients have systemic embolic symptoms prior to aneurysm repair (123,126–8). Examination may reveal an apical heave, third heart sound, and a pansystolic murmur if mitral regurgitation coexists. Echocardiography, radioisotope scanning, and angiography may be diagnostically useful, but generally differentiation with areas of post-infarction patchy thick scarring mixed with significant viable muscle and therefore non-aneurysmal myocardium is difficult. Ultimate diagnosis can only be made intraoperatively; localized dense pericardial adhesions may be seen and the thiness of the aneurysm wall is best seen when cardiopulmonary bypass is established with the aneurysmal segment collapsing into the cavity of the decompressed left ventricle. Thus Froehlich found that only 61% of preoperatively diagnosed LV aneurysm coming to operation required resection (129).

The natural history of LV aneurysms remains controversial. Table 11.7 (130–139) illustrates the reported long-term survival of a number of series over the last 5 decades. Although studies have reported very poor long-term survival, recent series have reported 5 year survival of over 60%. The most important determinant factor in survival appears to be the residual LV function

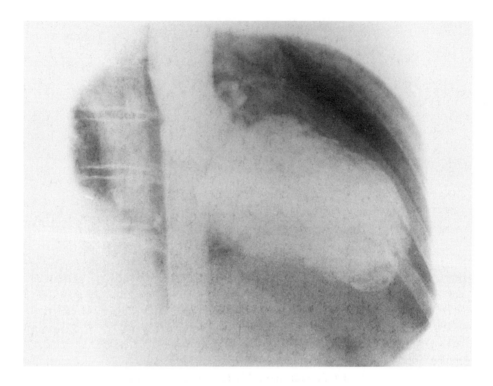

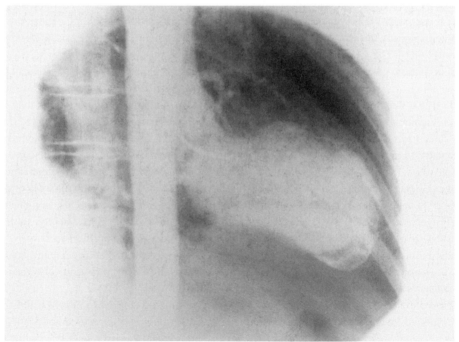

Fig. 11.4 Left ventricular aneurysm: (a) bulging contour during diastole; (b) dyskinetic movement during systole.

Table 11.7 Natural history of left ventricular aneurysm

Series	Year	Years follow up	Survival (%)
Schlicter et al. (130)	1954	5	12
Dubnow et al. (131)	1965	5	24
Nagle et al. (132)	1974	5	10
Schattenberg et al. (133)	1970	3	24
Bruschke et al. (134)	1973	10	18
Grondin et al. (135)	1979	5	90
Faxon et al. (136)	1982	5	71
Heras et al. (137)	1990	5	75
Shen et al. (138)	1992	5	68
Benediktsson et al. (139)	1994	5	70

rather than the presence of the aneurysm itself. This difference in survival rates may be due to variability in diagnostic criteria: Schlicter (130) diagnosed the condition at post mortem reporting a 5 year survival rate of 12% and Benediktsson (139) using left ventricular angiography reported a 5 year survival of 70%. In addition the medical treatment of the complications of LV aneurysms may have improved. It may also imply that the natural history of LV aneurysm is in itself changing. LV aneurysm have been associated with complete occlusion of the left anterior descending artery. Current successful revascularization with either thrombolysis or PTCA following acute myocardial infarction have led to the suspicion that the incidence of LV aneurysm may be decreasing. Current series of patients undergoing angiography following myocardial infarction have shown a prevalence of approximately 5% (139). Improved long-term survival may mean that the indications for prognostic surgery will have to be very carefully considered as long-term survival following aneurysmectomy have been shown to be better than conservative therapy by Faxon (136) in the CASS study; the reported 5 year survival has been approximately 60–70% (Table 11.8) (124,125,128,140–145).

Table 11.8 Operative mortality and long-term survival following left ventricular aneurysm surgery

Series	Year	Number of patients	Early mortality (%)	Years	Late survival (%)
Couper et al. (124)	1990	303	13	5	58
Baciewicz et al. (140)	1991	298	5	10	57
Komeda et al. (128)	1992	336	7	10	63
Kesler et al. (141)	1992	62	5	5	82
Elefteriades et al. (142)	1993	75	7	5	64
Stahle et al. (143)	1994	303	9	5	72
Samani et al. (125)	1994	120	17	5	65
Coltharp et al. (144)	1994	523	8	5	68
Mickleborough et al. (145)	1994	95	3	5	80

LV aneurysms that are small and asymptomatic are best left. When 10% of the ventricle contracts abnormally, there is a decrease in the ejection fraction. Congestive heart failure and cardiogenic shock occurs when respectively 25% and 40% of the LV is involved (146). The presence of an LV aneurysm causes an increase in the end diastolic pressure and volume with a resultant increase in tension and hence oxygen demand. Therefore the two predominant symptoms of patients undergoing LV aneurysm surgery are angina either in isolation or in combination with exertional dyspnoea with a significant proportion of patients in NYHA functional class III or IV. The extent to which the aneurysm solely causes these symptoms is uncertain as the great majority of patients have associated coronary artery disease and symptomatic relief may be attributable to a great extent to CABG alone. Furthermore, concurrent CABG of significant coronary artery disease have been shown to improve survival (147) and current trends have shown that most series perform approximately bypass surgery in over 80% of patients undergoing surgery for a LV aneurysm (124,140,144,145,148,149). Nevertheless in groups of patients undergoing aneurysmectomy without bypass surgery, studies of left ventricular function appears to improve, correlating with symptomatic improvement (125,142). Therefore patients with large aneurysms are best operated on together with associated bypass grafting as appropriate, but difficulty occurs when significant coronary artery disease occurs in association with a moderate aneurysm. In such cases the risk of an extended procedure would have to be carefully balanced against possible additional symptomatic relief by operating on the LV aneurysm. Combined aneurysmectomy with CABG with poor ventricular function have been associated with an operative mortality rate of greater than 50% (127).

The principles at operation is to excise or exclude the aneurysm and repair the subsequent ventriculotomy thus reducing LV end diastolic volume, tension, and oxygen demand by restoring LV geometry. Restoring the orientation of the muscle fibres is also important. Several techniques have been shown to be effective in aneurysm resection. The classic description of the procedure includes excision of the aneurysm leaving behind a rim of scar tissue to facilitate closure (150). Subsequently patch repair (151), inverted 'T' closure (128), purse-string closure (152), endoventricular circular plasty (153), and the endoaneurysmorraphy technique (154) have been used in an attempt to improve the resultant LV geometry. Although improve results have been reported, this has coincided with the improvement of LV aneurysm surgery generally although there is some suggesting that it may be better in patients with ejection fractions of less than 20% (128). There have been few trials directly comparing the various techniques; results have been conflicting (141,155) and individual series employing various techniques have produced very comparable results (Table 11.8). Overall, irrespective of operative technique the operative mortality has been 5–10% in the last 5 years (Table 11.8). This has remained unchanged since the previous decade and compares very favourably to operative mortality rates in excess of 20–30% in the very early attempts at LV aneurysmectomy. The strongest risk factors that determine outcome in LV aneurysm surgery have been consistently shown to be residual LV function and age of the patient. Many others factors such as aneurysm size, extensive coronary artery disease, and left main stem stenosis have also been identified but these are much less important. Following aneurysmectomy, improvement have been consistently shown in the left ventricular functional indices such as end diastolic and systolic volumes, ejection fraction, and regional wall movement which is related to the improvement in functional status seen. However, up to 17% of patients have been reported to have no benefit from an aneurysmectomy (125,148) suggesting that selection of patients remains very important. The greatest benefit occurs in the group with the lowest ejection fraction, which unfortunately also has the highest operative risk. Long-term survival following aneurysmectomy has frequently been quoted at between 60% and 80% at 5 years (Table 11.8), which is only slightly better than conservative therapy. However, owing to the variation in the definition of an LV aneurysm comparisons cannot be drawn and as yet no prospective randomized trial exists comparing the outcome between conservative and surgical treatment of patients with LV aneurysms.

Left ventricular free wall rupture

Left ventricular free wall rupture complicates approximately 8% of transmural myocardial infraction. Presentation is usually sudden collapse with electromechanical dissociation at day 3–5 post-infraction (156). Resuscitation and survival are unlikely and the diagnosis is often made at post mortem examination (157). The total number of patients undergoing surgical repair is therefore small.

Occasionally presentation is less acute and the diagnosis may be suspected in the presence of cardiac failure associated with signs of cardiac tamponade. Diagnosis can be confirmed with echocardiography and angiography, with surgical repair being the only feasible treatment option. Surgical repair usually involves closure with sutures reinforced with Teflon buttress, but Padro (159) has recently reported a 100% survival by using a sutureless technique and cyanoacrylate glue to attach a Teflon patch to the rupture site. Rarely, particularly in association with inferior infarcts, left ventricular rupture may be contained and the patient present at a much later stage with a chronic inferior false left ventricular aneurysm. The results derived from a number of series reviewed by Boolooki (160) shows the operative mortality to be approximately 35% in the group of patients who survive to be operated upon but the average number of 3.6 cases per report makes any valid conclusion difficult. Nevertheless, Lopez-Sendon (161) reported similar operative mortality of 24% in a series of 33 patients, approximately 50% of whom became long-term survivors. Therefore for the group that survive to operation the eventual outcome appears reasonable, considering the catastrophic nature of this complication, and it appears that a realistic way of reducing the overall mortality from this relatively common complication of acute myocardial infarction is to raise the level of clinical suspicion so that surgery may be undertaken as soon as possible.

References

1. Califf RM, Ohman EM. Thrombolytic therapy: overview of clinical trials. *Coronary Artery Disease* 1990;**1**:23.
2. Lavie CJ, Gersh BJ, Chesebro JH. Reperfusion in acute myocardial infarction. *Mayo Clinic Proc* 1990;**65**:549.
3. Schwartz F, Schuler G, Katus H *et al.* Intracoronary thrombolysis inacute myocardial infarction: duration of ischaemic as a major determinant of late result after recanalization. *Am J Cardiol* 1982;**50**:933.
4. Sheehan FH, Mathey DG, Schofer J *et al.* Factors that determine recovery of left ventricular function after thrombolysis in patients with acute myocardial infarction. *Circulation* 1985;**71**:1121.
5. Sheehan FH, Braunwald E, Canner P *et al.* The effect of intravenous thrombolytic therapy on left ventricular function: a report on tissue-type plasminogen activator and stroptokinase in the thrombolysis in myocardial infarction (TIMI Phase I) trial. *Circulation* 1987;**75**:817.

6. Kurnik PB, Courtois MR and Ludbrook PB. Diastolic stiffening induced by acute myocardial infarction is reduced by early reperfusion. *J Am Coll Cardiol* 1988;**12**:1029.

7. European Cooperative Study Group for Streptokinase Treatment in Acute Myocardial Infraction. Streptokinase in acute myocardial infraction. *N Engl J Med* 1979;**301**:797–802.

8. Gissi–Gruppo Italiano per lo Studio della Streptocninasai nell' Infarto Miocardico. Effectiveness of intravenous thrombolytic treatment of acute myocardial infarction. *Lancet* 1986;**1**:397.

9. ISIS 2 Collaborative Group. Randomized trial of intravenous streptokinase, oral aspirin, both, or neither among 17 187 cases of suspected acute myocardial infarction: ISIS 2. *Lancet* 1988;**2**:349.

10. Agress CM, Jacobs HI, Clark WG *et al.* Intravenous trypsin in experimental acute myocardial infarction (Abst). *J Pharmacol Exp Ther* 1952;**110**:1.

11. Verstrate M, Bory M, Brower RW *et al.* Randomized trial of intravenous recombinant tissue type plasminogen activator versus intravenous streptokinase in acute myocardial infarction. *Lancet* 1985;**1**:842–7.

12. TIMI Study Group. The Thrombolysis in Myocardial Infarction (TIMI) trial. *N Engl J Med* 1985;**312**:932–6.

13. Collen D. Coronary thrombolysis: streptokinase or recombinant tissue type plasminogen activator? *Ann Intern Med* 1990;**112**:529.

14. The International Study Group. In-hospital mortality and clinical course of 20 891 patients with suspected acute myocardial infarction randomized to altepase and streptokinase with or without heparin. *Lancet* 1990;**2**:71.

15. Anderson JL. Reperfusion, patency and reocclusion with anistreplase (APSAC) in acute myocardial infarction. *Am J Cardiol* 1989;**64**:12A.

16. Anderson JL, Rothbard RL, Hackworthy RA *et al.* Multicentre reperfusion trial of intravenous anisoylated plasminogen activator comples (APSAC) in acute myocardial infarction: controlled comparison with intracoronary streptokinase. *J Am Coll Cardiol* 1988;**11**:1153.

17. Serruys PW, Wijns W, Vab Denbrand M *et al.* Is transluminal coronary angioplasty mandatory after successful thrombolysis? Quantitative coronary angiography study. *Br Heart J* 1983;**50**:257–65.

18. Topol EJ, Califf RM, George BS *et al.* A randomized trial of immediate versus delayed elective angioplasty after intravenous tissue plasminogen activator in acute myocardial infarction. *N Engl J Med* 1987;**317**:501–88.

19. Rothaum DA, Linne Meier TJ, Landin RJ *et al.* Emergency percutaneous transluminal angioplasty in acute myocardial infarction: a three year study experience. *J Am Coll Cardiol* 1987;**10**:204–72.

20. Pepine CJ, Prida X, Hill JA *et al.* Percutaneous transluminal coronary angioplasty in acute myocardial infarction. *Am Heart J* 1984;**107**:820–2.

21. Simoons CJ, Betriu A, Col J *et al.* Thrombolysis with tissue plasminogen activator in acute myocardial infarction: no additional benefit from immediate percutaneous angioplasty. *Lancet* 1990;**1**:197–202.

22. TIMI Research Group: immediate versus delayed catheterization following thrombolytic therapy for acute myocardial infarction. *JAMA* 1988;**260**:2849–50.

23. DeWood MA, Spores J, Notske RW *et al.* Medical and surgical management of myocardial infarction. *Am J Cardiol* 1979;**44**:1356–64.

24. DeWood MA, Spores J, Berg R *et al.* Acute myocardial infarction: a decade of experience with surgical reperfusion in 701 patients. *Circulation* 1983;**68**(Suppl II)8–16.

25. Phillips SJ, Zed RH, Skinner RJ *et al.* Reperfusion protocol and the results in 738 patients with evolving myocardial infarction. *Ann Thorax Surg* 1986;**41**:119–25.

26. Naunheim KS, Kesler KA, Kanter KR *et al.* Coronary artery bypass for recurrent myocardial infarction. Predictors of mortality. *Circulation* 1988;**78**(Suppl K):I-122–8.

27. Floten HS, Ahmad A, Swanson JS *et al.* Long term survival after postinfarction bypass operation: early versus late operation. *Ann Thorac Surg* 1989;**48**:757–63.

28. Applebaum R, House R, Rademaker A *et al.* Coronary artery bypass grafting within thirty days of acute myocardial infarction. Early and late results in 406 patients. *J Thorac Cardiovasc Surg* 1991;**102**:745–52.

29. Lichtenstein SV, Abel JG, Salerno TA. Warm heart surgery and results of operation for recent myocardial infarction. *Ann Thorac Surg* 1991;**52**:455–8.

30. Sintek CF, Pfeffer TA, Khonsari S. Surgical revascularization after acute myocardial infarction. Does timing make a difference? *J Thorac Cardiovasc Surg* 1994;**107**:1317–21.

31. Mathey DG, Rodeward G, Rentrop P *et al.* Intracoronary streptokinase thrombolytic recanalization and subsequent surgical bypass of remaining atherosclerotic stenosis in acute myocardial infarction. *Am Heart J* 1981;**102**:1194–201.

32. Messmer BJ, Uebis R, Rieger C *et al.* Late results after intracoronary thrombolysis and early bypass grafting for acute myocardial infarction. *J Thorac Cardiovasc Surg* 1989;**87**:10–18.

33. Athanasuleas CL, Geer DA, Arciniegas JG *et al.* A reappraisal of surgical intervention for acute myocardial infarction. *J Thorac Cardiovasc Surg* 1987;**93**:405–14.

34. Stuart RS, Baumgartner WA, Soule L *et al.* Predictors of perioperative mortality in patients with unstable angina. *Circulation* 1988;**78**(Suppl I):I-163–5.

35. Deloche A, Fabiani JN, Camilleri JP *et al.* The effect of coronary artery reperfusion on the extent of myocardial infarction. *Am Heart J* 1977;**93**:358.

36. Kereiakes DJ. The role of emergency surgical revascularization in AMI. In: Topol EJ, ed. *Acute coronary intervention.* New York: AR Liss, Wiley, 1987.

37. Gruntzig A. Transluminal dilatation of coronary artery stenosis. *Lancet* 1978;**1**:263.

38. Holmes DR, Holubkov R, Vlietstra RE *et al.* Comparison of complications during percutaneous transluminal coronary angioplasty from 1977 to 1981 and from 1985 to 1986: the National Heart, Lung and Blood Institute percutaneous coronary angioplasty registry. *J Am Coll Cardiol* 1988;**12**:1149–55.

39. Bredlau CE, Roubin GS, Leimgruber PP, Douglas JS, King SB, Grunzig AR. In-hospital morbidity and mortality in patients undergoing elective coronary angioplasty. *Circulation* 1985;**72**:1044–52.

40. Baim DS, Ignatius EJ. Use of percutaneous transluminal coronary angioplasty: results of a current survey. *Am J Cardiol* 1988;**61**:3G–8G.

41. Greene MA, Gray LA Jr, Slater AD, Ganzel BL, Mavroudis C. Emergency aortocoronary artery bypass after failed angioplasty. *Ann Thorac Surg* 1991;**51**:194–9.

42. Sinclair IN, McCabe CH, Sipperly ME, Baim DS. Predictors, therapeutic options and long term outcome of abrupt reclosure. *Am J Cardiol* 1988;**61**:61G.

43. Atkins CW, Block PC. Surgical intervention for failed percutaneous transluminal coronary angioplasty. *Am J Cardiol* 1984;**53**:108C–11C.

44. Cowley MJ, Dorros G, Kelsey SF, Van Raden M, Detre KM. Emergency coronary artery bypass surgery after coronary angioplasty: the National Heart, Lung and Blood Institute's percutaneous transluminal coronary angioplasty registry experience. *Am J Cardiol* 1984;**53**:22C–6C.

45. Golding LAR, Loop FD, Hollman JL *et al*. Early results of emergency surgery after coronary angioplasty. *Circulation* 1986;**74**:III-26–9.

46. Killen DA, Hamaker WR, Reed WA. Coronary artery bypass following percutaneous transluminal coronary angioplasty. *Ann Thorac Surg* 1985;**40**:133–8.

47. Pelletier LC, Pardini A, Renkin J, David PR, Hebert Y, Bourassa MG: myocardial revascularization after failure of percutaneous transluminal angioplasty. *J Thorac Cardiovasc Surg* 1985;**90**:265–71.

48. Reul GJ, Cooley DA, Hallman GL *et al*. Coronary artery bypass for unsuccessful percutaneous transluminal coronary angioplasty. *J Thorac Cardiovasc Surg* 1984;**88**:685–94.

49. Roberts AJ, Faro RS, Rubin MR *et al*. Emergency coronary artery bypass graft surgery for threatened acute myocardial infarction related to coronary artery catheterisation. *Ann Thorac Surg* 1985;**39**:116–24.

50. Talley JD, Jones EL, Weintraub WS, King SB. Coronary artery bypass surgery after failed elective percutaneous transluminal coronary angioplasty. *Circulation* 1989;**79**:I-126–31.

51. Klepzig H, Kober G, Satter P, Kalternbach M. Analysis of 100 emergency aortocoronary bypass operation after percutaneous transluminal coronary angioplasty: Which patients are at risk for large infarctions. *Eur Heart J* 1991;**12**:946–51.

52. Kinoshita T, Makino S, Saito K, Fuji H. Emergency coronary bypass after failed coronary angioplasty. *Japanese J Thorac Surg* 1992;**45**:294–8.

53. Buffet P, Villemot JP, Danchin N, Amrein D *et al*. Emergency coronary surgery after transluminal angioplasty. Immediate results and long term outcome of 100 operations. *Archives des Maladies du Coeur et des Vaisseaux* 1992;**85**:17–23.

54. Gruentzig AR, Senning A, Siegenthaler WE. Nonoperative dilatation of coronary artery stenosis. Percutaneous transluminal coronary angioplasty. *N Engl J Med* 1979;**301**:61–8.

55. Powney JG, Bonser RS, Lentini S. Emergency coronary surgery after refractory cardiac arrest: a single centre experience. *Br Heart J* 1992;**67**:392–4.

56. Caes FL, Van Nooten GJ. Use of internal mammary artery for emergency grafting after failed coronary angioplasty. *Ann Thorac Surg* 1994;**57**:1295– 9.

57. Reddy SG, Roberts WC. Frequency of rupture of the left ventricular free wall or ventricular septum among necropsy cases of fatal acute myocardial infarction since introduction of coronary care units. *Am J Cardiol* 1989;**63**:906–11.

58. Brandt B, Wright CB, Ehrenhaft JL. Ventricular septal defect following myocardial infarction. *Ann Thorac Surg* 1979;**27**:580–9.

59. Hill JD, Larry D, Kerth WJ *et al*. Acquired ventricular septal defects. *J Thorac Cardiovasc Surg* 1975;**70**:440–50.

60. Swithinbank JM. Perforation of the interventricular septum after myocardial infarction. *Br Heart J* 1959;**21**:562.

61. Miyamoto AT, Lee ME, Kass RM *et al*. Postmyocardial infarction VSD. Improved outlook. *J Thorac Cardiovasc Surg* 1983;**86**:4–6.

62. Daggett WM, Buckley MJ, Akins CW *et al*. Improved results of surgical management of postinfarction ventricular septal rupture. *Ann Surg* 1982;**196**:269–77.

63. Fananapazier L, Bray CL, Dark JF, Moussalli H, Deiraniya AK, Lawson RAM. Right ventricular dysfunction and surgical outcome in postinfarction ventricular septal defect. *Eur Heart J* 1983;**4**:155–67.

64. Dellborg M, Held P, Swedberg K, Vedin A. Rupture of the myocardium. Occurrence and risk factors. *Br Heart J* 1985;**54**:11–16.

65. Skehan JD, Carey C, Norrell MS, de Belder M, Balcon R, Mills PG. Patterns of coronary artery disease in post-infarction ventricular septal ruptures. *Br Heart J* 1989;**62**:268.

66. Skillington PD, Davis RH, Luff AJ *et al.* Surgical treatment for infarct-related ventricular septal defects. *J Thorac Cardiovasc Surg* 1990;**99**:798–808.

67. Parry G, Goudevenos J, Adams PC, Reid DS. Septal rupture after myocardial infarction: is very early surgery really worthwhile. *Eur Heart J* 1992;**13**:373–82.

68. Helmcke F, Mahan EF, Nanda NC *et al.* Two-dimensional echocardiography and doppler color flow mapping in the diagnosis and prognosis of ventricular septal rupture. *Circulation* 1990;**81**:1775–83.

69. Smyllie JH, Sutherland GR, Geuskens R, Dawkins K, Conway N, Roelandt JR. Doppler color flow mapping in the diagnosis of ventricular septal rupture and acute mitral regurgitation after myocardial infarction. *J Am Coll Cardiol* 1990;**15**:1449–55.

70. Bansal RC, Eng AK, Shakudo M. Role of two-dimensional echocardiography, pulsed, continuous wave color flow doppler techniques in the assessment of ventricular septal rupture after myocardial infarction. *Am J Cardiol* 1990;**65**:852–60.

71. Blanche C, Khan SS, Matloff JM *et al.* Results of early repair of ventricular septal defect after acute myocardial infarction. *J Thorac Cardiovasc Surg* 1992;**104**:961–5.

72. Muehrcke DD, Daggett WM, Mortimer JB, Akins CW, Hilgenberg AD, Austen WG. Postinfarction ventricular septal defect repair: Effect of coronary artery bypass grafting. *Ann Thorac Surg* 1992;**54**:876–83.

73. Oyamada A, Queen FB. Spontaneous rupture of an interventricular septum following acute myocardial infarction with some clinicopathological observations of survival in five cases. Presented at the Pan-Pacific Pathology Congress, Tripler US Army Hospital, Honolulu, Hawaii, 12 October 1961.

74. Saunders RJ, Kern WH, Blount SG Jr. Perforation of the interventricular septum complicating myocardial infarction: A report of eight cases, one with cardiac catheterisation. *Am Heart J* 1956;**51**:736–48.

75. Lemery R, Smith HC, Giuliani ER, Gersh BJ. Prognosis in rupture of the ventricular septum after acute myocardial infarction and role of early surgical intervention. *Am J Cardiol* 1992;**70**:147–51.

76. Komeda M, Fremes SE, David TE. Surgical repair of postinfarction ventricular septal defect. *Circulation* 1990;**982**(suppl):IV-243–7.

77. Loisance DY, Cachera JP, Poulain H *et al.* Ventricular septal defect after acute myocardial infarction. *J Thorac Cardiovasc Surg* 1975;**70**:440–50.

78. Jones MT *et al.* Surgical repair of acquired ventricular septal defect. Determinants of early and late outcome. *J Thorac Cardiovasc Surg* 1987;**93**:680–6.

79. Deville C, Fontan F, Chevalier JM, Madonna F, Ebner A, Besse P. Surgery of post-infarction ventricular septal defects: Risk factors for hospital death and long-term survival. *Eur J Cardio-Thorac Surg* 1991;**5**:167–74.

80. Teo WS, Tong MC, Quek SS, Tan AT, Ong KK. Ventricular septal rupture in acute myocardial infarction. *Annals of the Academy of Medicine, Singapore* 1990;**19**:15–22.

81. Davies RH, Dawkins KD, Skillingon PD *et al*. Late functional results after surgical closure of acquired ventricular defect. *J Thorac Cardiovasc Surg* 1993;**106**:592–8.

82. Guiliani ER, Danielson GK, Pluth JR, Odyniec NA, Wallace RB. Postinfarction ventricular septal rupture. *Circular* 1974;**49**:455–9.

83. Held AC, Cole PL, Lipton B *et al*. Rupture of the interventricular septum complicating acute myocardial infarction: a multicentre analysis of clinical findings and outcome. *Am Heart J* 1988;**93**:1330–6.

84. Baillot R, Pelletier C, Trivino-Mavin J *et al*. Postinfarction VSD: delayed closure with prolonged mechanical circulatory support. *Ann Thor Surg* 1983;**35**:138–42.

85. Estrada-Quintero T, Uretsky BF, Murali S, Hardesty RL. Prolonged intraaortic balloon support for septal rupture after myocardial infarction. *Ann Thorac Surg* 1992;**53**:335–7.

86. Benton JP, Barker KS. Transcatheter closure of ventricular septal defect: a nonsurgical approach to the care of the patient with acute ventricular septal rupture. *Heart Lung* 1992;**21**:256–64.

87. Cooley DA, Belmonte BA, Zeis LB, Schur S. *et al*. 1957. Surgical repair of ruptured interventricular septum following acute myocardial infarction. *Surgery* **42**:930–7.

88. Hanson EC, Daggett WM. Surgery for complications of myocardial infarction. In: Wheatley DJ, ed. *Surgery for coronary artery disease* London: Chapman & Hall, 1986, pp. 503–22.

89. Koh Y, Kitanura N, Shuntoh K, Kawashima M, Tatebayashi T, Yamaguchi A. A successful transatrial repair of post-infarction ventricular septal defect. *Journal of the Japanese Association for Thoracic Surgery* 1992;**40**:1733–7.

90. Seguin JR, Frapier JM, Colson P, Chaptal PA. Fibrin sealant for early repair of acquired ventricular septal defect. *J Thorac Cardiovasc Surg* 1992;**104**:748–51.

91. Daggett WM. Surgical technique for early repair of posterior ventricular septal defects. *J Thorac Cardiovasc Surg* 1982;**84**:306–12.

92. Hendren WG, Nemec JJ, Lytle BW *et al*. Mitral valve repair for ischaemic mitral insufficiency. *Ann Thorac Surg* 1991;**52**:1246–52.

93. Kratz JM, Crawford FA, Sade RM, Crumbley AJ, Stroud MR. St Jude prosthesis for aortic and mitral valve replacement: a ten year experience. *Ann Thorac Surg* 1993;**56**:462–8.

94. Heikkila J. Mitral incompetence complicating acute myocardial infarction. *Br Heart J* 1967;**29**:162–9.

95. Loperfido F, Biasucci LM, Pennestri F *et al*. Pulsed doppler echocardiography analysis of mitral regurgitation after myocardial infarction. *Am J Cardiol* 1986;**58**:692–7.

96. Barzilai B, Davis VG, Stone PH, Jaffe AS and the MILIS Group. Prognostic significance of mitral regurgitation in acute myocardial infarction. *Am J Cardiol* 1990;**65**:1169–75.

97. Lehmann KG, Francis CK, Dodge HT and the TIMI Study Group. Mitral regurgitation in early myocardial infarction. *Ann Int Med* 1992;**117**:10–17.

98. Kranidis A, Koulouris S, Filippatos G, Sideris A, Anthopoulos L. Mitral regurgitation from pappillary muscle rupture: role of transesophageal echocardiography. *J Heart Valve Dis* 1993;**2**:529–32.

99. Tcheng JE, Jackman JD, Nelson CL *et al*. Outcome of patients sustaining acute ischaemic mitral regurgitation during myocardial infarction. *Ann Int Med* 1992;**177**:18–24.

100. Wei JY, Hutchins GM, Bulkley BH. Papillary muscle rupture and fatal acute myocardial infarction. *Ann Int Med* 1979;**90**:149–53.

101. Sanders RJ, Neubuerger KT, Ravin A. Rupture of papillary muscles: Occurrence of rupture of the posterior muscle and posterior myocardial infarction. *Dis Chest* 1957;**31**:316–23.

102. Miller DC, Stinson EB. Surgical management of acute mechanical defects secondary to myocardial infarction. *Am J Surg* 1981;**141**:677–83.

103. Radford MJ, Johnson RA, Buckley MJ *et al*. Survival following mitral valve replacement for mitral regurgitation due to coronary artery disease. *Circulation* 1979;**60**(suppl I):I39–47.

104. Tepe NA, Edmunds LH Jr. Operation for acute post-infarction mitral insufficiency and cardiogenic shock. *J Thorac Cardiovasc Surg* 1985;**89**:525–30.

105. Andrade IG, Cartier R, Panisi P, Ennabli K, Grondin CM. Factors influencing early and late survival in patients with combined mitral valve replacement and myocardial revascularisation and in those with isolated replacement. *Ann Thorac Surg* 1987;**44**:607–13.

106. David TE, Ho WC. The effect of preservation of chordae tendineae on mitral valve replacement for post-infarction mitral regurgitation. *Circulation* 1986;**74**:I-116–20.

107. Nishimura RA, Schaff HV, Shub C, Gersh BJ, Edwards WD, Tajik AJ. Papillary muscle rupture complicating acute myocardial infarction: Analysis of 17 patients. *Am J Cardiol* 1983;**57**:373–7.

108. Yadav KS, Ross JK, Monro JL, Shore DF. Study of the risk factors related to early mortality following combined mitral valve replacement and coronary artery bypass grafting. *J Thorac Cardiovasc Surg* 1985;**33**:16–19.

109. Rankin JS, Fenely MP, Hickey MSt J *et al*. A clinical comparison of mitral valve repair versus replacement in ischaemic mitral regurgitation. *J Thorac Cardiovasc Surg* 1988;**95**:165–77.

110. Defraigne JO, Lavigne JP, Remy D, Dekoster G, Limet R. Mitral valve replacement in postinfarction rupture of the papillary muscle. *Archives des Maladies du Coeur et des Vaisseaux* 1990;**83**:377–82.

111. Loisance DY, Deleuze P, Hillion ML, Cachera JP. Are there indications for reconstruction surgery in severe mitral regurgitation after acute myocardial infarction? *Eur J Cardiovasc Surg* 1990;**4**:394–7.

112. Reinfeld HB, Samet P, Hildner FJ. Resolution of congestive failure, mitral regurgitation, and angina after percutaneous transluminal coronary angioplasty of triple vessel disease. *Cathet Cardiovasc Diagn* 1985;**11**:273–7.

113. Heuser RR, Maddoux GL, Goss JE, Ramo BW, Raff GL, Shadoff N. Coronary angioplasty for acute mitral regurgitation due to myocardial infarction. *Ann Intern Med* 1987;**107**:852–5.

114. Shawl FA, Forman MB, Punja S, Goldbaum TS. Emergency coronary angioplasty in the treatment of acute ischaemic mitral regurgitation: Long term results in 5 cases. *J Am Coll Cardiol* 1989;**14**:986–91.

115. Kay JH, Zubiate P, Mendez MA, Vanstrom N, Yokoyama T, Gharavi M. Surgical treatment for mitral insufficiency secondary to coronary artery disease. *J Thorac Cardiovasc Surg* 1980;**79**:12–18.

116. Pinson CW, Cobanoglu A, Metzdorff, Grunkemeier GL, Kay PH, Starr A. Late surgical results for ischaemic mitral regurgitation. *J Thorac Cardiovasc Surg* 1984;**88**:663–72.

117. Czer LSC, Gray RJ, DeRobertis MA *et al*. Mitral valve replacement: Impact of coronary artery disease and determinants of prognosis after revascularisation. *Circulation* 1984;**70**:I198–207.

118. McGovern JA, Pennock JL, Campbell DB, Pierce WS, Waldhausen JA. Risk of mitral valve replacement and mitral valve replacement with coronary artery bypass. *Ann Thorac Surg* 1985;**39**:346–52.

119. Connolly MW, Gelbfish JS, Jacobowitz IJ *et al*. Surgical results for mitral regurgitation from coronary artery disease. *J Thorac Cardiovasc Surg* 1986;**91**:379–88.

120. Vidal V, Langanay T, Corbineau H *et al*. Mitral valve replacement in postinfarction mitral insufficiency. Immediate and long term results of a series of 39 surgically treated patients. *Archives des Maladies du Coeur et des Vaisseaux* 1991;**84**:1419–24.

121. Czer LSC, Maurer G, Trento A *et al*. Comparative efficacy of ring and suture annuloplasty for ischaemic mitral regurgitation. *Circulation* 1992;**86**(Suppl II):II46–52.

122. Cosgrove DM, Loop FD. Ventricular aneurysms. In: Wheatly DJ, ed. *Surgery of coronary artery disease*, London: Chapman & Hall, 1986:pp. 449–61.

123. Cosgrove DM, Loop FD, Irarrazaval MG, Groves LK, Taylor PC. Determination of long term survival after ventricular aneurysmectomy. *Ann Thorac Surg* 1978;**26**:357–63.

124. Couper GS, Bunton RW, Birjiniuk V *et al*. Relative risk of left ventricular aneurysmectomy in patients with akinetic scars versus true dyskinetic aneurysms. *Circulation* 1990;**82** (5 Suppl):IV248–56.

125. Samani NJ, Mauric AT, Nair S, Thompson J, De Bono DP. Ventricular aneurysmectomy: indications, operative findings and outcome at a single centre. *Quart J Med* 1994;**87**:41–8.

126. Rao G, Zikria EA, Miller WH *et al*. Experience with 60 consecutive ventricular aneurysm resections. *Circulation* 1974;**49**(Suppl 2):149–53.

127. Barrett-Boyes BG, White HD, Agnew TM, Pewberton JR, Wild C. The results of surgical treatment of left ventricular aneurysms: an assessment of the risk factors affecting early and late mortality. *J Thorac Cardiovasc Surg* 1984;**87**:87–98.

128. Komeda M, David TE, Malik A, Ivanov J, Sun Z. Operative risk and long term results of operation for left ventricular aneurysm. *Ann Thorac Surg* 1992;**53**:22–8.

129. Froehlich RT, Falsetti HL, Doty DB, Marcus ML. Prospective study of surgery for left ventricular aneurysm. *Am J Cardiol* 1980;**45**:923–31.

130. Schlichter J, Hellerstein HK, Katz LN. Aneurysm of the heart: correlative study of 102 proved cases. *Medicine* 1954;**33**:43–86.

131. Dubnow RE, Burchell HB, Titus JL. Postinfarction ventricular aneurysm. A clinicomorphological and electrocardiographic study of 80 cases. *Am Heart J* 1965;**70**:753–60.

132. Nagle RE, Williams DO. Natural history of ventricular aneurysm without surgical treatment (abstr.) *Br Heart J* 1974;**36**:1037.

133. Schattenberg TT, Giuliani ER, Campion BC, Danielson GK Jr. Postinfarction ventricular aneurysm. *Mayo Clin Proc* 1970;**45**:13–19.

134. Bruschke AV, Proudfit WL, Sones FM Jr. Progress study of 590 consecutive non-surgical cases of coronary disease followed five–nine years. II. Ventriculographic and other correlation. *Circulation* 1973;**47**:1154–63.

135. Grondin P, Kretz JG, Bical O *et al*. Natural history of saccular aneurysm of the left ventricle. *J Thorac Cardiovasc Surg* 1979;**77**:57–64.

136. Faxon DP, Ryan TJ, Davis *et al*. Prognostic significance of angiographically documented left ventricular aneurysm from the coronary artery surgery study (CASS). *Am J Cardiol* 1982;**50**:157–64.

137. Heras M, Sanz G, Betriu L, Mont L, De Flores T, Navarro-Lopez F. Does left ventricular aneurysm influence survival after acute myocardial infarction? *Eur Heart J* 1990;**11**:441–6.

138. Shen WF, Tribouilloy C, Mirode A, Dufosse H, Lesbre JP. Left ventricular aneurysm and prognosis in patients with first acute transmural anterior myocardial infarction and isolated left anterior descending artery disease. *Eur Heart J* 1992;**13**:39–44.

139. Benediktsson R, Eyjolfsson O, Thorgeirsson G. Natural history of chronic left ventricular aneurysm; a population based cohort study. *J Clin Epidemiol* 1991;**44**:1131–9.

140. Baciewicz PA, Weintraub WS, Jones EL *et al*. Late follow-up after repair of left ventricular aneurysm and (usually) associated coronary bypass grafting. *Am J Cardiol* 1991;**68**:193–200.

141. Kesler KA, Fiore AC, Naunheim KS *et al*. Anterior wall left ventricular aneurysm repair. A comparison of linear versus circular closure. *J Thorac Cardiovasc Surg* 1992;**103**:841–7.

142. Elefteriades JA, Solomon LW, Salazar AM, Batsford WP, Baldwin JC, Kopf GS. Linear left ventricular aneurysmectomy: modern imaging studies reveal improved morphology and function. *Ann Thorac Surg* 1993;**56**:242–50.

143. Stahle E, Bergstrom R, Nystrom SO, Edlund B, Sjogren I, Holmberg L. Surgical treatment of left ventricular aneurysm: assessment of risk factors for early and late mortality. *Eur J Cardiothorac Surg* 1994;**8**:67–73.

144. Coltharp WH, Hoff SJ, Stoney WS *et al*. Ventricular aneurysmectomy. A 25 year experience. *Ann Surg* 1994;**219**:707–13.

145. Mickleborough LL, Maruyama H, Liu P, Mohamed S. Results of left ventricular aneurysmectomy with a tailored scar excision and primary closure technique. *J Thorac Cardiovasc Surg* 1994;**107**:690–8.

146. Rackley CE, Russell RO, Mantle JA, Rogers WJ. Modern approach to the patient with acute myocardial infarction. *Curr Probl Cardiol* 1977;**1**:1–47.

147. Mills NL, Everson CT, Hockmuth DR. Technical advances in the treatment of left ventricular aneurysm. *Ann Thorac Surg* 1993;**55**:792–800.

148. Di Donato M, Barletta G, Maioli M *et al*. Early haemodynamic results of left ventricular reconstructive surgery for anterior wall left ventricular aneurysm. *Am J Cardiol* 1992;**69**:886–90.

149. Salati M, Di Biasi P, Paje A, Cialfi A, Bozzi G, Santoli C. Functional results of left ventricular reconstruction. *Ann Thorac Surg* 1993;**56**:316–22.

150. Cooley DA, Collins HA, Morris GC, Chapman DW. Ventricular aneurysm after myocardial infarction: Surgical excision with temporary cardiopulmonary bypass. *JAMA* 1958;**167**:557–60.

151. Daggett WM, Guyton RA, Mundth ED *et al*. Surgery for post-myocardial infarct ventricular septal defect. *Ann Surg* 1977;**186**:260–71.

152. Jatene AD. Left ventricular aneurysmectomy. *J Thorac Cardiovasc Surg* 1985;**89**:321–31.

153. Dor V, Saab M, Coste P, Kornaszewski M, Montiglio F. Left ventricular aneurysm: a new surgical approach. *J Thorac Cardiovasc Surg* 1989;**37**:11–19.

154. Cooley DA, Ventricular endoaneurysmorrhaphy; a simplified repair for extensive post infarction aneurysm *J Card Surg* 1989;**4**:200–5.

155. Cooley DA. Repair of post-infarction aneurysm of the left ventricle. In: Cooley DA, ed. *Cardiac Surgery: state of the art reviews*. Vol. 4, No 2, Philadelphia: Handley and Belfus 1990:p. 309.

156. Bates RJ, Beutler S, Resnekov L, Anagnostopoulos CE. Cardiac rupture. Challenge in diagnosis and management. *Am J Cardiol* 1977;**40**:429–37.

157. Martin RH, Almond CH, Saab S, Watson LE. True and false aneurysms of the left ventricle following myocardial infarction. *Ann J Med* 1977;**62**:418–24.

158. Vlodaver Z, Coe JI, Edwards JE. True and false left aneurysms: propensity for the latter to rupture. *Circulation* 1975;**51**:567–72.

159. Padro JM, Mesa JM, Silvestre J *et al.* Subacute cardiac rupture: repair with a sutureless technique. *Ann Thorac Surg* 1993;**55**:20–3.

160. Bolooki H. Emergency cardiac procedures in patients in cardiogenic shock due to complications of coronary artery disease. *Circulation* 1989;79(suppl I):I-137–48.

161. Lopez-Sendon J, Gonalez A, Lopez de Sa E *et al.* Diagnosis of subacute ventricular wall rupture after acute myocardial infarction: sensitivity of specificity of clinical, haemodynamic and echocardiographic criteria. *J Am Coll Cardiol* 1992;**19**:1145–53.

12 Alternative approaches for coronary artery bypass grafting

Steven S.L. Tsui and John J. Dunning

The past decade has seen a wave of enthusiasm for the use of limited access and minimally invasive techniques in the performance of surgical procedures. The rationale for using these approaches is to reduce the morbidity associated with surgical procedures, thereby minimizing the amount of time taken for patients to recover from their operations. This should in turn reduce the postoperative hospital stay and consequently enable an earlier return to normal for the patients. Cardiac surgery is no exception to this vogue. Over the recent years, many surgeons have developed ingenious methods, some of which are less invasive than the conventional approaches. Minimally invasive approaches have been described for most routine cardiac surgical procedures including coronary artery bypass grafting (CABG) valvular repairs and replacements.

Conventional CABG, which involves a median sternotomy incision and cardiopulmonary bypass, has excellent results with proven benefits from a number of prospective randomized clinical trials. It has been accepted as the treatment of choice over medical therapy for certain patient groups with advanced ischaemic heart disease because it provides improved long-term survival as well as superior symptomatic relief. Inevitably, an operation of this magnitude is accompanied by a small but definite risk of mortality and morbidity. Most of the risks are related to the use of cardiopulmonary bypass, inadequate myocardial protection, surgical incisions to access the heart, and harvesting of bypass conduits. In patients with less severe coronary artery disease who are unlikely to gain significant survival benefit from undergoing CABG, these risks may be more difficult to justify. Therefore, alternative means of coronary revascularization have been developed in the hope that myocardial ischaemia can be relieved without the attending risks of conventional CABG. These include balloon angioplasty, coronary atheromectomy, and stenting of coronary artery lesions. Although these trans-catheter procedures are reasonably efficacious with a lower morbidity and shorter recovery time than conventional CABG, there is continued concern over their long-term results (1,2). This has been the impetus for the development of more definitive procedures that can provide the excellent long-term results of standard CABG while minimizing the injuries associated with the conventional operation. Advances in surgical techniques and instrumentation have facilitated the performance of these procedures over the recent years. We will discuss some of the approaches that are in use or currently under development.

Historical perspectives

CABG without cardiopulmonary bypass was first successfully performed in Leningrad by Kolessov in 1964. The patient was a 45 year old man who had chronic angina. The operation

Table 12.1 Alternative approaches for coronary artery bypass grafting

- Minimal access incisions
    Mini-sternotomy incision
    Small anterior thoracotomy incision
    Video-assisted thoracoscopic access

- *Alternative methods for institution of CPB*
    Femoro-femoral cannulation for CPB
    Endovascular Cardiopulmonary Bypass System (Heartport Inc.)

- *CABG without cardiopulmonary bypass*
    No circulatory support
    Intra-aortic balloon pump
    Hemopump
    Jarvik Cannula Pump

- *Minimal access vein harvesting*
    Mayo vein dissector
    Endoscopic vein harvesting

involved a left thoracotomy incision and the left internal mammary artery (LIMA) was anastomosed to the circumflex branch of the left coronary artery on a beating heart without extracorporeal support (3,4). Other surgeons, including Garrett from Houston and Favaloro from the Cleveland Clinic, also described CABG without cardiopulmonary bypass using reversed saphenous veins (5,6). However, most surgeons abandoned these techniques in favour of CABG using cardiopulmonary bypass since this provided added safety, accuracy, and versatility (7).

Current alternative approaches

A multitude of different techniques have been described which enables direct coronary artery bypass (Table 12.1). These techniques can either be use singly or in combination with each other. They share the common goal of surgically bypassing coronary artery lesions whilst reducing the injurious effects of the operation on the body.

Minimal access incisions

A median sternotomy incision is without doubt the most versatile approach for multivessel CABG through a single incision. It enables easy harvesting of both internal mammary arteries and unrestricted access to all epicardial coronary arteries. However, some morbidity does exist from this incision. The most devastating complication is sternal wound dehiscence. Even with aggressive management, this is still accompanied by considerable mortality and morbidity.

A partial sternotomy incision can often provide exposure comparable to a full sternotomy. The patient is placed in the supine position and a skin incision is made from the level of the manubriosternal joint to the fifth costal cartilage. At either end of the incision, the skin is undermined to increase exposure of the underlying sternum. An oscillating saw is used to make the sternotomy which commences at the jugular notch in the midline and exits at the left fourth or fifth costosternal space. If difficulty is encountered with sternal spreading, a complete transverse sternotomy can be performed at this level (8). This incision allows good access to the right coronary artery (RCA) as well as the left anterior descending artery (LAD) and its diagonal branches.

To allow harvesting of the right gastroepiploic artery and exposure of the posterior descending branch of the right coronary artery, a lower midline incision extending into the epigastrium is used. The xiphisternum is excised and the peritoneum is entered. Elevation of the lower end of the sternum often facilitates exposure of the inferior surface of the heart, especially when pericardial adhesions are present from a previous sternotomy incision. Although the time necessary for a partial sternotomy to heal should be no different from a full sternotomy, it is thought to provide improved chest wall mechanics postoperatively and has the advantage that patients can resume activity earlier (8).

An alternative approach is via a small anterior thoracotomy incision. The patient is placed in the supine position with an anterolateral tilt of 20–30°. A submammary incision is made over the fourth intercostal space and the pleural cavity can be entered if necessary. This allows limited mobilization of the distal internal mammary artery (IMA). Early experience with this approach gave rise to concerns about kinking of the IMA on the chest wall when an insufficient length is mobilized. Possibility of the steal syndrome from patent first and second intercostal branches was also noted. With the use of a specially developed IMA retractor (Cardio Thoracic systems, Cupertino, CA), it is now possible to harvest the IMA from its origin to the level of the fifth costal cartilage (Fig. 12.1). It is sometimes necessary to excise a costal cartilage to avoid

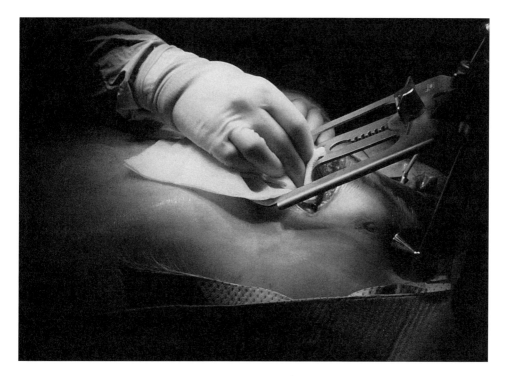

Fig. 12.1 Submammary incision with a special retractor in place for mobilization of the internal mammary artery pedicle. See also colour plate section (Plate 6).

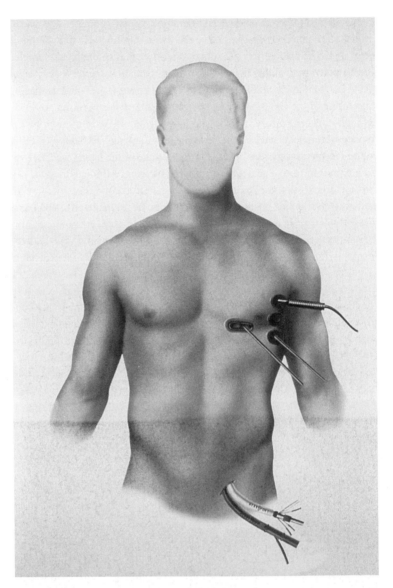

Fig. 12.2 Location of ports in the third, fourth and fifth intercostal spaces in the mid-axillary line for thoracoscopic mobilization of the internal mammary artery. Femoral arterial and venous cut-down for insertion of the Endovascular Cardiopulmonary Bypass System (Heartport Inc., Redwood City, CA). See also colour plate section (Plate 7).

excessive retraction of the intercostal space. On the left-hand side, a longitudinal incision can be made in the pericardium 1 cm lateral to the LIMA and the heart can be delivered into the wound by pericardial retraction stitches for exposure of the LAD. On the right-hand side, access and mobilization of the RIMA for grafting to the mid-RCA can be performed.

Video-assisted thoracoscopy can also be used for mobilization of the IMA. A double-lumen endotracheal tube is placed to allow single lung ventilation. A trocar is inserted in the fourth intercostal space in the mid or posterior axillary lines through which a standard 10 mm 0° thoracoscope is positioned. Further instrument ports are made in the third and fifth intercostal spaces

(Fig. 12.2). The IMA is visualized by video images and is mobilized from the subclavian vein to the level of the xiphoid process with diathermy and endoscopic ligaclips (9,10). If a small anterior thoracotomy is to be used for direct anastomosis of the IMA to the LAD, this incision can be used to facilitate thoracoscopic take down of the distal IMA (11). With experience, this part of the procedure can be completed within 20 minutes (12).

Alternative methods for CPB

When a median sternotomy incision is used for CABG, the institution of CPB via standard ascending aortic and right atrial cannulations is easily performed. However, when small anterior thoracotomy incisions are used, CBP is not so readily instituted. Surgeons who prefer to conduct coronary anastomosis on a non-beating heart via a small incision can use femoro-femoral cannulation for CPB. The Endovascular Cardiopulmonary Bypass System developed by Heartport Inc. (Redwood City, CA) is inserted by way of a femoral artery and vein cutdown. The right side of the heart is decompressed with an endopulmonary vent inserted via the internal jugular vein. The

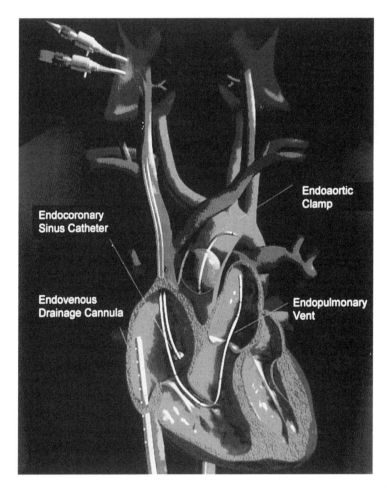

Fig. 12.3 The Endovascular Cardiopulmonary Bypass System developed by Heartport Inc. (Redwood City, CA). See also colour plate section (Plate 8).

ascending aorta can be occluded by an endoaortic balloon occlusion catheter. The central lumen of this endoaortic clamp is then used for the delivery of cardioplegic solution and for venting of the aortic root (11) (Fig. 12.3).

For those who prefer to perform coronary surgery on a fibrillating heart through a small anterior thoracotomy incision, hypothermic fibrillatory arrest (13) or electrically induced fibrillation can be used once the patient has been placed on femoro-femoral bypass. As the aorta is not cross clamped, the myocardium is continuously perfused. To prevent distention of the fibrillating heart, it is important to vent the left ventricular cavity with a suction catheter via a stab incision in the apex.

CABG without cardiopulmonary bypass

Although current methods of cardiopulmonary bypass are remarkably safe, it is widely recognized that numerous pathophysiological abnormalities do occur with the use of cardiopulmonary bypass. These changes result in injury to all organ systems in the body (14). They can arrange from common and self-limiting effects such as the generalized inflammatory response to more serious and permanent neurological injuries. Concerns over these problems have led to a resurgence of interest in CABG without cardiopulmonary bypass (CPB) during the 1980s. The avoidance of CPB may be particularly beneficial in high-risk patients such as those with renal failure, respiratory problems, advanced age, cerebrovascular accidents, and other systemic diseases.

Several series of CABG without CPB have been reported documenting the advantages of the technique (15–19). Most of these are performed via a standard median sternotomy incision, although some are performed via a left anterior thoracotomy incision. The LIMA is dissected simultaneously with harvesting of the long saphenous vein or other conduits as necessary. The pericardium is opened and traction sutures are applied to the edges of the pericardium to displace the heart anteriorly. Patients are usually heparinized with half the dose normally used for cardiopulmonary bypass (1.5–2.0 mg/kg). Sponges can be placed behind the heart to improve exposure of the target coronary artery. Fixation of the anastomotic site is achieved with deep stay sutures around the coronary artery proximal and distal to the site selected for the arteriotomy. The stay sutures can be snared with thin silicone tubing to facilitate a dry operative field. The anastomosis between the conduit and the coronary artery is then completed with standard techniques. In cases of multiple grafts, the coronary artery with the most severe stenosis or occlusion is bypassed first. In addition to the usual electrocardiogram and haemodynamic monitoring, continuous transoesophageal echocardiography is often used to detect segmental wall motion abnormality which may occur when snares are applied to non-occluded coronary arteries. These changes are usually transient and revert to normal when the anastomosis has been completed and the snares removed. Ischaemic preconditioning of the myocardium can be performed prior to snaring of the vessel for bypass grafting.

The main challenges in CABG without CPB are twofold. First, displacement of the heart for exposure of coronary arteries followed by their occlusion with snares may give rise to haemodynamic instability. In practice, this is only a problem during exposure of the marginal branches of the circumflex artery. This instability can be exacerbated by the use of drugs that reduce heart rate and contractility. Rapid fluid infusion with administration of vasocontrictors or inotropes usually stabilize the blood pressure. Otherwise, the heart can be returned to its normal position until an intra-aortic balloon pump is inserted for haemodynamic support (20). Other mechanical devices such as the Hemopump (Medtronic, Minneapolis, MN) (21) and the Jarvik Cannula

Pump (Jarvik Research, NY) (22) have been proposed as alternatives to CPB for CABG. Both of these devices can offload the left ventricle and provide non-pulsatile flows of up to 4.8 and 5.0 L/min respectively. The obvious advantage of these devices is the avoidance of exposure of blood to artificial surfaces of a pump oxygenator. However, both of these devices require careful positioning in the left ventricular cavity, traversing the aortic valve into the ascending aorta. Displacement of the device can occur with manipulation of the heart resulting in failure of support. Furthermore, there is the potential for damage to the aortic valve, mitral valve and to the left ventricle. It is therefore difficult to see how these devices in their current forms can replace CPB for CABG.

A simpler option is to bypass the left heart alone (23). Here, the left atrial appendage is cannulated and the oxygenated blood is drained and pumped back into the aorta. The advantage of this approach is that the heart can better tolerate the distortion required for exposure of the more posteriorly placed coronary branches while avoiding the need for an oxygenator.

The other challenge in CABG without CPB is the performance of coronary anastomosis on a beating heart. This can be facilitated by reductions in the systemic blood pressure and heart rate with drugs such as verapamil, esmolol and adenosine (10,24). Epicardial stay sutures are also routinely used on either side of the arteriotomy to reduce motion of the target vessel. Movement can be further reduced by specially developed coronary artery stabilizers such as those from CardioThoracic Systems, Inc. (Cupertino, CA) (Fig. 12.4). These instruments essentially consists of two parallel blades that are used to apply pressure on the surface of the heart either side of the target vessel. They are available either as a hand-held instrument or as an attachment to a full retractor system. Early experience suggests that they are both simple to use and effective (25).

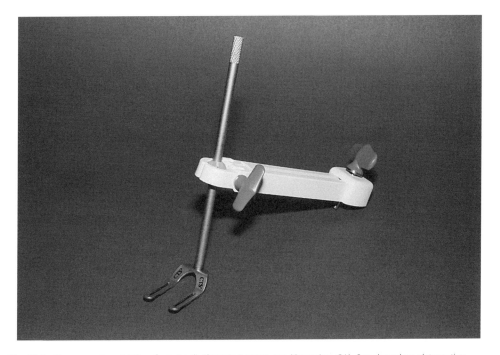

Fig. 12.4 Coronary artery stabilizer from CardioThoracic Systems, Inc. (Cupertino, CA). See also colour plate section (Plate 9).

Buffolo and associates reported on their experience with 1274 cases of CABG without CPB (24). Patients received an average of 1.7 grafts, the majority of which were to the LAD or the RCA. Mean hospital stay was 5.2 days compared with 9.6 days for patients operated on with CPB. The in-hospital mortality was 2.5%. In a subgroup of 30 patients studied prospectively, the patency rate of LIMA to LAD without CPB was 93.4% prior to hospital discharge. This was identical to a matched group of 30 patients in which the anastomosis was performed on CPB. The incidence of postoperative arrhythmias and pulmonary and neurological complications were all significantly lower in patients operated on without CPB compared with those operated on with CPB during the same period.

Minimal access vein harvesting

Long saphenous vein is the most commonly used conduit for CABG. However, open harvesting of the leg vein involves considerable soft tissue trauma. Pain, swelling, and wound infection are significant but frequently overlooked complications in the early postoperative period. Patients often experience more discomfort from the leg wound than from the sternotomy wound. Treatment of these complications prolongs hospital stay and sometimes require hospital re-admission. In order to reduce the length of the leg incision, other techniques have been developed for mobilization of the vein.

A Mayo dissector can be used to convert the single full-length incision to multiple shorter incisions separated by skin bridges. A 4 cm incision is made in the groin or over the medial maleolus where the long saphenous vein is identified. Once the correct plane has been entered, the ring portion of the dissector can be railroaded along the length of the vein. When the dissector encounters a side branch of the vein, resistance can be felt and the ring is pushed towards the surface of the skin. A further 2 cm incision is made over this point. The side branch is then ligated and divided. This process is repeated until a sufficient length of vein has been mobilized. In addition to reducing the postoperative discomfort, this technique can also reduce intraoperative blood loss compared with large open wounds. Identification of medium-sized to larger branches of the saphenous vein is usually not a problem as the dissector is passed along the vein. Smaller branches are sometimes avulsed and require stitch repair. However, with experience, the number can be kept to a minimum.

A further refinement of this technique is to include the use of an endoscope with video assistance. For this approach, a 5–6 cm incision is made at the level of the knee joint overlying the long saphenous vein. A transparent spoon-shaped dissector (Ethicon Endo Surgery, Louisville, KY) is placed over the end of a 30° endoscope (Fig. 12.5). The dissector is positioned on the surface of the vein. Under video guidance, the dissector is passed towards the groin and a tunnel is created superficial to the vein. A second device is then passed to retract this tunnel open. The vein is encircled with a modified Mayo vein dissector and tributaries of the vein can be divided between ligaclips under video guidance. A 3–4 cm incision is made in the groin to ligate and divide the vein at the saphenofemoral junction. A further length of vein can be mobilized by repeating the procedure from the knee to the medial maleolus. With this approach, the entire length of the long saphenous vein can be harvested with just three small incisions in less than 40 minutes. Closure of these small incisions can also be completed rapidly. Early experience suggests that quality of veins harvested with this approach is comparable to those harvested from open dissection. There is also a significant reduction in problems associated with leg wounds in the postoperative period. With practice, the vein can be divided endoscopically in the groin and at the ankle and the full length of vein can be harvested from a single incision around the knee joint.

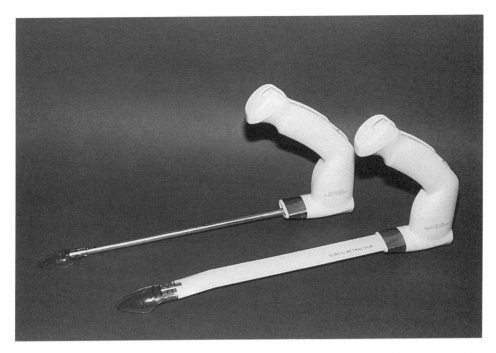

Fig. 12.5 Dissectors for endoscopic saphenous vein harvest (Ethicon Endo Surgery, Louisville, KY). See also colour plate section (Plate 10).

Discussion

The growing interest in minimally invasive coronary artery surgery can be measured by the large number of recent publications on the subject. However, the term 'minimally invasive' is not clearly defined. In fact, almost every alternative surgical approach to the conventional CABG has been so described by its protagonists. In our view, some of these alternative approaches are at least as invasive as conventional CABG, if not more so. Therefore, before we embrace all these new concepts and accept them into our own repertoire, we must examine each of these approaches carefully, bearing in mind what we are setting out to achieve in the first place.

By far the most widely used alternative approach to performing CABG is via a full or limited median sternotomy incision without CPB. Avoiding CPB obviously eliminates the risks of bypass-related complications. Both the left and right coronary arteries can be bypassed. Although it is more demanding to perform an accurate anastomosis on a beating heart, most experienced coronary surgeons can rapidly develop the skills required. After more than 10 years of experience with this approach, Benetti and associates claimed an impressive 3.1 grafts per patient with a 1% mortality (18). In recent years, they have managed to perform CABG without CPB on over 80% of their patients.

In patients with single-vessel disease limited to the LAD, bypass grafting using the LIMA can be performed via a left anterior thoracotomy on a beating heart (26,27). The LIMA can be harvested to a limited extent via the anterior thoracotomy incision alone (28) or in its entirety with the aid of a thoracoscope (9,29). In a report by Calafiore and associates where 162 patients were scheduled for this procedure, 7 cases (4.3%) had to be converted to a median sternotomy incision with or without CPB because the LAD was too small or could not be located with the thoracotomy incision; 9 patients (5.8%) required a re-operation for failure and the overall mortality was 0.6% (28).

Of the different approaches, sternotomy certainly seems to be the preferred method when learning to perform coronary anastomosis on a beating heart (30). The entire length of the coronary artery to be grafted can be visualized and the patient is readily placed on CPB should problems arise. As experience and confidence grow, the length of the incision can be gradually reduced. Eventually, a partial sternotomy or a small anterior thoracotomy approach can be used. Protagonists of each of these approaches claim that neither of these incisions are particularly painful in the postoperative period. However, there is the potential for chronic pain from damage to the intercostal nerve following a thoracotomy.

The use of stay sutures to minimize movement of the target vessel; drugs to reduce the heart rate and contractility; gas jets to provide a dry anastomotic field and the Coronary Artery Stabilizer from CardioThoracic Systems are all widely accepted means to facilitate an accurate anastomosis on a beating heart. The occasional patient may also require some form of haemodynamic support and the insertion of an intra-aortic balloon in these cases certainly seem to be very reasonable. However, it is harder to justify the use of other technologies such as the Hemopump and the Jarvik Cannula pump. The devices are quite invasive in their insertion and yet they cannot be relied upon to provide consistent haemodynamic support during manipulation of the heart. Left heart bypass without the use of an oxygenator may be a better alternative under these circumstances.

When difficulties are encountered with identifying target vessels through a small anterior thoracotomy approach, or when the artery is too small for anastomosis on a beating heart, it is normal practice to convert to a median sternotomy and the operation completed on CPB. The Endovascular Cardiopulmonary Bypass System developed by Heartport Inc. (Redwood City, CA) allows the performance of cardiopulmonary bypass and myocardial protection with cardioplegic arrest without conversion to a sternotomy. With a motionless heart, the vessel can be dissected out and the anastomosis can be performed under optimal conditions even through a small thoracotomy incision. As a means of bailing out difficult situations, Heartport certainly offers an alternative to an open conversion. However, it is debatable whether its routine use is truly less invasive than conventional CABG since the patients are exposed to all the potential risks of CPB. The same criticisms can be levelled at femoro-femoral bypass and hypothermic fibrillatory arrest.

The mortality and morbidity rates of reoperative CABG are higher than in primary CABG (31). The risks are mainly associated with reopening of the sternum and manipulation of the heart and the old grafts (32,33). Some of the alternative approaches that have been described are potentially useful for re-operative CABG especially if only one or two vessels have to be revascularized. In these cases, adhesions from the previous operation may be positively advantageous because they tend to reduce motion of the epicardial surface. Boonstra and associates reported on a series of six reoperations in which the LAD was re-grafted with a LIMA without CPB through a small anterior thoracotomy incision (34). The mean operation time was 86 minutes; mean postoperative hospital stay was 5.7 days with no mortality. In patients who require bypass grafting of the posterior descending branch of the RCA alone, an epigastric incision for harvesting of the right gastroepiploic artery and excision of the xiphisternum seems an attractive approach. This is particularly true in the presence of a patent LIMA graft from a previous operation.

With reduced postoperative hospital stay, approaches that are truly less invasive should also result in a certain amount of cost savings. However, this should be viewed as an added bonus of these approaches rather than as their prime objective.

Most of the techniques described are more demanding then conventional CABG and there is a steep initial learning curve. Bearing in mind that incomplete revascularization is an established determinant of early return of angina (35), technical difficulty cannot be used to justify inadequate revascularization. The temptation to bypass only what may seem to be the culprit lesion and leave less severe narrowings for angioplasty must be resisted. The fact that some of these alternative approaches are technically feasible is not justification for their widespread adoption if the quality of the anastomosis is compromised. With all these different approaches, we must demand studies directly comparing the new procedures with the standard operation (36). Angiographic follow-up will probably be necessary to convince both cardiologists and cardiac surgeons that comparable results can be achieved (37). Appropriate patient selection and proper training are necessary to ensure the success of these exciting developments.

References

1. Hamm C, Reimers J, Ischinger T, Rupprecht H, Berger J, Bleifield W. A randomized study of coronary angioplasty compared with bypass surgery in patients with symptomatic multi-vessel coronary disease. *N Engl J Med* 1994;**331**:1037–43.
2. King III S, Lembo N, Weintraub W *et al*. A randomized trial comparing coronary angioplasty with coronary bypass surgery: Emery Angioplasty versus Surgery Trial (EAST). *N Engl J Med* 1994;**331**:1044–50.
3. Kolessov V, Potashov L, Operatsii na venechugkh arteriiakh serdtsa. *Eksp Khir Anest* 1965;**2**:3–8.
4. Kolessov V. Mammary artery-coronary artery anastomosis as method of treatment for angina pectoris. *J Thorac Cardiovasc Surg* 1967;**54**:535–44.
5. Garrett H, Dennid E, Debakey M. Aorta-coronary bypass with saphenous vein graft: seven-year follow-up. *JAMA* 1973;**223**:792–4.
6. Favaloro R. Saphenous vein graft in the surgical treatment of coronary artery disease: operative technique. *J Thorac Cardiovasc Surg* 1969;**58**:178–85.
7. Loop F, Cosgrove D, Lytle B, Thurer R, An 11-year evolution of coronary artery surgery (1967–1978). *Ann Surg* 1979;**190**:444–55.
8. Arom K, Emery R. Mini-sternotomy for coronary bypass grafting. *Ann Thorac Surg* 1996;**61**:1271–2.
9. Benetti F, Ballester C. Use of thoracoscopy and a minimal thoracotomy, in mammary-coronary bypass to left anterior descending artery, without extracorporeal circulation. *J Cardiovasc Surg* 1995;**36**:159–61.
10. Acuff T, Landreneau R, Griffith B, Mack M. Minimally invasive coronary artery bypass grafting. *Ann Thorac Surg* 1996;**61**:135–7.
11. Stevens J, Burdon T, Peters W *et al*. Port-access coronary artery bypass grafting: a proposed surgical method. *J Thorac Cardiovasc Surg* 1996;**111**:567–73.
12. Lima L. In discussion: Left anterior descending coronary artery grafting via left anterior small thoracotomy without cardiopulmonary bypass. *Ann Thorac Surg* 1996;**61**:1664.
13. Lin P, Chang C, Chu J *et al*. Video-assisted coronary artery bypass grafting during hypothermic fibrillatory arrest. *Ann Thorac Surg* 1997;**63**:1113–7.

14. Kirklin J, Barratt-Boyes B. *Cardiac Surgery*, 2nd edn. Edinburgh, Churchill Livingstone, 1993, pp. 83–97, 210–21.

15. Archer R, Ott D, Parracicine R *et al.* Coronary revascularization without cardiopulmonary bypass. *Tex Heart Inst J* 1984;**11**:52–7.

16. Laborde F, Abdelmeguid I, Piwnica A. Aortocoronary bypass without extracorporeal circulation: Why and when? *Eur J Cardiothorac Surg* 1989;**3**:152–4.

17. Buffolo E, Andrade J, Branco I, Agviar L, Ribeiro E, Jatene A. Myocardial revascularization without extracorporeal circulation. *Eur J Cardiothorac Surg.* 1990;**4**:504–8.

18. Benetti F, Naselli G, Wood M, Geffner L. Direct myocardial revascularization without extracorporeal circulation. *Chest* 1991;**100**:312–16.

19. Pfister A, Zaki M, Garcia J *et al.* Coronary artery bypass without cardiopulmonary bypass. *Ann Thorac Surg* 1992;**54**:1085–92.

20. Moshkovitz Y, Lusky A, Mohr R. Coronary artery bypass without cardiopulmonary bypass: analysis of short-term and mid-term outcome in 220 patients. *J Thorac Cardiovasc Surg* 1995;**110**:979–87.

21. Lonn U, Peterzen B, Granfeldt H, Casmir H. Coronary artery operation with support of the Hemoshield cardiac assist system. *Ann Thorac Surg* 1994;**58**:519–23.

22. Jarvik R, Macris M, Marnis S, Robinson J, Frazier O. Cannula pumps for less invasive coronary surgery. In: *Proceedings of the First International Teleconference on Least Invasive Coronary Surgery*. Oxford: Oxford Heart Centre, 1996.

23. Lick S, Conti V, Zwisxhenberger J, Kurusz M. Simple technique of left heart bypass. *Ann Thorac Surg* 1996;**61**:1555–6.

24. Buffolo E, de Andrade J, Branco J, Teles C, Aguiar L, Gomes W. Coronary artery bypass without cardiopulmonary bypass. *Ann Thorac Surg* 1996;**61**:63–6.

25. Shennib H, Lee A, Akin J. Safe and effective method of stabilization for coronary artery bypass grafting on the beating heart. *Ann Thorac Surg* 1997;**63**:988–92.

26. Subramanian V, Stelzer P. Clinical experience with minimally invasive coronary artery bypass grafting. *Eur J Cardiothorac Surg* 1995.

27. Stanbridge RDL, Symons G, Banwell P. Minimal access surgery for coronary artery revascularization. *Lancet*, 1995;**346**:837.

28. Calafiore A, Giammarco G, Teodori G *et al.* Left anterior descending coronary artery grafting via left anterior small thoracotomy without cardiopulmonary bypass. *Ann Thorac Surg* 1996;**61**:1658–65.

29. Acuff T, Landreneau R, Griffith B, Mack M. Minimally invasive coronary artery bypass grafting. *Ann Thorac Surg* 1996;**61**:135–7.

30. Arom K, Emery R. Mini-sternotomy for coronary artery bypass grafting. *Ann Thorac Surg* 1996;**61**:1271–2.

31. Edwards F, Clark R, Schwartz M. Coronary artery bypass grafting: the Society of Thoracic Surgeons national database experience. *Ann Thorac Surg* 1994;**57**:12–19.

32. Fanning W, Kakos G, Williams TJ. Reoperative coronary bypass grafting without cardiopulmonary bypass. *Ann Thorac Surg* 1993;**55**:486–9.

33. He G, Acuff T, Ryan W, He Y, Mack M. Determinants of operative mortality in reoperative coronary artery bypass grafting.
J Thorac Cardiovasc Surg 1995;**110**:971–8.

34. Boonstra P, Grandjean J, Mariani A. Reoperative coronary bypass grafting without cardiopulmonary bypass through a small thoracotomy. *Ann Thorac Surg* 1997;**63**:405–7.

35. Buda A, MacDonald I, Anderson M, Strauss H, David T, Berman N. Long-term results following coronary bypass operation: importance of preoperative factors and complete revascularization. *J Thorac Cardiovasc Surg* 1981;**82**:383–9.

36. Ullyot D. In invited commentary: video-assisted coronary artery bypass grafting during hypothermic fibrillatory arrest. *Ann Thorac Surg* 1997;**63**:1117.

37. Westaby S, Benetti F. Less invasion coronary surgery: consensus from the Oxford Meeting. *Ann Thorac Surg* 1996;**62**:924–31.

13 Vascular biology of coronary artery bypass grafts: pathophysiology of graft failure and strategies for its prevention

Alan J. Bryan and Gianni D. Angelini

During the 25 years that have elapsed since the introduction of coronary artery bypass grafting (CABG) it has been clear that graft patency is one of the primary determinants of clinical outcome. In the early 1980s, the unsatisfactory late results with saphenous vein became obvious, with up to 50% of grafts occluded at 10 years, and a significant proportion of the remainder diseased. Subsequently, the superior clinical results reported using the left internal thoracic artery to graft the left anterior descending coronary artery (2) led to its routine use (3). These two observations have clearly shown that the biological characteristics and long-term behaviour of a particular conduit may profoundly influence late clinical outcome.

Despite a logical increase in the use of arterial conduits, saphenous vein grafts continue to be widely used (4). An improved understanding of the cellular mechanisms underlying graft failure is essential for the development of new strategies to improve late patency. Current developments in molecular biology offer the exciting prospect of increased insight into the biology of the vessel wall, and the potential for genetic modulation of its behaviour. Knowledge of the characteristics which specifically enhance patency may also help to predict the performance of newer arterial conduits (5).

The evolution of CABG has been predominantly based on clinical observation. However, clinical outcome can now be explained by our improved understanding of the biology of the endothelium and vascular smooth muscle cell. Such knowledge is essential to the development and application of new approaches to improve early and late outcome after CABG.

Pathophysiology of graft failure

Saphenous vein grafts implanted into the arterial circulation undergo a series of pathophysiological changes which, in part, represent adaptation to systemic pressure. These cellular and morphological changes have been clearly defined from studies of both human pathological specimens (6) and time course experiments in comparable animal models (7).

Early occlusions within the first month after operation occur in 8–18% of saphenous vein grafts and are almost always thrombotic. These may be attributed partly to grafting small or severely diseased vessels leading to low flow and subsequent thrombosis (8–10). In addition, endothelial loss and damage to the media resulting from surgical preparation, including excessive intraluminal pressure distension, may promote early graft thrombosis (11–13). Mural thrombus has also been demonstrated angiographically in asymptomatic patients in the early postoperative period (14), and was evident in 75% of vein grafts obtained within 24 hours of operation (15).

Loss of endothelium eliminates the physical and electrostatic barrier separating platelets from subendothelial collagen, binding to which initiates platelet activation. Loss of endothelial cells or impairment of their function leads to reduced production of prostacyclin (16), and nitric oxide (17) and intrinsic fibrinolytic activity (18), which act to inhibit platelet activation and adhesion and thrombus formation. Platelet activation stimulates synthesis of thromboxane A_2 and release of clear granule components including serotonin and ATP and α granule components including platelet-derived growth factor (PDGF), platelet factor IV, fibrinogen, fibronectin, von Willebrand factor, and β-thromboglobulin (19). These agents act together to produce vasoconstriction, further platelet aggregation and hence further thrombin and fibrin generation. These are the mechanisms which occur in thrombotic occlusion and particularly where vein graft flow is limited by an inadequate distal coronary circulation (Fig. 13.1).

Within a few days of implantation, even when endothelial continuity is preserved, medial thickening occurs secondary to vascular smooth muscle cell (VSMC) hyperplasia (13,20). These changes are the immediate response of the vessel wall to 'injury' and are caused by release of growth factors, e.g. PDGF, fibroblast growth factor (FGF) from platelets, monocytes, and elimination of the inhibitory effects of the intact endothelium. This is followed for several weeks by a phase in which VSMCs undergo a change from a contractile to a proliferative phenotype (21) and

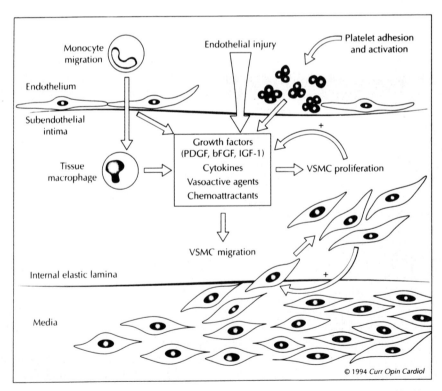

Fig. 13.1 Biochemical and cellular mediators of intimal proliferation after endothelial injury (bFGF, basic fibroblast growth factor; PDGF, platelet derived growth factor; VSMC, vascular smooth muscle cell; IGF-1, insulin like growth factor-1) (reproduced with permission from reference 41).

then migrate from the media through the internal elastic lamina into the intima. A phase of rapid intimal proliferation then follows. The hypothesis that the degree of early VSMC proliferation is related to platelet deposition (22) is supported by its reduction in an animal model made thrombocytopaenic (23). However, intimal proliferation continues well after endothelial regeneration and termination of platelet activation, suggesting that the autocrine and paracrine influence of the endothelium and VSMCs are important (24).

Intimal proliferation continues for many months and experimental work supports the view that the degree of late intimal hyperplasia is not influenced by the severity of the endothelial injury at the time of implantation (7). By 1 year after implantation the luminal diameter of saphenous vein grafts may have been reduced by 25%, primarily by intimal thickening (25). During this later phase there are marked increases in the connective tissue matrix consequent on the secretory activity of the VSMCs and fibroblasts with further thickening of both the media and intima (7). Beyond the first month, vein graft occlusion also results from thrombosis, but this is increasingly superimposed on a graft lumen narrowed by intimal proliferation (Fig. 13.2).

Between the first and fourth years after implantation, changes occurring are limited, with an occlusion rate of only 2% per year (1). There is less cellular activity, and the ratio of lumen to wall thickness stabilizes. There may be an increase in the lipid content and number of foam cells which may be precursors of atherosclerosis. Atherosclerotic changes are seen at 3 years and accelerate beyond 5 years with the appearance of mature lipid-laden atherosclerotic plaques, when the rate of graft occlusion is around 5% per year (1). The appearance of the atherosclerotic process in vein grafts is very similar to that seen in arteries (15,26). Overall, it may be more

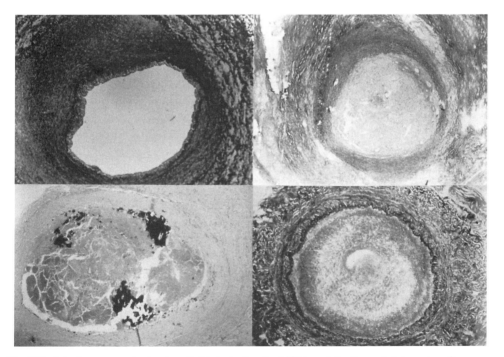

Fig. 13.2 Late changes occurring in vein grafts (clockwise from top left) (a) myointimal hyperplasia in a vein graft, (b) thrombotic occlusion of a vein graft with neovascularisation of thrombus, (c) occluded vein graft with calcification, (d) marked myointimal hyperplasia with severe luminal encroachment.

friable and diffuse, but rarely calcified and may result in aneurysmal dilatation, plaque rupture, and superimposed thrombus leading to sudden graft occlusion and clinical ischaemic events (27). By 10 years approximately 50% of grafts are occluded and a majority of the remainder have evidence of significant vein graft disease (1).

In comparison, 95% of internal thoracic artery grafts to the left anterior descending coronary artery are patent at 10 years (2). The occlusions that occur are predominantly early failures relating to surgical technique or poor quality distal coronary circulation or, in the case of free grafts, technical problems associated with the proximal aortic anastomosis. As a general observation, arterial grafts appear protected from intimal hyperplasia, atherosclerotic change, and late graft failure.

Aetiological considerations

Vein characteristics

Recent work has shown that saphenous vein grafts with reduced compliance or with pre-existing intimal hyperplasia, or other histological abnormalities, have an increased incidence of early graft failure and late stenosis (28–30). The presence of subendothelial spindle shaped cells greater than five layers thick was associated with a poor outcome (30). In addition, cultured, isolated VSMCs from patients developing vein graft stenoses due to intimal hyperplasia have been shown to exhibit decreased sensitivity to inhibition by heparin when cultured *in vitro*, suggesting differences in VSMC growth regulation between individuals (31,32). In an organ culture of human saphenous vein, intimal hyperplasia was greater in samples with greater pre-exiting intimal thickening (33). The finding that autologous arm vein yields unsatisfactory results (34) suggests that other characteristics of the vein used may be an important determinant of early patency. These influences may well be important but fail to explain the differing susceptibility of individual vein grafts taken from adjacent portions of the saphenous vein to atherosclerotic change.

Other investigators have suggested that venous valves in reversed vein grafts are a site of stenosis and clot formation and have advocated the use of non-reversed saphenous vein and valvotomy prior to vein implantation (35–37). In support of this Molina (37) has reported an impressive overall patency of 90% with a mean follow-up of 19 months in a small series of patients undergoing CABG. Despite this, scientifically convincing evidence to support these hypotheses has not been forthcoming and few surgeons employ such techniques.

Surgical preparation

Surgical preparation of saphenous vein for CABG traditionally involves exposure, dissection, and intraluminal distension to overcome spasm and test side-branch ligation. This may result in loss of endothelium and functional damage to the vessel wall (11,12,16,38–40). The changes that may occur during surgical preparation produce a prothrombotic environment (41) and act as a trigger for early intimal hyperplasia (42). It is suggested that this injury may be a contributing factor to early graft failure and there is good evidence from animal studies to support this hypothesis (13).

Storage temperature and solutions have also been implicated in the aetiology of endothelial injury (43). Some investigators have found that saline solutions may cause increased endothelial damage (44,45). However, others have condemned blood-based solutions because of the intraluminal platelet/fibrin thrombi observed (14). Optimal preparation and storage solutions have been formulated and their use advocated (46,47). Overall the nature, temperature, and duration of storage have effects of uncertain importance and discussion regarding the relative merits of different solutions in terms of the morphological, biochemical, and physiological behaviour of vein continues without consensus (48–50).

It seems therefore that damage to the saphenous vein during its preparation by a number of mechanisms produces detrimental effects which favour early thrombotic occlusion and trigger early intimal hyperplasia but may not influence the degree of late intimal hyperplasia or late graft failure. It has been disappointing to record that few surgeons actually appear to pay particular attention to these aspects in their practice (51).

Surgical technique and the coronary circulation

Although biological characteristics of particular conduits are important, it is self-evident that excellent patency can only be achieved by high technical standards of surgery. Indeed, it has been shown that there is a significant difference in operative mortality between individual surgeons which may not be explained by patient-related variables (52) and the best results are achieved by those surgeons and institutions performing coronary artery surgery in sufficient volume to develop and maintain their expertise (52,53). Bex *et al.* (54) have also elegantly highlighted that art is as much a part of surgery as science, and this cannot be masked however complex the statistical analysis. Grondin and Thornton (27) have identified technical errors which may lead to perfusion of only the proximal or distal limb of the anastomosis, the former leading more commonly to graft occlusion than the latter (25). It is clear from early data that as experience increases technical faults become less frequent and the rate of graft attrition reduces (55).

Appropriate selection of optimal grafting sites influences patency, particularly in vein grafts where poor distal run-off leads to reduced early patency (10). It is not surprising therefore to find in major studies that vein grafts to arteries less than 1.5 mm, occluded arteries, and those supplying infarcted areas of myocardium have a reduced early patency (9,56). Grafts to the LAD also have a patency greater than those to the circumflex and right coronary systems.

Haemodynamic influences

It is generally accepted that transplantation of vein into the arterial circulation stimulates VSMC proliferation, suggesting that some degree of intimal thickening is inevitable. The stimulus to proliferation appears to be wall tension which has been elegantly demonstrated in a number of animal models (57,58). The mechanism by which such haemodynamic changes induce VSMC proliferation is only now being elucidated. Endothelial cells respond to stretching forces and this may be transduced by a stretch activated channel on the cell surface (59,60). Shear stress has been shown to induce endothelial cell gene transcription of PDGF which is mediated by protein kinase C, a mechanism by which haemodynamic change is transformed into cellular response (61). As will be discussed later, it would seem that methods aimed at reducing wall tension by external stenting should be fully evaluated.

Local and systemic humoral influences

The realization that the behaviour of the VSMC is central to a number of vascular pathologies has led to intense research in understanding the paracrine and autocrine influences which modulate its proliferative activity. Many different stimuli interact to produce intimal hyperplasia, and a range of growth factors are important in mediating VSMC proliferation. Growth factors are known to be released by blood components, platelets, macrophages, and endothelial cells and VSMCs themselves. They act to stimulate cell proliferation by signal transduction by activation of cell surface receptors leading to activation of intracellular second messenger systems, e.g. cAMP, tyrosine kinase, which converts VSMCs to a proliferative phenotype.

Platelet-derived growth factor (PDGF)

The first of this group of polypeptides to be described (62) was originally shown to be released from aggregating platelets, through it is now known to be released from endothelial cells, macrophages, and VSMCs (63). PDGF is chemotactic to monocytes and macrophages, but is both chemotactic and mitogenic to VSMCs. It is undoubtedly important in the early vessel wall response to injury and stimulates the migration and proliferation of medial SMCs after injury (64), probably by separate pathways (65). Transfer of the PDGF BB isomer gene to the arterial wall has confirmed the importance of PDGF as a stimulus to VSMC proliferation (66). Experimental localization of PDGF to the neointimal layer in porcine vein grafts (67) and its continuing presence after endothelial regeneration suggests secretion by endothelial cells or VSMCs and supports a role for PDGF in the late phase of ongoing intimal hyperplasia in vein grafts.

Fibroblast growth factor (FGF)

The activity of this growth factor is due to two proteins, acidic (aFGF) and basic (bFGF). Both are potent mitogens for a variety of cells, including endothelial and VSMCs (63,68). It is synthesized by endothelial and VSMCs and monocytes and is bound within the vessel wall to basement membrane and extracellular matrix and released in response to vessel wall injury. The localization of bFGF expression in the experimental work available suggests that bFGF is more important in terms of vascular responses to injury (63). In experimental models of arterial injury, exogeneously administered bFGF caused VSMC proliferation in the presence of endothelial injury (69) and antibody to bFGF inhibited VSMC proliferation but did not reduce the overall degree of intimal thickening (70). Furthermore, recent data has shown that direct gene transfer of aFGF, to the vessel wall produced intimal hyperplasia in a porcine model, confirming its role in VSMC proliferation (67). It also seems likely that bFGF has a role in re-establishing an endothelial lining in denuded vessels (68). Currently, however, its importance in vein graft disease in humans remains to be established.

Other growth factors

A number of other growth factors and their receptors, have been identified, which may be important in intimal hyperplasia but as yet their place is undefined. These include insulin-like growth factor (IGF-1) (69,70), transforming growth factor (TGF) a and b, epidermal growth factor (EGF) and connective tissue growth factor (CTGF) (63,70).

Cytokines and vasoconstrictors

A variety of vasoactive substances, including serotonin, angiotensin, and endothelin-1 may also have mitogenic effects, some of which have been shown *in vitro* and *in vivo*. Whether this is a direct action or mediated by other growth factors remains undefined. Endothelial cells are also a source of growth inhibitors and inactivators. Nitric oxide and prostacyclin have direct inhibitory effects on VSMC proliferation, mediated by cGMP and cAMP which in addition to their antithrombotic effects may explain at least in part the importance of endothelial function in maintaining vascular graft patency (71).

A further group of proteins, the cytokines (interleukins, monocyte chemotactic and activating and tumour necrosis factor, etc.) which are known to mediate immune and inflammatory responses involved in intercellular signalling between leukocytes, endothelial cells, and VSMCs may play a part in intimal hyperplasia in vein grafts (70).

Early response genes

VSMCs express early response genes (e.g. c-*myc*, c-*myb*, c-*fos*) after growth factor stimulation and they are important in initiating proliferation. The expression of these proto-oncogenes is thought to be involved in the signal transduction pathways leading to cell division but may not be an essential prerequisite. It represents a further level at which VSMC proliferation might be modulated.

Lipid metabolism

In the presence of an atherogenic lipoprotein pattern, lipid deposition occurs in association with the development of atheroma. In primate models of vein grafts rapid lipid uptake after implantation has been observed even with normal serum lipid profiles (72,73). However, this has not been a striking finding in other animal models fed a non-hypercholesterolaemic diet (7). Autologous vein grafts in animals fed a hypercholesterolaemic diet, however, are particularly susceptible to the development of atheromatous lesions (74,75), and lipid and cholesterol accumulation appears to parallel the early development of intimal hyperplasia (73).

Patients who have disordered lipid/cholesterol metabolism undergoing CABG are at increased risk of vein graft atherosclerosis and occlusion leading to further intervention (76). In patients with atherosclerotic grafts, total serum cholesterol and triglycerides are higher than in those with vein grafts apparently free of disease (76,77). In addition, high density lipoprotein cholesterol (HDL) is lower and low density lipoprotein cholesterol (LDL) is higher in patients with atherosclerotic grafts (76). A further clinical study has demonstrated an association between serum lipoprotein A levels and an increased risk of saphenous vein graft stenosis (77). It is also possible that the association between hypercoagulability and high triglyceride levels may be implicated in the late risk of graft thrombosis (78). Overall the data suggest that the relationship between disordered lipid profile and late graft failure is strong, even in comparison to other atherogenic factors such as smoking (79). Arterial grafts, particularly the internal thoracic artery, are apparently intrinsically protected from accelerated atherosclerosis caused by dyslipidaemias although their influence on late degenerative changes in other arterial grafts is as yet unknown.

Biological advantages of arterial grafts

It comes as no surprise that autologous arteries function better than vein as arterial replacements. In comparing the biological properties of different conduits, a number of characteristics would seem to be important: the potential for development of atherosclerotic change, the vasomotor and intrinsic antithrombotic properties, and the ability of the conduit to respond to the changing requirements of the coronary circulation (71). It must be recognized that the overall suitability of a vessel as a conduit is not dependent only on its biological characteristics. A conduit which is technically difficult to harvest and prepare or implant may occlude early, despite excellent biological characteristics which would predict optimal late patency (80).

Endothelial function and morphology is central to several aspects of vascular function and plays an important role in regulating vascular tone, blood/vessel wall interactions, and VSMC control. Endothelial production of vasoactive substances like nitric oxide and prostacyclin is much less in saphenous vein than in internal thoracic artery (71,81,82) and may be further reduced by vein preparation (17). Internal thoracic artery grafts exhibit more marked endothelium-dependent relaxation and inhibition of platelet aggregation, characteristics which might favour graft patency (71). Similarly, nitric oxide and prostacyclin are thought to exert direct inhibitory effects on VSMC proliferation mediated via cGMP and cAMP and this may in part explain the lack of intimal proliferation observed in arterial grafts after implantation. Haemodynamic factors inevitably play a part and it has been shown that proliferation of VSMCs from saphenous vein in response to pulsatile stretch also appears markedly greater than arterial VSMCs (83) and may reflect a difference in response to growth factors such as PDGF (84). These differences have been confirmed in an organ culture model, where intimal proliferation was significantly increased in surgically prepared vein compared to the internal thoracic artery and fresh saphenous vein, suggesting greater vulnerability of the vein to injury (33). Flow characteristics, in particular velocity, may be a more important influence on graft patency than absolute flow. Flow patterns in venous and internal thoracic artery grafts are very different, with higher flow velocities and maximal shear rates in the latter (85).

There are therefore a number of biological and haemodynamic differences which may explain the superior performance in the long term and freedom from disease of internal thoracic artery grafts. The clinical evaluation of other arterial conduits will reveal whether they will give similar long-term results. Although there are differences in the histological characteristics and physiological behaviour of the inferior epigastric and gastoepiploic arteries, their long-term results have been predicted to lie between those of internal thoracic artery and saphenous vein grafts (5).

Therapeutic strategies to improve vein graft patency

Early failure

Efforts to maintain early graft patency centre around surgical techniques at the time of implantation which maintain the structural and functional integrity of the conduit and, in the case of saphenous vein, on the appropriate use of anti-thrombotic therapy (24). These early interventions are aimed at reducing platelet activation and adhesion and other mechanisms which may favour acute thrombosis.

Surgical technique

Surgical injury may be prevented by minimizing mechanical trauma and avoiding overdistension (43). Early methods of minimizing distension pressure included the use of a pressure-limiting balloon (12). More recently a number of techniques have been proposed involving simple modifications of the bypass circuit that rely only on the arterial pressure of the patient to distend the vein (86,87) (Fig. 13.3) or performing proximal anastomoses first (39). These studies have

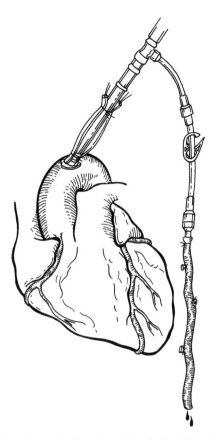

Fig. 13.3 Simple modifications of the bypass circuit have been devised to limit distension to arterial pressure (reproduced with permission from reference 86).

shown that morphological and functional injury to vein grafts at the time of implantation can be avoided (86) and that, at least in animal models, this leads to improvements in early patency (13).

From the point of view of arterial grafts, early patency of internal thoracic artery grafts to the left anterior descending coronary artery is extremely high (92–95%) (88). Although diathermy injury, hydrostatic dilatation, and the application of vascular clips may lead to morphological and functional injury and should be avoided, evidence that early patency is compromised to a significant degree by these mechanisms is lacking.

Anti-thrombotic therapy

Anti-thrombotic therapy is widely used for improving early vein graft patency. The original trials in the early 1980s demonstrated the efficacy of aspirin and dipyridamole (89) in improving graft patency at up to 1 year after operation. Since that time a large number of trials have been carried out and worthwhile meta-analyses have been presented (90–92). Aspirin at a dose of 325 mg/day represents the lowest dose with a consistent antithrombotic effect. This should be commenced in the very early postoperative period, since preoperative treatment is associated with increased bleeding and does not produce any additional therapeutic benefit (93). Although originally dipyridamole was perceived to convey additional benefit in combination with aspirin, current consensus suggests it has no additional benefit (90) and few cardiac surgeons in the UK currently prescribe it (4). Other anti-platelet agents have been shown to be as effective as aspirin (94), and oral anticoagulants appear to be as effective as anti-platelet agents, but not more so, and their use has been associated with more bleeding complications (90,95,96). In the UK anticoagulants have been used preferentially in patients requiring coronary endarterectomy (51), although the limited data available do not support this practice, and indeed aspirin may be more effective in this situation (97–99). The possible additive benefits of anticoagulation and anti-platelet therapy are poorly defined and it has been suggested that further work in this area would be of value (90). Overall, at least in the medium term, prolongation of aspirin therapy beyond the first year does not appear to reduce the incidence of late vein graft failure (100,101). Nevertheless, there may be good reason to continue aspirin indefinitely, given its proven rate as secondary prevention against cardiovascular events (101).

Aspirin has been shown to have no effect on maintaining internal thoracic artery graft patency to the left anterior descending coronary artery (88). The overall high patency rate for arterial grafts and the low late attrition rate mean that further studies may be irrational and impracticable.

Late graft failure

Late vein graft failure is secondary to intimal hyperplasia, the development of graft atherosclerosis and late thrombosis. Advances in the understanding of VSMC proliferation and intimal hyperplasia have allowed the development and evaluation of a number of potential therapies (70,102).

Advances in graft imaging also offer the prospect of improved graft surveillance in the context of evaluating new therapies in the clinical arena. Quantitative angiography has traditionally been the methodology for evaluating changes in coronary artery disease and bypass grafts, though its inability to image concentric luminal narrowing and intramural disease have been recognized (103). For this reason, intravascular ultrasound may be a major advance in the clinical evaluation of intimal hyperplasia and anti-atherosclerotic agents (106).

Late failure of arterial grafts is very unusual, given their relative immunity to atherosclerosis and graft disease with 10 year patency rates in excess of 90%. For this reason the main strategy that surgeons have adopted has been to take advantage of the favourable biological characteristics of arterial grafts, whenever possible, to minimize the use of vein grafts (105).

Pharmacological therapy

A variety of agents have been tested in animal models and a much smaller number in clinical trials (70). Heparin and its low molecular weight derivatives, despite theoretical potential, and a demonstrable effect on inhibition of VSMC proliferation *in vitro* (102), have been disappointing in both organ culture (105) and animal models of vein grafts (106,107).

Calcium channel blockers, angiopeptin, and anticholinesterase (ACE) inhibitors all appear to retard intimal hyperplasia in animal models of vein grafts (24). Angiopeptin almost certainly acts locally by a direct effect on VSMC proliferation, but it is possible that the other two groups of agent may exert their influence by systemic haemodynamic effects. In a clinical study, nifedipine significantly reduced the incidence of new lesion formation in vein grafts up to 1 year after operation (108). However, the recent demonstration that calcium antagonists inhibit VSMC proliferation due to PDGF but not wall tension suggests their effects on this process may be limited (109).

ACE inhibitors and angiopeptin are as yet untested clinically in graft disease. ACE inhibitors after angioplasty appear unhelpful but angiopeptin post-angioplasty does reduce restenosis (70), and would be worthy of evaluation in vein grafts. New agents which inhibit the Na^+–H^+ exchanger, a membrane transport protein which is activated by growth factors as an early event when VSMCs enter the cell cycle, appear effective in animal models of arterial injury (110,111) and again should be evaluated further.

The combination of colestipol and niacin therapy has been shown to reduce the incidence of new lesion formation in vein grafts, presumably by a reduction in LDL and increase in HDL (112). National Institutes of Health trials are currently underway to evaluate a combination of aspirin and lipid therapy (101) and a 3-hydroxy-3-methyglutaryl coenzyme A reductase inhibitor (79) for the prevention of vein graft atherosclerosis.

External vessel supports

The importance of wall tension in the adaptation of vein grafts to the arterial circulation has already been mentioned. The concept of vessel wall stenting to limit these effects and potentially diminish intimal hyperplasia would seen to be reasonable. A reduction in intimal hyperplasia by external vessel wall stenting has been demonstrated (113) though this has not been found by all workers (114). Two further studies have suggested a protective effect for vein grafts by this strategy (115,116) though there is as yet no general agreement.

Photodynamic therapy

Photodynamic therapy is a novel approach to prevention of intimal hyperplasia. It uses the ability of light-excitable photosensitizers to produce injury to targeted cells when activated by the appropriate wavelength of light. This has been shown to be an effective inhibitor of intimal hyperplasia in an animal model of arterial injury (117) and in an *in vitro* culture of VSMCs (118). Further information on this approach is awaited, though techniques of light exposure may prove too cumbersome for practical clinical use.

Molecular biological approaches

Advances in molecular biological techniques have led to the development of a new group of strategies currently being applied to the inhibition of intimal hyperplasia (70). Much of this work has been focused on responses to arterial injury with reference to angioplasty restenosis. Delivery of agents may be a problem (119) although the use of these techniques with vein grafts offers a unique opportunity for application of topical therapy at the time of implantation. A variety of different approaches are possible (Fig. 13.4).

Antibody-specific inhibition

Specific antibodies raised to growth factors have been used in models of arterial injury directed against both PDGF and bFGF. A polyclonal anti-PDGF IgG reduced intimal hyperplasia after balloon injury in the carotid artery of rats, but this appeared to be by preventing VSMC migration rather than proliferation (120). Similarly, antibodies to bFGF apparently reduced VSMC proliferation but not the overall degree of intimal hyperplasia (121).

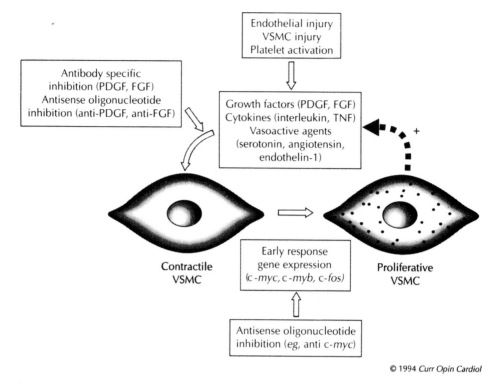

© 1994 *Curr Opin Cardiol*

Fig. 13.4 Potential molecular biological strategies for inhibiting the proliferation of vascular smooth muscle cells (VSMCs): (FGF, fibroblast growth factor; PDGF, platelet derived growth factor; TNF, tumour necrosis factor). (reproduced with permission from reference 41).

A different approach is based on the concept that cell binding to matrix is thought to be mediated by cell surface receptors called integrins. A monoclonal antibody to an integrin ($\alpha v \beta 3$) and an integrin receptor antagonist have been used to inhibit VSMC migration *in vitro* (122). Thus integrins may be important in cell migration induced by growth factors, but also small peptide receptor binding site antagonists may be a potentially worthwhile new class of therapeutic agent.

The main defect in any strategy directed against a specific growth factor is that given the multiple paracrine influences on intimal hyperplasia, inhibition of a single growth factor is unlikely to result in anything more than partial suppression.

Antisense oligonucleotide inhibition

This involves the development of antisense oligonucleotides with complementary base sequences which will bind to a specific mRNA and in so doing inhibit its translation (70). In cultures of VSMCs and endothelial cells antisense oligonucleotides to mRNA for PDGF-A, bFGF, and TGF-B, introduced using liposome mediated transfection, appeared to effectively block production of these factors (123). Studies in cultured VSMCs have demonstrated that c-*myc*, c-*fos* and c-*myb* proto-oncogenes are activated after various mitogenic stimuli. This has raised the possibility that nuclear proto-oncogene expression is a final common pathway for diverse mitogenic signals making it an attractive therapeutic target. Antisense oligonucleotides to both c-*myc* and c-

myb proto-oncogenes have been shown to inhibit VSMC proliferation both *in vivo* and *in vitro* (124,125). Other proteins implicated in smooth muscle cell proliferation, like proliferating cell nuclear antigen (PCNA) and non-muscle myosin heavy chain (NMMHC), have also been inhibited by antisense technology (126). The proliferation of VSMCs derived from human saphenous vein can be inhibited by c-*myc* oligonucleotide inhibition (127) and these strategies are currently under evaluation in animal models of vein grafts.

Gene therapy

Gene therapy is a rapidly developing area with the potential for treatment of a range of vascular diseases (128). There are several different approaches.

Direct gene transfer

Genes are directly transferred into vascular cells in this technique. Viral vectors such as adenovirus can be used to introduce new genetic material and in animal models gene transfer to the arterial wall with effective expression at up to 5 months has been demonstrated (66,67,128–130). A disadvantage of this technique is the inability to target genes to specific cells, and the relative inefficiency of gene transfer and expression *in vivo* (128).

Cell-mediated gene transfer

Involves *in vitro* modification of a cell line with sunsequent *in vivo* implantation. Delivery vehicles still represent a problem although vascular grafts lined with genetically modified endothelial cells have been successfully created (131).

In addition, autologous endothelial cells have been modified *in vitro* using recombinant retroviruses, with evidence of effective repopulation by modified endothelial cells 1–14 days after arterial injury in an animal model (132). Effective viral transfer of vascular cell adhesion molecules (VCAM-1) which may inhibit intimal hyperplasia by blocking endothelial monocyte adhesion, has been demonstrated in carotid artery vein grafts in an animal model with a high level of *in vivo* expression at 3 days (133).

Although these techniques are as yet in their infancy they hold great promise. In addition, the implantation of specific genes has been used to further clarify their influences on VSMC proliferation (66,129,130).

Summary

The biological characteristics of coronary artery bypass conduits have a profound influence on early and late patency and clinical outcome. Basic science and clinical research have allowed definition of the pathophysiology and natural history of vein graft failure and identified the favourable characteristics of arterial grafts.

Current clinical strategies are based on increasing use of arterial grafts. Nevertheless saphenous vein is still a widely used conduit and late vein graft failure represents a significant clinical and economic problem. A variety of pharmacological therapies have been evaluated and lipid lowering agents have been shown to be effective in delaying the progression of graft disease. A better understanding of the role of growth factors and gene expression by vascular smooth muscle cells in the genesis and progression of intimal hyperplasia is essential. We believe that basic science holds the key to the development and evaluation of new approaches to achieve the goal of improving late clinical outcome of patients with ischaemic heart disease.

Acknowledgements

The authors acknowledge the support of the British Heart Foundation, the Garfield Weston Trust and the National Heart Research Fund.

References

1. Campeau L, Enjalbert M, Lesperance J, Vaislic C, Grondin CM, Bourassa MG. Atherosclerosis and late closure of aortocoronary saphenous vein grafts: sequential angiographic studies 2 Weeks, 1 year, 5–7 years and 10–12 years after surgery. *Circulation* 1983;**68**(II):1–9.
2. Loop FD, Lytle BW, Cosgrove DM *et al*. Influence of the internal mammary artery graft on 10 year survival and other cardiac events. *N Engl J Med* 1986;**314**:1–6.
3. Kirklin JW *et al*. [ACC/AMA Task Force on Assessment of Diagnostic and Therapeutic Cardiovascular Procedures] Guidelines and indications for coronary artery bypass graft surgery. *J Am Coll Cardiol* 1991;**17**:543–89.
4. Izzat MB, West RR, Bryan AJ, Angelini GD. Coronary artery bypass surgery: current practice in the United Kingdom. *Br Heart J* 1994;**71**:382–5.
5. van Son JAM, Smedts F. Histology of arterial conduits as a predictor of their long term patency as coronary bypass conduits. *Eur J Cardiothorac Surg* 1993;**7**:277–8.
6. Cox JL, Chiasson DA, Gotlieb AI. Stranger in a strange land: the pathogenesis of saphenous vein graft stenosis. *Prog Cardiovasc Dis* 1991;**34**:45–68.
7. Angelini GD, Bryan AJ, Williams HMJ *et al*. Time course of medial and intimal thickening in pig venous arterial grafts: relationship to endothelial injury and cholesterol accumulation. *J Thorac Cardiovasc Surg* 1992;**103**:1093–103.
8. Grondin CM, Lepage G, Castonguay YR, Meere C, Grondin P. Aortocoronary bypass graft. Initial blood flow through the graft and early postoperative patency. *Circulation* 1971;**44**:815–19.
9. Cataldo G, Braga M, Pirotta N *et al*. on behalf of Studio Indobufene nel Bypass Aortocoronarico [SINBA]. Factors influencing 1-year patency of coronary artery saphenous vein grafts. *Circulation* 1993;**88**[II]:93–8.
10. Paz MA, Lupon J, Bosch X *et al*. and the GESIC Study Group. Predictors of early saphenous vein aortocoronary bypass graft occlusion. *Ann Thorac Surg* 1993;**56**:1101–6.
11. Ramos JR, Berger K, Mansfield PB, Sauvage LR. Histological fate and endothelial changes of distended and non-distended vein grafts. *Ann Surg* 1976;**183**:205–28.
12. Bonchek LE. Prevention of endothelial damage during preparation of saphenous veins for bypass grafting. *J Thorac Cardiovasc Surg* 1980;**79**:911–15.
13. Angelini GD, Bryan AJ, Williams HMJ, Morgan R, Newby AC. Distension promotes platelet and leucocyte adhesion and reduces short term patency in pig arteriovenous bypass grafts. *J Thorac Cardiovasc Surg* 1990;**99**:433–9.
14. Catinella FP, Cunningham JN Jr, Srungaram RK *et al*. The factors influencing early patency of coronary artery bypass vein grafts. Correlation of angiographic and ultrastructural findings. *J Thorac Cardiovasc Surg* 1982;**83**:686–700.

15. Bulkley BH, Hutchins GM. Accelerated atherosclerosis: a morphological study in 97 saphenous vein grafts. *Circulation* 1977;**55**:163–9.

16. Angelini GD, Breckenridge IM, Psaila JV *et al*. Preparation of human saphenous vein for coronary artery bypass grafting impairs its capacity to produce prostacyclin. *Cardiovasc Res* 1987;**21**:28–33.

17. Angelini GD, Christie M, Bryan AJ, Lewis MJ. Preparation of human saphenous vein for coronary artery bypass grafting impairs its capacity to release endothelium derived relaxant factor. *Ann Thorac Surg* 1989;**48**:417–20.

18. Underwood MJ, More R, Weeraseena N, Firmin RK, DeBono DP. The effect of surgical preparation and *in vitro* distension on the intrinsic fibrinolytic activity of human saphenous vein. *Eur J Vasc Surg* 1993;**7**:518–22.

19. Jang IK, Fuster V. Mechanisms of plaque formation and occlusion in venous coronary bypass grafts. In: Luscher T, Turina M, Braunwald E, eds. *Coronary artery graft disease: mechanisms and prevention*. Berlin: Springer Verlag, 1994; pp. 42–52.

20. Davies MG, Klyachkin ML, Dalen H, Massey MF, Svendsen E, Hagen PO. The integrity of experimental vein graft endothelium–implications on the etiology of early graft failure. *Eur J Vasc Surg* 1993;**7**:156–65.

21. Quist WC, Haudenschild CC, LoGerfo FW. Qualitative microscopy of implanted vein grafts: effects of graft integrity on morphologic fate. *J Thorac Cardiovasc Surg* 1992;**103**:671–7.

22. Clowes AW, Reidy MA, Clowes WM. Kinetics of cellular proliferation after arterial injury. I. Smooth muscle growth in the absence of endothelium. *Lab Invest* 1983;**49**:327–33.

23. Friedman RJ, Stemerman MB, Wenz B *et al*. The effect of thrombocytopaenia on experimental arteriosclerotic lesion formation in rabbit. *J Clin Invest* 1977;**60**:1191–201.

24. Angelini GD. Saphenous vein graft failure: etiologic considerations and strategies for prevention. *Curr Opin Cardiol* 1992;**7**:939–44.

25. Grondin CM, Lesperance J, Bourassa MG, Pasternac A, Campeau L, Grondin P. Serial angiographic evaluation in 60 consecutive patients with aortocoronary artery vein grafts 2 weeks, 1 year and 3 years after operation. *J Thorac Cardiovasc Surg* 1974;**67**:1–6.

26. Unni KK, Kottke BA, Titus JL, Frye RL, Wallace RB, Brown AL. Pathologic changes in aortocoronary saphenous vein grafts. *Am J Cardiol* 1974;**34**:526–32.

27. Grondin CM, Thornton JC (1994) The natural history of saphenous vein grafts. In: Luscher T, Turina M, Braunwald E. eds. *Coronary Artery Graft Disease; Mechanisms and Prevention*. Berlin Springer-Verlag; 1994; pp. 3–16

28. Davies AH, Magee TR, Baird RN, Sheffield E, Horrocks M. Vein compliance: a preoperative indicator of vein morphology and of veins at risk of vascular graft stenosis. *Br J Surg* 1992;**79**:1019–21.

29. Panetta TF, Marin ML, Veith FJ *et al*. Unsuspected preexisting saphenous vein disease. An unrecognised cause of vein bypass failure. *J Vasc Surg* 1992;**15**:102–12.

30. Marin ML, Veith FJ, Panetta TF *et al*. Saphenous vein biopsy: a predictor of vein graft failure. *J Vasc Surg* 1993;**18**:407–15.

31. Chan P, Munro E, Patel M *et al*. Cellular biology of human itimal hyperplastic stenosis. *Eur J Vasc Surg* 1993;**7**:129–35.

32. Chan P, Patel M, Betteridge L, Munro E *et al*. Abnormal growth regulation of vascular smooth muscle cells by heparin in patients with restenosis. *Lancet* 1993;**341**:341–2.

33. Holt CM, Francis SE, Newby AC *et al*. Comparison of response to injury in organ culture of human saphenous vein and internal mammary artery. *Ann Thorac Surg* 1993;**55**:1522–8.

34. Foster ED, Kranc MAT. Alternative conduits for aortocoronary bypass grafting. *Circulation* 1989;**79**(Suppl I):34–39.

35. Mills NL, Ochsner JL. Valvulotomy of valves in the saphenous vein graft before coronary artery bypass. *J Thorac Cardiovasc Surg* 1976;**71**:878–9.

36. Mills NL. Saphenous vein graft valves: 'the bad guys'. *Ann Thorac Surg* 1989;**48**:613–14.

37. Molina JE. Non-reversed saphenous vein grafts for coronary artery bypass grafting. *Ann Thorac Surg* 1989;**48**:624–7.

38. Angelini GD, Breckenridge IM, Butchart EG *et al.* Metabolic damage to human saphenous vein during preparation for coronary artery bypass grafting. *Cardiovasc Res* 1985;**19**:326–34.

39. Angelini GD, Breckenridge IM, Williams HM, Newby AC. A surgical preparative technique for coronary bypass grafts of human saphenous vein which preserves medial and endothelial functional integrity. *J Thorac Cardiovasc Surg* 1987;**94**:393–8.

40. Angelini GD, Passani SL, Breckenridge IM, Newby AC. Nature and pressure dependence of damage induced by disension of human saphenous vein coronary artery bypass grafts. *Cardiovasc Res* 1987;**21**:902–7.

41. Bryan AJ, Angelini GD. The biology of saphenous vein graft occlusion: etiology and strategies for prevention. *Curr Opin Cardiol* 1994;**9**:641–9.

42. Soyombo AA, Angelini GD, Bryan AJ, Newby AC. Surgical preparation induces injury and promotes smooth muscle cell proliferation in a culture of human saphenous vein. *Cardiovasc Res* 1993;**27**:1961–7.

43. Zilla P, von Oppell U, Deutsch M. The endothelium: a key to the future. *J Card Surg* 1993;**8**:32–60.

44. Barner HB, Fischer VW. Endothelial preservation in human saphenous vein harvested for coronary grafting. *J Thorac Cardiovasc Surg* 1990;**100**:148–9.

45. Gundry SR, Jones M, Ishihara T, Ferrans VJ. Intraoperative trauma to human saphenous veins: scanning electron microscopic comparison of preparation techniques. *Ann Thorac Surg* 1980;**30**:40–6.

46. LoGerfo FW, Quist WC, Crawshaw HM, Haudenschild CC. An improved technique for preservation of endothelial morphology in vein grafts. *Surgery* 1981;**90**:1015–24.

47. Gundry SR, Jones M, Ishihara T, Ferrans VJ. Optimal preparation techniques for human saphenous vein grafts. *Surgery* 1980;**88**:785–94.

48. Chester AH, O'Neil GS, Tadjkarimi S, Borland JAA, Yacoub M. Effect of perioperative storage solution on the vascular reactivity of the human saphenous vein. *Eur J Cardiothorac Surg* 1993;**7**:399–404.

49. Santoli E, DiMattia D, Boldorini R, Mingoli A, Tosoni A, Santoli C. University of Wisconsin solution and human saphenous vein graft preservation: preliminary anatomic report. *Eur J Cardiothorac Surg* 1993;**7**:548–52.

50. Zerkowski HR, Knocks M, Konerding MA *et al.* Endothelial damage of the venous graft in CABG. *Eur J Cardiothorac Surg* 1993;**7**:376–82.

51. Angelini GD, Bryan AJ, West RR, Newby AC, Breckenridge IM. Coronary artery bypass surgery: current practice in the United Kingdom. *Thorax* 1989;**44**:721–4.

52. O'Connor GT, Plume SK, Olmstead EM *et al.* A regional prospective study on in-hospital mortality associated with coronary artery bypass grafting. *JAMA* 1991;**266**:803–9.

53. Hannan EL, O'Donnell JF, Kilburn H JR, Bernard HR, Yazici A. Investigation of the relationship between volume and mortality for surgical procedures performed in New York state hospitals. *JAMA* 1989;**262**:503–10.

54. Bex JP, Latini L, Durandy Y. The art of cardiac surgery: critical analysis of the limits of statistics in cardiac surgery. *J Cardiac Surg* 1994;**9**:288–91.

55. Campeau L, Crochet D, Lesperance J, Bourassa MG, Grondin CM. Postoperative changes in aortocoronary saphenous vein grafts revised: angiographic studies at two weeks and at one year in two series of consecutive patients. *Circulation* 1975;**52**(Suppl I):369–377.

56. Bernal JM, Rabasa JM, Echevarria JR, Pajaron A, Revuelta JM. A multivariate analysis of factors affecting early coronary artery bypass patency. *Coronary Artery Disease* 1991;**2**:713–16.

57. Schwartz LB, O'Donohue MK, Purut CM, Mikat EM, Hagen PO, McCann RL. Myointimal thickening in experimental vein grafts is dependent on wall tension. *J Vasc Surg* 1992;**15**:176–86.

58. Galt SW, Zwolak RM, Wagner RJ, Gilbertson JJ. Differential responses of arteries and vein grafts to blood flow reduction. *J Vasc Surg* 1993;**17**:563–70.

59. Lansman JB, Hallam TJ, Rink TJ. Single activated ion channels in vascular endothelial cells as mechanotransducers. *Nature* 1987;**325**:811–13.

60. Rubanyi GM, Freay AD, Kauser K, Johns A, Harder DR. Mechanoreception by the endothelium: mediators and mechanisms of pressure and flow induced vascular responses. *Blood Vessels* 1990;**27**:246–57.

61. Hsieh H-J, Li N-Q, Frangos JA. Shear stress induced platelet derived growth factor gene expression in human endothelial cells is mediated by protein kinase C. *J Cell Physiol* 1992;**150**:552–8.

62. Ross R, Glomset J, Kariya B, Harker L *et al*. A platelet dependent serum factor stimulating the proliferation of arterial smooth muscle cells *in vitro*. *Proc Natl Acad Sci USA* 1974;**71**:1207–10.

63. Newby AC, George SJ. Proposed roles for growth factors in mediating smooth muscle proliferation in vascular pathologies. *Cardiovasc Res* 1993;**27**:1173–83.

64. Jawien A, Bowen-Pope DF, Lindner V, Schwartz SM, Clowes AW. Platelet derived growth factor promotes smooth muscle cell migration and intimal thickening in a rat model of balloon angioplasty. *J Clin Invest* 1992;**89**:507–11.

65. Bornfeldt KE, Raines EW, Nakano T, Graves LM, Krebs EG, Ross R. Insulin like growth factor-1 and platelet derived growth factor BB induce directed migration of human arterial smooth muscle cells via signalling pathways that are distinct from those of proliferation. *J Clin Invest* 1994;**93**:1266–74.

66. Nabel EG, Yang Z, Liptay S *et al*. Recombinant platelet derived growth factor B gene expression in porcine arteries induces intimal hyperplasia *in vivo*. *J Clin Invest* 1993;**91**:1822–9.

67. Nabel EG, Plautz G, Nabel GJ. Site specific gene expression *in vivo* by direct gene transfer into the arterial wall. *Science* 1990;**249**:1285–8.

67. Francis SE, Hunter S, Holt CM *et al*. Release of platelet derived growth factor activity from pig venous arterial grafts. *J Thorac Cardiovasc Surg* 1994;**108**:540–8.

68. Hughes S, Hall PA. Overview of the fibroblast growth factor and receptor families: complexity, functional diversity and implications for future cardiovascular research. *Cardiovasc Res* 1993;**27**:1199–203.

68. Lindner V, Reidy HA. Expression of basic fibroblast growth factor and its receptor by smooth muscle cells and endothelium in injured rat arteries: an En face study. *Circulation Res* 1993;**73**:589–95.

69. Edelmann ER, Nugent MA, Smith LT, Karnovsky MJ. Basic fibroblast growth factor enhances the coupling of intimal hyperplasia and proliferation of vasa vasorum in injured rat arteries. *J Clin Invest* 1992;**89**:465–73.

69. Sidawy AN, Hakim FS, Neville RF, Korman LY. Autoradiographic mapping and characterization of insulin like growth factor-1 receptor binding in human greater saphenous vein. *J Vasc Surg* 1993;**18**:947–53.

70. Foegh ML, Virmani R. Molecular biology of intimal proliferation. In: Yacoub M, Pepper J, eds. *Annual of Cardiac Surgery*. London: Current Science 1994:pp. 63–6.

70. Olson NE, Chao S, Lindner V, Reidy MA. Intimal smooth muscle cell proliferation after balloon injury: the role of basic fibroblast growth factor. *Am J Pathol* 1992;**140**:1017–23.

71. Yang Z, Luscher TF. Basic cellular mechanisms of coronary bypass graft disease. *Eur Ht J* 1993;**14**(Suppl I):193–7.

72. Boerboom LE, Bonchek LI, Kissebah AH *et al*. Effect of surgical trauma on tissue lipids in primate vein grafts: relation to plasma lipids. *Circulation* **62**(II):II42–II47.

73. Boerboom LE, Olinger GN, Lui T-Z, Rodriguez E, Ferrans V, Kissebah AH. Histologic, morphometric and biochemical evaluation of vein bypass grafts in a non-human primate model: sequential changes within the first three months. *J Thorac Cardiovasc Surg* 1990;**99**:97–106.

74. Scott HW, Morgan CV, Bolasny M *et al* (1970). Experimental atherosclerosis in autogenous venous grafts. *Arch Surg* 1970;**101**:677–81.

75. Landymore RW, Kinley CE, Cameron CA. Intimal hyperplasia in autogenous vein grafts used for arterial bypass. A canine model. *Cardiovasc Res* 1985;**19**:589–92.

76. Campeau L, Enjalbert M, Lesperance J *et al*. The relationship of risk factors to the development of atherosclerosis in saphenous vein bypass grafts and the progression of disease in the native circulation: a study 10 years after aorto-coronary bypass surgery. *N Engl J Med* 1984;**311**:1329–32.

77. Hoff HF, Beck GJ, Skibinski CI *et al*. Serum Lp[a] level as a predictor of vein graft stenosis after coronary artery bypass surgery in patients. *Circulation* 1988;**77**:1238–44.

77. Fox MH, Gruchow HW, Barboriak JJ *et al*. Risk factors among patients undergoing repeat aorto-coronary bypass procedures. *J Thorac Cardiovasc Surg* 1987;**93**:56–61.

78. Simpson HCR, Meade TW, Stirling Y *et al*. Hypertriglyceridemia and hypercoagulability. *Lancet* 1983;**1**:786–9.

79. Drexel H, Amann FW. Lipids and lipid lowering drugs and graft function. In: Luscher T, Turina M, Braunwald E. eds. *Coronary artery graft disease; mechanisms and prevention*. Berlin: Springer-Verlag, 1994, pp. 247–58.

80. Perrault LP, Carrier M, Hebert Y, Cartier R, Leclere Y, Pelletier LC. Early experience with the inferior epigastric artery in coronary artery bypass grafting. A word of caution. *J Thorac Cardiovasc Surg* 1991;**106**:928–30.

81. Subramanian VA, Hernandez Y, Rtack-Goldman K, Grabowski EF, Weksler BB. Prostacyclin production by internal mammary artery as a factor in coronary artery bypass grafts. *Surgery* 1986;**100**:376–83.

82. Chua YL, Pearson PJ, Evora PRB, Schaff HV. Detection of intraluminal release of endothelium-derived relaxing factor from human saphenous vein. *Circulation* 1993;**88**:[Part 2]:128–32.

83. Predel HG, Yang Z, Von Segesser L, Turina M, Buhler FR, Luscher TF. Implications of pulsatile stretch on growth of saphenous vein and mammary artery smooth muscle. *Lancet* 1992;**340**:878–9.

84. Yang Z, Von Segesser L, Stulz P, Turina M, Luscher TF. Pulsatile stretch and platelet-derived growth factor (PDGF). Important mechanism for coronary venous bypass graft disease. *Circulation* 1992;**86**:1–84(A).

85. Bach RG, Kern MJ, Donohue TJ, Aguirre FV, Caracciolo EA. Comparison of phasic blood flow velocity characteristics of arterial and venous coronary artery bypass conduits. *Circulation* 1993;**88**[Part 2]:133–140.

86. Angelini GD, Bryan AJ, Hunter S, Newby AC. A surgical technique that preserves human saphenous vein functional integrity. *Ann Thorac Surg* 1992;**53**:871–4.

87. Waters DJ, Thomsen TA. Saphenous vein preparation for coronary artery bypass grafting using a cardioplegia delivery set. *Ann Thorac Surg* 1993;**56**:385–6.

88. Goldman S, Copeland J, Moritz T *et al.* Internal mammary artery and saphenous vein graft patency; effects of aspirin. *Circulation* 1990;**82**(Suppl IV):237–42.

89. Chesebro JH, Clements IP, Fuster V *et al.* A platelet inhibitor drug trial in coronary artery bypass operations. Benefit of perioperative dipyridamole and aspirin therapy on early post-operative vein graft patency. *N Engl J med* 1982;**307**:73–8.

90. Fremes SE, Levinton C, Naylor CD, Chen E, Christakis GT, Goldman BS. Optimal antithrombotic therapy following aortocoronary bypass: a meta-analysis. *Eur J Cardiothorac Surg* 1993;**7**:169–80.

91. Antiplatelet Triallists Collaboration. Collaborative overview of randomised trials of antiplatelet therapy – II-Maintenance of vascular graft or arterial patency by antiplatelet therapy. *B M J* 1994;**308**:159–68.

92. Chesebro JH, Meyer BJ, Fernando-Ortiz A, Jang IK, Fuster V. Antiplatelet drugs. In: Luscher TF, Turina M, Braunwald E, eds. *Coronary artery graft disease; mechanisms and preventions.* Springer-Verlag, Berlin, 1994, pp. 276–98.

93. Gavaghan TP, Gebski V, Baron DW. Immediate postoperative aspirin improves vein graft patency early and later after coronary artery bypass graft surgery. A placebo controlled ran-domised study. *Circulation* 1991;**83**:1526–33.

94. Rajah SM, Nair U, Rees M *et al.* Effects of antiplatelet therapy with Ibobufen or aspirin-dipyridamole on graft patency one year after coronary artery bypass grafting. *J Thorac Cardiovasc Surg* 1994;**107**:1146–53.

95. Pfisterer M. Anticoagulant and antiplatelet drugs to prevent aortocoronary vein graft occlu-sion in: *Coronary Artery Graft Disease; Mechanisms and Prevention.* Eds Luscher T, Turina M, Braunwald E. Springer Verlag, Berlin; 299–311.

96. Van Der Meer J, Hillege HL, Kootstra GJ *et al.* for the CABADAS Group. Prevention of one year vein graft occlusion after aortocoronary bypass surgery: a comparison of low dose aspirin, low dose aspirin and dipyridamole, and oral anticoagulants. *Lancet* 1993;**342**:257–64.

97. Weber MAJ, Hasford J, Taillens C *et al.* Low dose aspirin versus anticoagulants for preven-tion of coronary graft occlusion. *Am J Cardiol* 1990;**66**:1464–8.

98. Pfisterer M, Burkart F, Jockers G *et al.* Trial of low-dose aspirin plus dipyridamole versus anticoagulants for prevention of aortocoronary vein graft occlusion. *Lancet* 1989;**1**:1–7.

99. Yli-Mayry S, Huikuri HV, Korhonen VR *et al.* Efficacy and safety of anticoagulant therapy started pre-operatively in preventing coronary vein graft occlusion. *Eur Ht J* 1992;**13**:1259–64.

100. Goldman S, Copeland J, Moritz T *et al.* and the Department of Veterans Affairs Cooperative Study Group. Long term graft patency [3 Years] after coronary artery surgery. Effects of aspirin: results of a VA cooperative study. *Circulation* 1994;**89**:1138–43.

101. Fuster V, Dyken ML, Vokonas PS, Hennekens C (AHA Medical/Scientific Statement). Aspirin as a therapeutic agent in cardiovascular disease. *Circulation* 1993;**87**:659–75.

102. Weissberg PL, Grainger DJ, Shanahan CM, Metcalfe JC. Approaches to the development of selective inhibitors of vascular smooth muscle proliferation. *Cardiovasc Res* 1993;**27**:1191–8.

103. Lichtlen PR, Hausmann H. Coronary angiography in the diagnosis of graft failure in: *Coronary Artery Graft Disease; Mechanisms and Prevention.* Eds Luscher T, Turina M, Braunwald E. Springer Verlag, Berlin; 144–171.

104. Waller BF, Pinkerton CA, Slack JD. Intravascular ultrasound: a histological study of vessels during life. The new gold standard for vascular imaging. *Circulation* 1992;**85**:2305–10.

105. Angelini GD, Bryan AJ. Extending the use of arterial conduits in myocardial revascularisation. *Br Heart J* 1992;**68**:161–2.

105. Francis SE, Holt CM, Taylor T, Gadsdon P, Angelini GD. Heparin and neointimal thickening in an organ culture of human saphenous vein. *Atherosclerosis* 1992;**93**:155–6.

106. Cambria RP, Ivarsson BL, Fallon JT, Abbott WM. Heparin fails to suppress intimal proliferation in experimental vein grafts. *Surgery* 1992;**111**:424–9.

107. Wilson NV, Salisbury JR, Kakkar VV. The effect of low molecular weight heparin on intimal hyperplasia in vein grafts. *Eur J Vasc Surg* 1994;**8**:60–4.

108. Gotlieb SO, Brunker JA, Mellito ED *et al.* Effect of Nifedipine on the development of coronary bypass graft stenoses in high risk patients. A randomised double blind placebo controlled trial. *Circulation* 1989;**80**:[Suppl 2]28.

109. Yang Z, Noll G, Luscher TF. Calcium antagonists differently inhibit proliferation of human coronary smooth muscle cells in response to pulsatile stretch and platelet derived growth factor. *Circulation* 1993;**88**:832–6.

110. Kranzhofer R, Schirmer J, Schomig A *et al.* Suppression of neointimal thickening and smooth muscle cell proliferation after arterial injury in the rat by inhibitors of Na$^+$–H$^+$ Exchange. *Circ Res* 1993;**73**:264–8.

111. Mitsuka M, Nagoe M, Berk BC. Na$^+$–H$^+$ Exchange inhibitors decrease neointimal formation after rat carotid injury. *Circulation Res* 1993;**73**:269–75.

112. Cashin-Hemphill L, Mack WJ, Pogoda JM, San Marco ME, Blankenhorn DH, Azen SP. Beneficial effects of colestopol+niacin on coronary atherosclerosis: a 4 year follow up. *JAMA* 1992;**264**:3013–17.

113. Kohler TR, Kirkman TR, Clowes AW. The effect of rigid external support on vein graft adaptation to the arterial circulation. *J Vasc Surg* 1989;**9**:277–85.

114. Violaris AG, Newby AC, Angelini GD. Effects of external stenting on wall thickening in arteriovenous bypass grafts. *Ann Thorac Surg* 1993;**55**:667–71.

115. Zweep HP, Satoh S, van der Lei B *et al.* Autologous vein supported with a biodegradable prosthesis for arterial grafting. *Ann Thorac Surg* 1993;**55**:427–33.

116. Batellier J, Wassef M, Merial R, Duriez M, Tedgui A. Protection from atherosclerosis in vein grafts by a rigid external support. *Arteriosclerosis and Thrombosis* 1993;**13**:379–84.

117. Ortu P, La Muraglia GM, Roberts G, Flotte T, Hasan T. Photodynamic therapy of arteries. A novel approach for treatment of experimental intimal hyperplasia. *Circulation* 1992;**85**:1189–96.

118. March KL, Patton BL, Wilensky RL, Hathaway DR (1993). 8-Methoxypsoralen and long-wave ultraviolet irradiation are a novel antiproliferative combination for vascular smooth muscle. *Circulation* 1993;**87**:184–91.

119. Rogers C, Karnovsky MJ, Edelman ER. Inhibition of experimental neointimal hyperplasia and thrombosis depends on the type of vascular injury and the site of drug administration. *Circulation* 1993;**88**:1215–21.

120. Ferns GA, Raines EW, Sprugel KH, Motani AS, Reidy MA, Ross R. Inhibition of neointimal smooth muscle accumulation after angioplasty by an antibody to PDGF. *Science* 1991;**253**:1129–32.

121. Lindner V, Reidy MA. Proliferation of smooth muscle cells after vascular injury is inhibited by an antibody against basic fibroblast growth factor. *Proc Natl Acad Sci USA* 1991;**88**:3739–43.

122. Choi ET, Engel L, Callow AD *et al.* Inhibition of neointimal hyperplasia by blocking $\alpha v \beta_3$ integrin with a small peptide fragment Gpen GRGDSPCA. *J Vasc Surg* 1994;**19**:125–34.

123. Dzau VJ, Pratt RE. Antisense technology to block autocrine growth factors. *J Vasc Surg* 1992;**15**:934–35.

124. Simons M, Edelman ER, DeKeyser J-L, Langer R, Rosenberg RD. Antisense c-*myb* oligonucleotides inhibit arterial smooth muscle cell accumulation *in vivo*. *Nature* 1992;**359**:67–70.

125. Bennett MR, Anglin S, McEwan JR, Jagoe R, Newby AC, Evan GI. Inhibition of vascular smooth muscle cell proliferation *in vitro* and *in vivo* by c-*myc* antisense oligonucleotides. *J Clin Invest* 1994;**93**:820–8.

126. Simons M, Rosenberg RD. Antisense nonmuscle myosin heavy chain and c-*myb* oligonucleotides suppress smooth muscle cell proliferation *in vitro*. *Circulation* 1992;**70**:835–43.

127. Shi Y, Hutchinson HG, Hall DJ, Zalewski A. Down regulation of c-*myc* expression by antisense oligonucleotides inhibits proliferation of human smooth muscle cells. *Circulation* 1993;**88**:1190–95.

128. Nabel EG, Pompili VJ, Plautz GE, Nabel GJ. Gene transfer and vascular disease. *Cardiovasc Res* 1994;**28**:445–55.

129. Nabel EG, Shum L, Pompili VJ *et al.* Direct gene transfer of transforming growth factor B_1 into arteries stimulates fibrocellular hyperplasia. *Proc Natl Acad Sci USA* 1993;**90**:1054–63.

130. Nabel EG, Yang Z-Y, Plautz G *et al.* Recombinant fibroblast growth fctor-1 promotes intimal hyperplasia and angiogenesis in arteries *in vivo*. *Nature* 1993;**362**:844–6.

131. Wilson JM, Birinyi LK, Salomon RN, Libby P, Callow AD, Mulligan RC. Implantation of vascular grafts lined with genetically modified endothelial cells. Science 1989;**244**:1344–6.

132. Conte MS, Birinyi LK, Miyata T *et al.* Efficient repopulation of denuded rabbit arteries with autologous genetically modified endothelial cells. *Circulation* 1994;**23**:2161–9.

133. Chen SJ, Wilson JM, Muller DWM. Adenovirus mediated gene transfer of soluble vascular adhesion molecule to porcine interposition vein grafts. *Circulation* 1994;**89**:1922–8.
    Weintraub WS, Jones EL, Craver JM, Guyton RA. Frequency of repeat coronary bypass or coronary angioplasty after coronary artery bypass surgery using saphenous venous grafts. *Am J Cardiol* 1994;**73**:103–12.

14 Cardiac transplantation for ischaemic heart disease

Andrew Murday

Cardiac transplantation offers patients with end-stage cardiac disease the prospect of increased life expectancy and a return to a good functional life. This prospect is available only at some risk to the potential transplant recipient. Cardiac transplantation carries a relatively high operative mortality. In addition to this there is a considerable practical burden for the recipient and their supporters resulting from continued dependency upon immunosuppressive drugs and the concomitant frequent hospital attendance for the supervision of these regiments. There is also the ongoing risk of postoperative morbidity resulting from the dual hazards of rejection and infection. Finally, there is a definitive time-limited prognosis following cardiac transplantation.

The decision to recommend to a patient a particular course of therapy usually depends upon a balance of the risks and benefits accruing from such a course of action. An additional and crucial factor when considering cardiac transplantation is the scarcity of organ donors. Currently in the UK there are approximately 300 heart donors each year. With a rapid and welcome reduction in road traffic accident deaths, the number of donors has probably reached a peak and is almost certainly destined to fall in the coming years. This pattern is mirrored throughout the world. The consequent restriction in transplant activity means that a substantial number of patients die while awaiting transplantation. For most programs, the waiting list mortality amounts to about 20%.

It is only possible to provide a very rough estimate of the total number of patients who might benefit from cardiac transplantation. It probably amounts to several thousand people each year. Nonetheless, the enormous shortfall between supply and demand of donor organs requires rationing on a grand scale. Those responsible for cardiac transplant programs must therefore take on a dual responsibility involving not only the securing of the best possible outcome for each individual transplant recipient, but also striving for the best possible outcome for each heart that is donated.

Contraindications to heart transplantation

Ideally, patients undergoing cardiac transplantation should be expected to return to normal or near-normal activities after the procedure. In practical terms, both the perioperative and postoperative outcomes for cardiac transplant recipients are dependent upon risks that can be reduced by excluding patients with certain pre-existing factors. All of these are relative and some of them, such as age, are arbitrary (Table 14.1) and vary from one programme to another. Nonetheless they provide a framework upon which those responsible for deciding which patients may be

Table 14.1 A list of relative contraindications to cardiac transplantation

Age greater than 60 years
Pulmonary vascular resistance greater than 3 Wood units
Irreversible renal failure (creatinine clearance <40 ml/min)
Irreversible hepatic failure
Acute severe hypotension with anuria
Symptomatic or severe asymptomatic peripheral or cerebral vascular disease
Severe chronic obstructive airways disease
Active infection
Undiagnosed radiographic pulmonary lesions
Pulmonary failure
Severe hypertension, i.e. diastolic pressure > 105 mm Hg on full medication.
Inability to comply with medical therapy
Drug addiction
Peptic ulceration
Osteoporosis
Previous neoplastic disease

accepted for cardiac transplantation, can begin to ensure the best possible outcome for each donated organ. One of the hardest parts of running a cardiac transplant service is to be faced in the clinic with a patient who falls well outside the accepted criteria, and having to deflate their and their families' only hope of long-term survival. This can be reduced by avoiding referral of such patients in the first place.

What constitutes inoperable coronary artery disease?

Apart from non-cardiac co-morbidity, the two most important factors when considering operability of a patient presenting with ischaemic heart disease are the state of the coronary arteries and the function of the left ventricle. A patient with good ventricular function and 'operable' vessels presents no problem; they should undergo myocardial revascularization when indicated. There is though a point for each cardiac surgeon when either the ventricular function is too poor, or the vessels are too diseased, for the risk of myocardial revascularization to be justified. Often the two circumstances coexist. Diffuse coronary artery disease and left ventricular dysfunction are both incremental risk factors for perioperative death during coronary artery surgery. However, the risk very rarely approaches that of cardiac transplantation. Nonetheless, there is no point in putting a patient through a surgical procedure if there is little likelihood of benefit.

There are now many reports in the literature of patients undergoing successful surgical revascularization with poor left ventricular function (1–4). Although many surgeons would not consider a left ventricular ejection fraction of under 30% as being anything particularly unusual in their practice, it is now well established that coronary artery bypass surgery (CABG) in such patients can be carried out with low risk of perioperative death. Furthermore, there is good evidence that myocardial contractility improves with improvement in myocardial blood supply. This had been established before the advent of positron emission tomography and single photon emission tomography. However, by identifying hibernating myocardium, these new techniques allow for accurate preoperative prediction of the likelihood of improvement in myocardial function after revascularization (5–10).

At least for myocardial contractility there are some methods for measuring the degree of dysfunction, and the amount of improvement after intervention. By its very nature, the degree of diffuseness of coronary atherosclerosis does not lend itself to simple measurement. It should therefore not be surprising that the number of opinions as to when coronary arteries become inoperable equates approximately to the number of cardiac surgeons whose opinions are sought. Nonetheless, the literature supports the view that coronary endarterectomy can be performed with a low risk of both perioperative myocardial infarct and mortality (11,12). Furthermore, although not as good as non-endarterectomized vessels, long-term graft patency can be achieved when endarterectomy is confined to those vessels that are truly ungraftable by other means and that subtend a coronary bed of reasonable size (13).

What simple set of rules can be formulated for the decision as to whether a patient with ischaemic heart disease is inoperable? First, I believe that patients who present with angina as a symptom should almost always be offered conventional surgery whatever the measured left ventricular function. There remain those patients with little in the way of angina, but suffering symptomatically from cardiac failure as a result of ischaemic myocardial disease. Poor ejection fraction itself, however measured, is not a useful guide of the potential merit of myocardial revascularization. What should be demonstrated is proof of reversible ischaemia.

In the absence of angina, formal exercise testing has two values. First, it may demonstrate exercise-related electrocardiographic changes. Second, when combined with oxygen consumption and carbon dioxide exhalation measurements, one can derive a value for maximal oxygen consumption at the point of onset of anaerobic metabolism. Providing the anaerobic threshold is reached, this value (V_{O_2max}) provides a measure of the ability of the circulation to provide tissues with oxygenated blood. It is a relatively sensitive and repeatable measure of cardiac reserve. Beyond that, assessment of the degree to which myocardial dysfunction is the result of hibernating myocardium, and therefore potentially reversible by revascularization, should be carried out in order that the potential benefit of revascularization can estimated.

Those patients who have already undergone surgical myocardial revascularization, but have persistent or recurrent symptoms, present a somewhat different problem. Despite reports from single units of low mortality for redo CABG procedures, the 30-day mortality in the whole of the UK for repeat operation is 9.2%, considerably higher than the 30-day mortality for first-time operations of 2.4% (United Kingdom Cardiac Surgical Register 1992). This incremental risk must push the management strategy decision more towards transplantation.

Results of heart transplantation for ischaemic heart disease

The most recent data from the cardiac surgical register of the Society of Cardiothoracic Surgeons of Great Britain and Ireland reveals that the 30-day mortality for all heart transplantation procedures was 19% in 1992. The International Society for Heart and Lung Transplantation (ISHLT) maintains a registry to which any unit throughout the world may provide data. This registry has accumulated a database comprising over 25 000 patients. Currently, the 1 year survival after first-time heart transplantation is 80%. These figures should be compared with a 30 day mortality for all isolated CABG operations in the UK of 2.4% (United Kingdom Cardiac Surgical Register

1992). For most transplant programs approximately 1 in 5 patients put on the waiting list will die before they can be transplanted. This presents an additional risk for patients accepted for heart transplantation while they wait for a suitable donor organ to become available.

Beyond the first year after transplantation, the commonest cause of graft failure and death is allograft vascular disease. This process, which is common to all solid organ transplants, results in diffuse intimal thickening of the graft vasculature, and is probably a manifestation of repeated endothelial damage, largely immunological in aetiology. According to the ISHLT figures the annual rate of mortality after the first year is fairly constant at about 3% per annum. Thus overall 10 year survival after cardiac transplantation is approximately 55%. There is now quite strong evidence from follow-up of several large series of transplant patients that allograft vascular disease is more likely to develop in patients whose original cardiac disease was ischaemic in aetiology (14,15).

Alternative strategies

Some centres have accumulated an experience using heterotopic cardiac transplantation. The Harefield group have reported a series of patients who underwent heterotopic cardiac transplantation together with adjunctive operation on the recipient heart (16). Of 28 patients, 20 underwent CABG and aneurysmectomy, 5 CABG, and 3 aneurysmectomy. The 1 year and 5 year actuarial survival rate were 79% and 63%. It remains the case that no other unit is currently accumulating the experience of the Harefield Hospital group with respect to heterotopic cardiac transplantation.

Emergency cardiac transplantation

A proportion of patients who suffer extensive myocardial infarction survive, dependent upon either pharmacological or mechanical support or a combination of both. These patients with a very limited life expectancy present a dilemma for their carers, in that often their only prospect of long-term survival is some form of cardiac replacement. Currently, heart transplantation is the only effective form of therapy. This situation may change in the future with the possible advent of satisfactory long-term mechanical heart replacement devices or readily available transgenic xenografts. The current generation of mechanical cardiac replacement devices offers only temporary support.

Until mechanical devices, or xenografts, provide satisfactory long-term cardiac replacement therapy, the only practical proposition for the patient in or on the verge of cardiogenic shock is temporary support followed as soon as possible by cardiac transplantation. In order to give these patients their best chance, they would need priority in terms of access to donor organs. This in turn would deprive those patients, not in such a critical condition, but for whom nonetheless the wait for a donor involves a risk of death. Surprisingly, the medium-term result of cardiac transplantation following a period of mechanical support, providing renal, hepatic, and other system failure have not supervened, are comparable to results following transplantation in the more stable situation (17). Donor organs are a finite and extremely limited resource. There are more than enough stable potential recipients for the number of donor organs available. It is therefore questionable to entertain the possibility of supporting very unstable patients in the hope of carrying out transplantation. Indeed, in the UK the 'urgent' category for waiting patients was abandoned several years ago, although it still exists in various forms in the US and other countries.

The moral dilemma

The cost of the first year of care for a patient undergoing cardiac transplantation is approximately 10 times the cost of a patient undergoing CABG surgery. According to the Cardiac Surgical Registry, in 1992 some 300 CABG operations were carried out for each million of population in the UK. This level of activity is approximately one quarter of that achieved in the US, and less than half of that in either France or Germany. Given that these resource restraints exist, and that as a result many individuals in the UK must forego the opportunity to have a proven effective intervention for their ischaemic heart disease, does it make sense to maintain a cardiac transplant service? The alternative would be to redirect the money currently devoted to cardiac transplantation to provide resources for an additional 3000 patients to have coronary artery surgery.

Summary

No trial exists, nor is there the prospect of one being carried out, in which patients with end-stage ischaemic heart disease have been randomized either to myocardial revascularization or to cardiac transplantation. The restriction in the numbers of patients undergoing cardiac transplantation, imposed by the small number of suitable donor organs, means that only a very small number of patients can benefit from the treatment. Every effort should be made to treat patients by non-transplant modalities, and this means revascularization whenever possible. There are very few circumstances when surgical myocardial revascularization is not possible, and it should always be considered as the management of choice rather than transplantation for ischaemic cardiomyopathy. In exceptional circumstances, when a patient presents with NYHA grade IV heart failure symptoms despite maximal medical therapy and when there is no evidence of reversible ischaemia, cardiac transplantation should be considered.

References

1. Shumakov VI, Kazakov EN, Senchenko OR *et al*. Surgical tactics in patients with ischaemic heart disease, extensive cicatricial myocardial lesions and circulatory insufficiency. *Grudnaia i Serdechno-Sosudistaia Khirurgiia* 1991;**12**:27–32.
2. Sanchez JA, Smith CR, Drusin RE, Reisen DS, Malm JR, Rose EA. High-risk reparative surgery. A neglected alternative to heart transplantation. *Circulation* 1990;**82**:IV302–5.
3. Dreyfus G, Duboc D, Blasco A *et al*. Coronary surgery can be an alternative to heart transplantation in selected patients with end-stage ischaemic heart disease. *European Journal of Cardiothoracic Surgery* 1993;**7**:482–7.
4. Tashiro T, Todo K, Haruta Y *et al*. Coronary artery bypass surgery in patients with poor left ventricular function. *Japanese Journal of Thoracic Surgery* 1993;**46**:385–90.
5. Takeishi Y, Tono-oka I, Kubota I *et al*. Functional recovery of hibernating myocardium after coronary bypass surgery: does it coincide with improvement in perfusion? *American Heart Journal* 1991;**122**:665–70.
6. Oxelbark S, Mannting F, Morgan MG, Henze A. Revascularization of infarcted myocardial. Effect on myocardial perfusion assessed with quantified T1-201 SPECT technique. *Scandinavian Journal of Thoracic and Cardiovascular* 1991;**25**:89–95.

 7. Lucignani G, Paolinin G, Landoni C *et al*. Presurgical identification of hibernating myocardial by combined use of technitium-99m hexakis 2-methoxyisobutylisonitrile single photon emission tomography and fluorine- 18 fluoro-2-deoxy-D-glucose positron emission tomography in patients with coronary artery disease. *European Journal of Nuclear Medicine* 1992;**19**:874–81.
 8. Carrel T, Jenni R, Haubold-Reuter S, Von Schulthess G, Pasic M, Turina M. Improvement of severely reduced left ventricular function after surgical revascularisation in patients with preoperative myocardial infarction. *European Journal of Cardiothoracic Surgery* 1992;**6**:479–84.
 9. Rahimtoola SH. The hibernating myocardium in ischaemia and congestive heart failure. *European Heart Journal* 1993;**14**:A22–A26.
10. Alfieri O, La Canna G, Giubbini R, Pardini A, Zogno M, Fucci C. Recovery of myocardial function. The ultimate target of coronary revascularisation. *European Journal of Cardiothoracic Surgery* 1993;**7**:325–30.
11. Johnston RH, Garcia-Rinaldi R, Wall MJ. Coronary artery endarterectomy: a method of myocardial preservation. *Texas Medicine* 1993;**89**:56–9.
12. Christakis GT, Rao V, Fremes SE, Chen E, Naylor CD, Goldman BS. Does coronary endarterectomy adversely affect the results of bypass surgery? *Journal of Cardiac Surgery* 1993;**8**:72–78.
13. Chaptal PA, Seguin JR, Frapier JM, Malak M, Grolleau R. Coronary revascularisation by long endarterectomy and reconstruction. *Annales de Chirurgie* 1991;**45**:653–6.
14. Sharples LD, Caine N, Mullins P *et al*. Risk factor analysis for the major hazards following heart transplantation: rejection, infection, and coronary occlusive disease. *Transplantation* 1991;**52**:244–52.
15. Frimpong-Boateng K, Haverich A, Schafers HJ *et al*. Results of orthotopic heart transplantation for ischaemic cardiomyopathy. *European Journal of Cardiothoracic Surgery* 1987;**1**:98–103.
16. Ridley PD, Khagani A, Musumeci F *et al*. Heterotopic heart transplantation and recipient heart operation in ischaemic heart disease. *Annals of Thoracic Surgery* 1992;**54**:333–7.
17. Farrar DJ, Hill JD. Univentricular and biventricular Thoratec VAD support as a bridge to transplantation. *Annals of Thoracic Surgery* 1993;**55**:276–82.

15 Long-term survival following coronary artery bypass grafts

Tom Treasure and Nicola Batrick

Coronary artery bypass grafting (CABG) is 30 years old and enormous numbers of operations have been performed over the last 20 years. It has probably been studied more extensively than any other surgical procedure and yet, when we come to review the long-term results, there are substantial gaps in our knowledge. Several problems confound any attempt to interpret the effects of the operation on the long term outcome for the patient.

Coronary artery disease has a long natural history. It is unpredictable in its progression but, in many cases, runs a remarkably benign course. We know that coronary plaques are common in young men. Soldiers in the Korean War, by definition previously fit young men killed in battle, were found to have a substantial incidence of coronary plaques; over two-third had obvious plaques at an average age of 22 years. The incidence was less in the victims of the Vietnam War, with a reduction in the number and severity of coronary lesions between these two conflicts. This may be the first evidence that an epidemic of coronary artery disease, the seeds of which were sown in the years after the Second World War, is on the decline. Perhaps the origins of the epidemic of coronary artery disease go back even further, to fetal life. There are cogent arguments to suggest that the relatively sparse diet of many pregnant mothers in the early years of the twentieth century, followed by the plentiful diet of the postwar years, rich in animal fats, was just the combination of circumstances that led to a steady rise of coronary artery disease during the 1950s and 1960s and which is now working its way up the age groups as the epidemic declines.

We know that the relationship between the presence of coronary plaques, their severity, and the occurrence of angina is extremely variable. Finally, the relationship of coronary lesions to the incidence of infarction and death is extremely varied and unpredictable (1); not only is the pathological substrate changing with time, but its relationship to clinical manifestations is haphazard.

Surgical practice, both in the selection of cases and the type of operation performed, has changed steadily. Worse ventricles and older people undergo surgery now compared with 20 years ago, and more artery grafts and extensive revascularization are employed. Many of the series reporting results 10–20 years after surgery divide the data according to numbers of vessels involved with substantial numbers of single and double vessel disease. Cases with fewer vessels diseased appear infrequently in surgical series. Between the uncertainties of the pathological process and the evolution of surgical practice, it is difficult to ascribe changes in survival appropriately to changing risk factors, medical management or operation.

Many studies have investigated the results of coronary artery bypass grafts, but for the purposes of this chapter we will largely confine ourselves to results 10 years or more after surgery. Data is available for as much as 20 years follow-up of purely saphenous vein drafts, but in looking at survival figures we have to note change in practice and in this case the likely effect of the increase in use of the internal mammary artery (IMA) from the mid 1980s. It is generally believed that the long-term results improved in the era following increased IMA usage. This makes all the interpretation of data sets from the 1970s difficult.

Techniques of myocardial preservation, anaesthesia and intensive care strategies have improved dramatically with time, undoubtedly affecting the immediate, and probably intermediate and long-term effects of coronary bypass surgery. The long-term follow up of IMA grafts is shorter, since the IMA was not clearly accepted or established as an alternative conduit until the 1980s. Thus, there are few large scale studies extending to more than 10 years of follow-up and for other arterial conduits there is little data at or beyond 5 years.

Internal mammary artery grafts

There is clearly documented evidence in the form of retrospective data analysis to support the use of the IMA as the conduit of choice in the majority of patients, especially to left anterior descending artery lesions. Indeed, it is widely accepted as a superior conduit to saphenous vein in terms of its patency rate at long-term follow-up and its long-term results in respect of anginal relief and long-term survival. However, there is no strong evidence that patency in the first days or weeks is better with an IMA. Any difference in early patency is more likely to be a surgical selection. It is likely that a surgeon would bias the outcome by ensuring that an IMA was not wasted on precarious, ragged, or poor run-off vessels. This is unprovable on the available evidence, but that is our reading of it.

By 5 years there is such a large difference that most people are completely convinced that the benefit is attributable to the inherent superiority of the IMA over vein. Furthermore, IMAs patent at that time and beyond can be seen to enlarge and serve larger territories whereas the only change seen in the vein graft is deterioration. It is known that the saphenous vein graft is prone to developing progressive intimal hyperplasia and that there is an increasing rate of attrition with time. Okies *et al.* (2) in comparing their series of saphenous vein drafts with IMA grafts found significantly increasing annual attrition rates in their vein grafts. They report an increase of atherosclerotic changes from 16% in the first 5–7 year period, compared to 36% in the 7–12 years follow-up ($p < 0.01$). Actual graft closure increased from 10% to 26% in these two periods ($p < 0.02$). Other angiographic studies have shown a 2% per year vein graft attrition rate in years 1–7 postoperatively, which increases to 5% per year from year 7 to year 12. The number of vein grafts that are patent and of a normal appearance at 10 years is 38–45% (3).

Much of the relevant work on the IMA has been carried out by the Cleveland Clinic (4) who are able to provide retrospective analysis of data with up to 20 years follow-up from their early practice from 1971–73, at a time when the vessel was not routinely used as an alternative conduit to vein by most centres. They clearly demonstrated in matched groups in the treatment of isolated left anterior descending artery (LAD) lesions that use of the IMA conferred not only a significant survival advantage, but also significantly better intervention-free survival. They then extended their initial work to encompass their practice in the period up to the end of the 1970s (1971–79) (3) in which they were able to compare large numbers of patients receiving IMA ± saphenous vein grafting (SVG)(2306) with a patient population receiving only vein grafts ($n = 3625$). From this, they confirmed their earlier findings of significantly increased survival in the IMA group: 86.6% compared to 75.9% in the SVG group ($p = 0.0001$ by univariate analysis). Cameron *et al.*

(5) performed 15 year follow-up of over 500 patients receiving IMA grafts (5% received double IMA) compared with 216 patients receiving vein grafts only. A number of variable factors were analysed. The survival rate at 15 years were 40.2% in the SVG group but 67.3% in those receiving IMAs, principally to LAD lesions (510/532). When the recurrence of angina was assessed it was seen that in both the SVG and IMA group the recurrence rate at 15 years was of the order of 73%. Event-free survival at 10 years, i.e. freedom from angina, infarction, reoperation, and death was 22.7% and 39% in the SVG and IMA group respectively.

Evidence of patency

When examining data on patency of grafts, it is important to take into consideration that most studies are of relatively small numbers of grafts and that mostly the restudies are undertaken in symptomatic patients.

Lytle and colleagues from the Cleveland Clinic (6) produced one of the most comprehensive assessments of IMA versus SVG by reviewing serial arteriograms in 501 patients (a mixture of symptomatic and asymptomatic patients) and comparing the findings in two distinct time periods: up to 5 years and 5–12 years. Patency in the first study group (i.e. up to 5 years) showed 82% of vein grafts studied were patent, 5% were stenotic or irregular, and 13% were occluded. In comparison, 97% (136/140) IMA grafts were patent with only 3% occluded or stenosed. Of the vein grafts patent in the first study group, 55% remained patent, 18% were stenotic or irregular, and 26% were occluded in the second phase of the study. However, of the IMA grafts patent in the first study group, 96% were unchanged and only 4% were occluded by up to 12 years follow-up, thus clearly demonstrating that IMA grafts are relatively free of atherosclerosis at up to 12 years postoperatively and that their late patency is superior to that of SVG. The attrition rate of vein grafts exceeded that of mammaries ($p < 0.0001$), but particularly important is that the difference becomes increasingly marked with time beyond 5–7 years because of almost no failures of established IMA grafts.

Angiographic studies were also carried out in a proportion of patients at 10 years in the early Cleveland study (4). In the SVG group 32 patients were studied with a graft occlusion rate of 50% and with 12% of remaining patent grafts having a greater than 50% stenosis. This compared to a 10% occlusion rate in the 29 patients in the IMA group re-studied, who had only a 3% rate of greater than 50% stenosis.

It would of course be of great interest and benefit to examine the improved patency of the IMA in terms of relief of symptoms, freedom from infarction, preservation of left ventricular function, freedom from further intervention, and survival. However, there is not sufficient data in the series reviewed to enable us to address many of these issues. Why does use of the IMA on LAD lesions produce such a favourable influence on long-term survival figures and cause a significant reduction in late morbidity?

Sequential arteriograms of IMAs have shown that frequently the IMA increases in size with time, thereby adapting its flow to the necessary oxygen demands, and indeed it does not appear to be as susceptible to atherosclerotic changes as coronary arteries or other vessels (3).

Histologically, we know that is the only peripheral artery that is elastic and it has been proposed that the IMA is protected from the changes that other vessels are subjected to because of the smaller number of fenestrations in its internal elastic lamina that prevent migration of smooth muscle cells into the subintimal plane initiating subintimal thickening (7).

Controversy still remains over whether use of both mammary vessels confers an advantage to the patient in the long term. A report from Green's group suggested that the results of double IMA were much superior, with only 33% recurrence of angina at 13 years compared with 73% in those with LIMA only, but the data set included only 38 patients with BIMA (5). The question was addressed by Fiore and co-workers in 1990 (8). Although initial reports from the team suggested a survival advantage in the double IMA group at 15 years, they modified the claim when data were subsequently re-analysed by Kirklin and Blackstone (9). However, their data did show a statistically significant advantage in the double IMA group when freedom from recurrent angina and myocardial infarction was analysed ($p < 0.025$ for both).

In an attempt to move towards complete arterial revascularization, other conduits are being assessed including the gastroploeic artery and the inferior epigastric artery. The radial artery is also being reassessed as an alternative conduit, despite its poor results when originally investigated in the 1970s. There are no long-term follow-up results beyond 3–5 years on the function and patency of these grafts, but early results are encouraging with patency rates of greater than 90% at 3–5 years follow-up of the gastroepiploic artery.

Freedom from angina

It is interesting that despite the extensive analysis on longevity after coronary surgery, few of the studies fail to give data on the freedom from angina at 10 or 15 years survival, or any indication of the quality of life following surgery.

Schaff's data from the Mayo Clinic (10) showed that more than half of the patients had some recurrence of their angina by the tenth year of follow-up. A fifth had a diagnosed myocardial infarction within that time and 11% had undergone further coronary surgery. The analysis is based upon the 355/500 who were alive at the time of the review; of these, 69% reported that they were improved although nearly half (46%) had cardiac symptoms. There were several predictors of likely return of angina. One was the number of vessels diseased; it is not surprising that there was a greater likelihood of increase of angina and of subsequent myocardial infarction with more vessels diseased ($p = 0.06$). This employs a simple but robust coronary disease stratification and, for the group, the worse pathology results in the worse symptoms.

Although we have discussed above the problem of the relatively poor association between number, site, and severity of coronary plaques, severity of angina, and risk of infarction in the prediction of outcome for an individual, it would be surprising if there were poor association between severity of disease and outcome for a group. However, the p value is 0.06, which would stand not up to conventional criteria for 'proof'.

Leaving vessels ungrafted is also associated with less good outcome in that recurrence of angina was higher at 52% if one vessel was left ungrafted and 68% if two were left ungrafted. This again is not surprising, since angina is due to poor perfusion and coronary surgery relieves it. The sceptic could argue that the cases in whom the surgeon left ungrafted vessels must have had particularly difficult distal vessels, and thus the pattern of disease determined outcome. The survival figures for this Mayo Clinic series show a clear relationship between 10 year survival and number of vessels diseased (90%, 75% and 60% for one-, two-, and three-vessel disease respectively). In non-randomized CASS, surgery largely neutralized the differential survival effect of the extent of coronary disease (12) bringing them to rather similar survival, at least up to 5 years.

In a report from Baylor, Lawrie and colleagues (11) provide us with some data on work status and angina relief in patients 10–14 years post-CABG and subsequently in 1991 (13) at 15–20 years. They followed over 1000 patients, initially finding that 49% were asymptomatic at 10–14 years and 38% were improved compared with their preoperative status. They showed an increasing need for anti-anginal medication, when comparing medication requirements at 10 years with those at 10–14 years. Those requiring beta-blockage rose from 36% to 68% and use of vasodilators increased from 49% to 56%. In the 10–14 year follow-up, for 885 patients questioned, 46% were carrying out the same or more work but 24% were unable to work.

In a later paper, examining 1698 patients up to 15–20 years post-bypass surgery, Lawrie *et al.* (13) provided similar data for 332 patients who were followed up for 16–20 years post-saphenous vein CABG. Of the surviving patients, 67% were asymptomatic and 26% were improved. Only 2% had worse angina than preoperatively. Figures on work status revealed 26% were able to carry out the same amount of work but 69% were carrying out less or no work, although this must clearly reflect the ageing of some of the population into retirement.

The VA study (14) which reviewed its patients according to angina score and intention to treat score, showed that these scores were much lower at 5 years in the surgical treatment group although at 10 years there was no significant differences between groups. The actual figures quoted free of angina at 10 years are surprisingly poor, 6% versus 5% (medicine versus surgery) and very different from other studies. This is a reminder that we may draw confusing inferences from any retrospective analysis of clinical data if we are overlook the influence of case mix, surgical skill, learning curve, and the era effect. At the time the study was first published there was anxiety about whether the surgical limb of the trial was representative of contemporary practice and it is certainly unlike present coronary surgery in many respects.

Van Brussel (15) quotes freedom from angina figures similar to those of both Lawrie and Schaff in his study of 428 patients receiving SVG in a comparable era; 52% at 10 years and 27% at 5 years.

Factors affecting long-term survival

Are there preoperative determinants that can be isolated as predictors of long-term survival? Many of the authors already discussed have investigated this, and clear evidence is available to suggest that left ventricular function, age and metabolic factors such as diabetes are of most importance.

Left ventricular dysfunction has been found by many to be a factor that can be directly related to poor long-term survival and, indeed, increased perioperative risk. However, it must be remembered that poor left ventricular function is not a contraindication to surgery as many of these patients have poor results in the short and long term with medical treatment.

Johnson *et al.* (16) studied the factors that affected long-term survival in over 6000 patients undergoing CABG. It was clear that severe left ventricular dysfunction at the time of surgery was the dominant factor affecting long-term survival. The 10 year survival decreased from 79% in patients with normal left ventricular function to 49% in those classified as having severe left ventricular dysfunction (i.e. ejection fraction less than 40%). These survival figures dropped to 59% and 28% respectively at 15 years.

Van Brussel *et al.* (15) also found in his study of 428 patients at 15 years post-CABG that by Cox regressional analysis abnormal left ventricular function was an independent predictor of poor late survival.

Table 15.1 Relationship of survival to left ventricular function

Source	Left ventricular function classification	10 year survival
Johnson *et al*. 1989 (16)	Normal vs < 40%	79% vs 49%
Lawrie *et al*. 1991 (13)	Normal vs	70% vs 55%
	LVEDP > 15 mm Hg	
Cosgrove *et al*. 1985 (18)	Normal or severe	84% vs 54%

Lawrie *et al*. (11) classified the bypass graft patients they reviewed into either good or poor left ventricular function (good left ventricular function meaning LVEDP < 15 mm Hg with no akinetic or aneursymal segments on ventriculography). The survival probability at 10 years for good left ventricular function was 70% compared with 55% for those with poor left ventricular function, thus attaining statistical significance.

The CASS trial (17) randomized its patients according to left ventricular function and found that those patients with an ejection fraction between 0.35 and 0.5 who had been randomized to surgery had a survival advantage at 10 years compared to those treated medically (80% survival versus 59% survival.)

Cosgrove *et al*. (18) reviewed data from a large series at the Cleveland Clinic in order to elucidate preoperative determinants of long-term survival. They quote an actuarial survival rate for those with severe left ventricular impairment at 10 years of 54% compared to 84% in those with normal function (Table 15.1). They also found that advancing age was the single most important determinant affecting long-term survival. Age was of particular relevance in the over 60 year old group, where it was the most significant risk factor, but in those patients receiving surgery under the age of 50 it had no prognostic significance. Johnson's (16) findings support this, showing that actuarial survival at 10 years in patients under 45 years is 78% dropping to 60% in patients aged 65–70 years. It is therefore important that age is taken into consideration whenever a specific risk factor is considered.

Metabolic factors affecting survival

Metabolic factors such as diabetes mellitus and hypercholesterolaemia are contributary factors to development of coronary artery disease, but what effect do they have on the degeneration of bypass grafts and the long-term survival of patients who undergo CABG? Lawrie *et al*. in 1987 (11) found that only severely elevated serum cholesterol levels (total >6 mmol/l) were predictive of vein graft degeneration.

In 1991 the same group conducted Kaplan–Meier analyses of the influence of total plasma cholesterol and triglycerides on 20 year survival probablities (13). They found that there were no significant differences in survival at 20 years and that therefore total cholesterol or triglycerides were not predictive of survival. Lytle *et al*. (6) conducted serial arteriograms in patients undergoing coronary surgery and found that hypercholesterolaemia was associated with progression of stenosis or occlusion in vein grafts ($p < 0.006$), but that the influence on the overall 10 year survival figures was slight. Van Brussel (15) looked at preprocedural independent risk factors that were predictive of myocardial infarction following CABGs and reports that an elevated serum triglyceride was one. Recent data from 3 studies suggest should pay more attention to cholesterols ***.

Lawrie *et al.* (19) also investigated the influence of diabetes mellitus on the long-term survival on 212 diabetic patients undergoing CABG in 1968–73 (8% insulin dependent). They found that the severity of the diabetes preoperatively influenced the long-term survival, the overall survival probability at 15 years being 53% in non diabetics, 33% in those patients receiving oral hypoglycaemics and 19% in the insulin dependent group.

Survival in women

More controversial than the influence of left ventricular function, age, etc. on long-term results of CABG is the effect of the patient's sex on likelihood of survival. Original work, mainly based on data from surgery carried out in the 1970s, has suggested that CABGs in women were of reduced efficacy, with higher short-term and long-term mortalities and less symptomatic relief in the long term. However, more recent data from the CASS Registry goes some way to countering this. The different endpoints examined by the various groups makes direct comparison of this data difficult, and for this reason we have included below a brief synopsis of what we consider to be the most important studies.

Bolooki *et al.* (20) published findings from a small series (*n* = 260, 13% female) of early results on surgery performed from 1969 to 1973. He found that operative mortality and 4 year follow-up of functional status were worse in women than in men.

Douglas *et al.* In 1981 (21) reviewed data in their practice of CABG carried out from 1973 to 1979 on 492 women compared to 2663 men with follow-up for 78 months. They found that at follow-up of 21 months, significantly more men were asymptomatic (70% versus 52%, (*p* < 0.001) and that men achieved a higher activity level. They suggested that this difference between the sexes may be in part due to the smaller coronary vessels in females making incomplete revascularization more likely and also graft flow less certain. However, this was unlikely to be the entire explanation as late symptomatic results of patients who were completely revascularized and matched (for baseline characteristics) also showed 71% men versus 53% women were asymptomatic (*p* < 0.001). SVG patency was greater in men than in women 86% versus 74%: (*p* < 0.001); however, these figures were based on re-studies carried out in predominantly symptomatic patients and the overall patency rate might be different if all grafts were restudied.

In 1986 Richardson (22) published data on 256 women out of 1089 patients undergoing CABG during the period 1978–85 in Alabama. Again long-term data is only available to 5 years, but they report a cumulative survival rate of 91% for men and 82% for women (*p* = 0.008). Event-free survival overall was 61% at 5 years. For men it was 67% at 5 years and for women 43% (*p* = 0.03).

However, Tyras' (23) in 1978 reported that 5 year survival was *not* significantly different between men and women in their series of 1541 patients (15.6% women). They also report a favourably high incidence of anginal relief in women 70% at 5 years being asymptomatic and 22% markedly improved having either class 1 or class 2 angina (Canadian Heart Association classification.).

Killen *et al.* (24) reviewed 385 female patients (14.6% of their total experience) from a 6 year period in the early 1970s. They compared actuarial survival between men and women and also expected survival with an age- and sex-matched general population. The study showed that actuarial survival in women was equal to that of men following CABG — 75% at 10 years. However, CABG in women did not confer to them a 'normal age matched survival pattern' as it did in men.

The Coronary Artery Surgery Study (CASS) Registry provides the longest follow-up of male and female patients at 15 years, as published as an abstract in *Circulation Supplement 1992*. These authors found that survival (including operative mortality) in those randomized to the surgical group was 50% for men versus 47% for women at 15 years, which was not statistically significant.

Left main stem lesions

It is generally accepted that the presence of a significant left main stem lesion demonstrated angiographically is an indication for priority surgery, but what effect does the presence of a lesion at this site have on long-term survival following surgery? Yusuf and co-workers (25) reviewed patient data from seven of the randomized trials that compared surgical versus medical treatment in stable coronary heart disease, including the VA trial (14), CASS (17), and the European Study (26). They found that in general those patients randomized to surgery had a significantly lower mortality and that the risk reduction was greater in patients with left main stem disease undergoing surgery than those patients with three-vessel disease at 5 year follow-up. The data are inadequate to draw a firm conclusion but it is probable that, once operated, the outlook for these patients resembles that for those with three-vessel disease.

Long-term survival in patients undergoing acute coronary artery surgery

The controversy of timing of CABG surgery following acute myocardial infarction still continues, but what are the long-term results in this particular patient population? Some answers have been provided by Floten *et al.* In 1989 (27) and by Applebaum in 1991 (28). Floten quotes 10 year survival at 70% for all patients in his study undergoing CABG within 30 days of myocardial infarction. This survival is independent of the actual timing of the surgery (ranging from less than 24 hours to 15–30 days), and although there was a difference in initial operative mortality between the groups, this difference was not statistically significant. Applebaum's data extends to only 5 year follow-up on 406 patients, again undergoing surgery within 30 days of an acute myocardial infarction. His survival figure at 5 years was 84%.

Randomized trials

There have been several large scale studies that were principally designed to compare the strategies of initial surgical management versus medical management in the treatment of coronary artery disease in a prospective randomized fashion, and these are frequently quoted when providing data on long-term follow-up: the CASS study (17), the VA Coronary Artery Bypass Surgery Study Group (14), and the European Coronary Surgery Study Group (26). All three trials provide valuable data, but there are several important factors that have to be taken into account when interpreting their long-term survival results.

As previously stated, these were randomized trials, each patient being allocated to one of two initial treatment groups, either medicine or surgery. It is important to take into consideration the cross-over rate from the medical treatment group to surgical intervention that occurred during the follow-up period. These rates are of a similar magnitude in all three subjects: of the order of 40% during the variable follow-up periods. Obviously, the high cross-over rate makes interpretation of late results difficult since any disadvantage of intention to treat medically is ameliorated when there is such a high cross-over to the surgical group.

Again, as with all studies, the era effect must be considered. The CASS trial was conducted on patients undergoing surgery between 1975 and 1979, the VA study was initiated in 1972, and the European study between 1973 and 1976. Of particular note is that, reflecting the surgical practice of that time, the number of IMA grafts used was very low in comparison with later practice after the efficacy of the IMA graft had been proven.

The interpretation of the CASS data has to be viewed in the light of the exclusion criteria applied to the 24 959 enrolled on the register. Of these only 2099 were eligible and only 780 eventually were randomized. Excluded from the trial were patients with a poor left ventricle (ejection fraction less than 0.35), patients over 65 years old, patients with left main stem lesions greater than 70%, and patients with angina of severity class 3 or 4 (Canadian Cardiovascular Society).

The CASS 10 year follow-up reports no statistically significant cumulative survival in those patients with an initial medical management compared to those randomized to surgical treatment (79% versus 82%), although, as previously quoted, those with poor left ventricular function showed a survival advantage in the surgical group.

The VA Study Group report on their data up to 18 years of follow-up and conclude that although there may have been an advantage in the surgically treated group in the initial follow up, these benefits were only transient. They found that there was a significant survival advantage with surgical therapy at 7 years (77% surgery versus 70% medicine, $p = 0.043$) but that by 11 years the survival rates were identical in the two groups at 58% and by final review at 18 years the cumulative survival rate was 33% versus 30% for medicine and surgery respectively ($p = 0.06$).

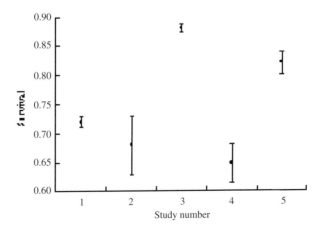

Fig. 15.1 Survival 10 years post coronary artery bypass grafts. Values are expressed as survival ±70% confidence interval. Data from five studies: 1, Smith *et al.* (26); 2, Yusuf *et al.* (25); 3, Alderman *et al.* (17); 4, Loop *et al.* (3); 5, VA Study (14).

However, in the report of the European study data up to 8 years follow-up, published in 1982, survival was improved significantly by surgery in all the population considered, in those with three-vessel disease, and non-significantly in those with left stem lesions. We have compared 70% confidence limits for 10 year survival in five of the trials that provide data for survival at this time — see Fig. 15.1. The majority of these trials are concerned with surgery carried out in the early part of the 1970s and hence provide data primarily for SVG, although there are a small number of arterial conduits in the CASS registry data. The long-term result are summarized in Yusuf *et al.*'s meta-analysis of these three large and some other smaller trials (25).

References

1. Patterson DHL, Treasure T. The culprit coronary artery lesion. *Lancet* 1991;**338**:1379–80.
2. Okies JE, Scott Page U, Bigelow JC, Krause AH, Saloman NW. The left internal mammary artery: the graft of choice. *Circulation* 1984;**70**:1-213–21.
3. Loop FD, Lytle BW, Cosgrove DM *et al*. Influence of the internal mammary artery graft on 10 year survival and other cardiac events. *New England Journal of Medicine* 1986;**314**:1–7.
4. Boylan MJ, Lytle BW, Loop FD *et al*. Surgical treatment of isolated left anterior descending coronary stenosis. Comparison of left internal mammary artery and venous autograft at 18 to 20 years of follow-up. *Journal of Thoracic and Cardiovascular Surgery* 1994;**107**:657–62.
5. Cameron A, Kemp HG, Green GE. Bypass surgery with the internal mammary artery graft: 15 year follow up. *Circulation* 1986;**74**:3-30–6.
6. Lytle BW, Loop FD, Cosgrove DM, Ratliff NB, Easley K, Taylor PC. Long term (5 to 12 years) serial studies of internal mammary artery and saphenous vein coronary bypass grafts. *Journal of Thoracic and Cardiovascular Surgery* 1985;**89**:248–58.
7. Sims FH. Discontinuities in the internal elastic lamina: a comparison of coronary and internal mammary arteries. *Aretery* 1985;**13**:127–43.
8. Naunheim KS, Barner HB, Fiore AC. 1990. Results of internal thoracic artery grafting over 15 years: single versus double grafts. 1992 update. *Annals of Thoracic Surgery* 1992;**53**:716–18.
9. Naunheim KS, Barner HB, Fiore AC. 1992 Update: Results of internal thoracic artery grafting over 15 years: single versus double grafts. *Annals of Thoracic Surgery* 1992;**53**:716–18.
10. Schaff HV, Gersh MB, Pluth JR *et al*. Survival and functional status after coronary artery bypass grafting: results 10 to 12 years after surgery in 500 patients. *Circulation* 1983;**68**:200–5.
11. Lawrie GM, Morris GC, Baron A, Norton J, Glaeser DH. Determinants of survival 10 to 14 years after coronary bypass: Analysis of pre operative variables in 1448 patients. *Annals of Thoracic Surgery* 1987;**44**:180–5.
12. Myers WO, Schaff HV, Gersh BJ *et al*. Improved survival of surgically treated patients with triple vessel coronary artery disease and severe angina pectoris. A report from the Coronary Artery Surgery Study (CASS) registry. *Journal of Thoracic and Cardiovascular Surgery* 1989;**97**:487–95.
13. Lawrie GM, Morris GC, Earle N. Long term results of coronary bypass surgery. Analysis of 1698 patients followed 15 to 20 years. *Ann Surg* 1991;**213**:377–85.
14. The VA Coronary Artery Bypass Surgery Cooperative Study Group (Peduzzi P). Eighteen year follow up in the Veterans Affairs cooperative study of coronary artery bypass surgery for stable angina. *Circulation* 1992;**86**:121–30.

15. Van Brussel BL, Plokker T, Ernst MPG *et al*. Venous coronary artery bypass surgery: A 15 year follow up study. *Circulation* 1993;**88**:2-87–92.

16. Johnson WD, Brenowitz JB, Kayser KL. Factors influencing long term (10 year to 15 year) survival after successful coronary artery bypass surgery. *Annals of Thoracic Surgery* 1989;**48**:19–25.

17. Alderman EL, Bourassa MG, Cohen LS *et al*. Ten-year follow-up of survival and myocardial infarction in the randomized Coronary Artery Surgery Study [see comments]. *Circulation* 1990;**82**:1629–46.

18. Cosgrove DM, Loop FD, Lytle BW *et al*. Determinants of 10 year survival after primary myocardial revascularization. *Ann Surg* 1985;**202**:480–9.

19. Lawrie GM, Morris GCJ, Glaeser DH. Influence of diabetes mellitus on the results of coronary bypass surgery. Follow up of 212 diabetic patients 10 to 15 years after surgery. *JAMA* 1986;**256**:2967–70.

20. Bolooki H, Vargas A, Green R, Kaiser GA, Ghahramani A. Results of direct coronary artery surgery in women. *Journal of Thoracic and Cardiovascular Surgery* 1975;**69**:271–7.

21. Douglas JS, King SB, Jones EL, Craver JM, Bradford JM, Hatcher CR. Reduced efficacy of coronary bypass surgery in women. *Circulating* 1981;**64**:2-11–16.

22. Richardson JV, Cyrus RJ. Reduced efficacy of coronary artery bypass grafting in women. *Annals of Thoracic Surgery* 1986;**42**:s16–21.

23. Tyras DH, Barner HB, Kaiser GC, Codd JE, Laks H, William VL. Myocardial Revascularisation in Women. *Annals of Thoracic Surgery* 1978;**25**:449–53.

24. Killen DA, Reed WA, Arnold M, McCallister BD, Bell HH. Coronary artery bypass in women: Long term survival. *Annals of Thoracic Surgery* 1982;**34**:559–63.

25. Yusuf S, Zucker D, Peduzzi P *et al*. Effect of coronary artery bypass graft surgery on survival: overview of 10 year results from randomised trials by the Coronary Artery Bypass Graft Surgery Trialists Collaboration. *Lancet* 1994;**344**:562–70.

26. European Coronary Artery Study Group. Long term results of prospective study of coronary artery bypass surgery in stable angina pectoris. *Lancet* 1982;1174–80.

27. Floten HS, Ahmad A, Swanson JS *et al*. Long term survival after post infarction bypass operation: Early versus late operation. *Annals of Thoracic Surgery* 1989;**48**:757–63.

28. Applebaum R, House R, Rademaker A *et al*. Coronary artery bypass grafting within thirty days of acute myocardial infarction. Early and late results in 406 patients. *Journal of Thoracic and Cardiovascular Surgery* 1991;**102**:745–52.

16 Epidemiology of coronary artery bypass surgery

John N. Newton

Introduced 30 years ago (1), coronary artery bypass grafting (CABG) is now widely adopted yet still to some extent controversial (2–4).

In this chapter, the pattern of use of CABG surgery is described, principally in the US and the UK, and the question of what constitute an appropriate level of intervention is considered. Statistics on coronary artery surgery are remarkable because of dramatic changes in surgical rates, and in the patient population, over the last two decades and because of obvious variation in surgical rates between countries, and between different areas of the same country.

Statistics on CABG activity

Information has been collected on procedures performed in the UK since 1977 by the Society of Thoracic and Cardiovascular Surgeons (5). This is maintained by the society for the benefit of its members in the form of the UK Cardiac Surgical Register. Private operations are included, but only if performed in NHS hospitals. A special study of the availability of CABG in four British regions was also commissioned by the national Clinical Standards Advisory Group (6) and has been updated (7). The European Academy of Sciences and Arts founded an Institute for Cardiac Survey in 1990. The Institute, based in Salzburg, was set up to monitor the development of cardiac interventions in Europe. The European and the UK registries rely on returns received from cardiac surgical units, or national registers in the latter case, and do not collect demographic or clinical data on the patients treated. More informative but less complete data are available from the National Hospital Discharge Survey in the United States (8). These are collected annually by the National Center for Health Statistics from a sample of US hospitals and include information on the patients' age, sex, race, area of residence, and other procedures or diagnoses. Similar data are available for all hospital discharges in Canada, for example from the Hospital Medical Records Institute in Ontario (9). In Table 16.1, non-age-adjusted rates of coronary artery surgery are given for the UK, the US, and Canada from 1981 to 1992.

Trends in CABG surgical rates

United States

Uptake of the new technique in the US was extremely rapid. As early as 1972 over 400 American hospitals were undertaking CABGs on a regular basis (10). By 1982 it was estimated

Table 16.1 Rates of coronary artery bypass surgery in the United Kingdom, United States and Ontario (1981–94): bypass grafts per million population per year

Year	UK[a]	US[b]	Ontario[c]
1981	106	694	321
1982	128	735	360
1983	167	810	396
1984	186	794	379
1985	208	851	406
1986	212	952	438
1987	225	1010	454
1988	217	1042	473
1989	245	1061	480
1990	277	1058	506
1991	301	1058	566
1992	365		
1993	396		
1994	417		
1995	425		

Sources: [a]UK Cardiac Surgical Register; [b]National Center for Health Statistics; [c]Statistics Canada.

that approximately one million operations had been performed on American citizens — at the same time a total of only 1300 patients had been entered into the randomized trials. It is hardly surprising that this exponential growth in activity led to concern that a whole health care industry was being built up around the operation (11). The expansion of cardiac surgical facilities across the US in the first decade of CABG surgery may have been necessary to achieve access for the national population. The continued growth that took place in the second decade looked as if it was driven more by the interests of the hospitals than the interests of their patients. By 1988 there were over 800 hospitals in the US with CABG programmes. Bypass surgery had become part of the national culture; failure to offer it was thought to condemn hospital to second-rate status.

It has been shown in a study from New York (12) that the availability of cardiac services in a hospital increases the likelihood of patients who present with an acute myocardial infarction subsequently undergoing CABG (odds ratio = 2.52 (1.95–3.24). However, the rate of bypass surgery in the US increased much more in the 1980s than could be accounted for simply by the increased number of hospitals undertaking the operations (see Table 16.1). Some surgeons believe that the increased competition for this lucrative work has led to less selective use of bypass surgery (10). Published data from case series tends to show the opposite, i.e. more extensive coronary disease among those undergoing CABG now than in the past (13). There now appear to be more patients with triple-vessel disease, left ventricular dysfunction, or unstable angina, and fewer with single-vessel disease. The publication of results from trials of CABG showing benefits in these groups of patients may have had an effect. Whether the published reports (which are from teaching centres) represent practice in the smaller community hospitals is also unknown.

The greater availability of invasive diagnostic tests, and a greater propensity to use them in a wider range of patients, has been an important factor influencing the CABG rate. The expansion of diagnostic facilities would have increased the number of patients found to be suitable for bypass surgery even if criteria for surgery did not change. The National Hospital Discharge Survey showed three times as many coronary arteriography procedures in 1986 as in 1979 (14). Another important cause of the rise in surgical rates was greater public awareness of the benefits and low risks of coronary surgery, especially among older Americans. The biggest single change in cardiac surgical practice in the US has been the increasing age of the bypass population. Older patients, even octagenarians, (15), are now less likely to accept the disability and handicap of chronic stable angina despite improvements in medical therapy. These patients are much more likely to be considered suitable for investigations with a view to coronary surgery than they were 15 years ago. In the Cleveland Clinic the median age of patients undergoing their first bypass operation rose from 56 in 1979 to 64 in 1988 and the proportion of patients over 70 rose from 4% to 30% in the same period. Nationally, 41% of patients were over 65 in 1986 compared with 23% in 1979.

Other trends reported from the Cleveland Clinic, which seem to represent general trends in practice, include an increase in the proportion of women in the patient population, from 12% to 22%. This may be partly as a result of the more even sex distribution of ischaemic heart disease (IHD) in older patients, but may also represent a reduction in the sex bias in favour of males (16). There was also an increase in the proportion of bypass operations that were repeats, from 6.8% in 1980 to 23.4% in 1988, and an increase in the number of patients who had previously had coronary angioplasty.

In the last few years the rise in CABG rates in the US has levelled off (Table 16.1). This may reflect increasing financial constraints as a result of the prospective payment systems widely introduced by funding agencies (17) and the influence of Health Maintenance Organizations. A fixed reimbursement for the procedure is a disincentive to expand the patient population yet

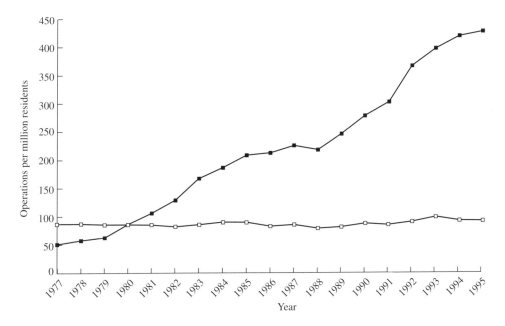

Fig. 16.1   Rates of bypass and valve operations performed in NHS hospitals in the UK, 1977–84. □, valve operations; ◆, CABGs (including operations performed with another procedure).

Table 16.2 Coronary artery bypass operations and cardiac value operations in the UK (1977–91)

Year	CABG alone	CABG with other procedure	Valve surgery
1977	2297	584	4832
1978	2653	537	4873
1979	2918	620	4791
1980	4057	802	4814
1981	5130	839	4762
1982	6008	1224	4652
1983	8332	1111	4811
1984	9433	1120	5026
1985	10667	1133	5073
1986	10767	1243	4633
1987	11521	1299	4755
1988	11113	1306	4447
1989	12648	1342	4571
1990	14431	1536	4924
1991	15659	1641	4828
1992	19241	1963	5164
1993	21031	2037	5653
1994	22056	2282	5229
1995	22475	2362	5234

Source = UK Cardiac Surgical Register.

further to those groups who are likely to be more costly to treat, for example the very elderly or those who are a poor surgical risk for other reasons.

United Kingdom

Figure 16.1 shows the steady increase in the crude rate of CABG surgery in the UK since 1980. By contrast the rate of valve replacement has remained remarkably stable over the same period. By 1991, over 141 000 bypass procedures had been performed in the UK of which 12% were bypass grafts undertaken at the same time as another procedure such as a valve replacement (see Table 16.2). There has been an impressive reduction in hospital mortality over this period, from around 6% before 1980 to 2.5% in 1990 for CABG performed alone. Unlike the US this increase in bypass activity has been achieved without a massive increase in the number of cardiac surgical centres. The number of consultant cardiac surgeons in the UK increased only from 110 in 1979 to 126 in 1990 (6). The number of cardiologists increased more, from 223 to 323 between 1980 and 1990. This reflects, firstly, the need for an integrated medical and surgical service with the capacity to investigate patients before surgery and, secondly, the growth in alternative methods of management, especially percutaneous transluminal coronary angioplasty (PTCA).

Although still increasing, the CABG rate in the UK remains extremely low compared with the US, Canada, and a number of other countries. The CABG rate in Australia was 2.4 times that in

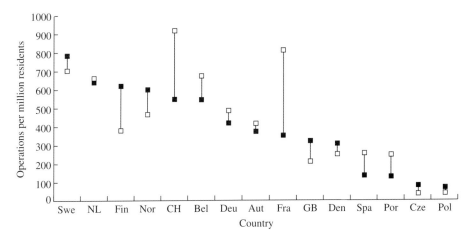

Fig. 16.2 Coronary artery surgery rates in European countries in 1992, crude (■) and adjusted (□) for standard mortality rates for ischaemic heart disease under 65 years in each country relative to the European average (source: European Institute for Cardiac Survey and World Health Organization).

the UK in 1990 (18). Figure 16.2 shows the bypass surgery rate in the UK relative to other European countries in 1992. There were 445 surgical units performing CABG operations in Europe in that year for a population of 510 million people (19). Thus, the average European unit covers a larger population (1.15 million) than its American counterpart and performs more operations (over 300 CABGs per year). The UK CABG rate in 1992 was above the European mean rate of 263 bypass grafts per million population. However, the UK had a distinctly low rate compared with most European countries of comparable prosperity, despite having a relatively high incidence of IHD. In Figure 16.2 the CABG rate is shown for a number of European countries after adjustment using the age-standardized mortality from IHD in people under 65 years in each country (20). For example, the adjusted rate for France is higher than the crude rate for that country because IHD is a relatively uncommon cause of premature mortality; for Britain the opposite is true.

It is possible that British doctors have systematically different views of the place of CABG surgery in the management of IHD compared with doctors in countries with higher CABG rates. This explanation for the difference between rates of bypass surgery in the UK and the US has been investigated. In a study of 386 American CABG patients, the appropriateness of surgery in each case was judged according to standards generated by groups of American and British doctors (21). The British doctors' standards led to 35% of the American operations being deemed definitely inappropriate, and only 41% definitely appropriate, compared with 13% and 62% respectively using the standards of US experts. These differences, although clinically important and statistically significant, would, however, only partially account for the difference between activity rates in the two countries. Nor is apparently inappropriate surgery confined to the US. A similar research group considered 319 British CABG patients (22,23). At the much lower overall activity level found in the Trent Region of the UK in 1987, it was still the case that 16% of procedures were inappropriate by British standards. At least 7% would even be considered inappropriate for CABG by the more interventionist American doctors.

Changes in surgical practice, and in the patient population, in the UK have been similar in direction if not in extent to those in the US. Cardiac centres that have monitored activity in detail have shown a steady increase in referrals for investigation by angiography which matches the increase in CABG surgery (24). More elderly patients are also being referred. The mean age of patients investigated in one centre rose from 52 to 59 between 1979 and 1988 (24). The proportion of bypass patients who were female increased to 18% in the same centre, a level comparable with the US. The CSAG study, performed in four British regions, also found that the mean age of patients undergoing revascularization procedures had increased by 6 months every year between 1987 and 1992 (25). The mean age of CABG patients was 59.4 years in 1992. The audit of bypass surgery in Trent in 1987 and 1988 showed that only 17% of patients were over 65 (23). In a series of patients investigated in Scotland at about the same time, only 4.6% of those having coronary angiograms were over 70 (26). These proportions must seem astoundingly low to American surgeons, half of whose patients are now likely to be over 65. The prevalence of symptomatic angina rises exponentially with age and angiographic studies show a high prevalence of left main stem stenosis and three-vessel disease in older patients. Such patients, particularly those aged between 65 and 75, should be considered good candidates for bypass surgery as most would expect to live long enough to benefit from the advantages of CABG over medical therapy (27). The operation frequently brings relief from the symptoms of angina and thereby improves autonomy, an important goal for older people.

The extent to which CABG surgery in the UK can be monitored is severely limited by the lack of appropriate routine data on activity. The UK Cardiac Surgical Register, although complete and valuable in other ways, does not allow analysis of trends in the composition of the patient population. Analysis of activity rates by regional centre can be misleading because many patients travel outside their region of residence to receive treatment and so denominator populations are uncertain. The national Hospital Episode System (HES), currently based on routine returns from NHS Trusts to Regional Health Authorities, should provide information on the age, sex, residence, and diagnoses of patients undergoing surgery. Unfortunately, doubts about the accuracy of operation coding are sufficient to prevent its use in practice until improvements have been made. In any cases the HES system, like the UK Cardiac Surgery Register, does not cover surgery performed in private hospitals and would therefore be substantially incomplete. Between 4% and 22% of bypass grafts were found to have been performed in private hospitals in the CSAG study of four different regions of the UK (6).

Impact of PTCA on CABG rates

When CABG was introduced no alternative method of revascularization was available. Percutaneous transluminal coronary angioplasty (PTCA) became popular very rapidly in the US from 1982 onwards, and is now performed more commonly there than CABG. The number of PTCA procedures performed per million population in European and North American countries in 1990 is given in Table 16.3. In the UK in 1990 there were 46 centres each undertaking more than 50 PTCA procedures a year (28).

PTCA has been shown to be safe and effective in alleviating the symptoms of angina in patients with amenable coronary artery stenoses. The demand for PTCA has continued to rise despite the lack (at the time) of published evidence that PTCA improves survival compared with medical therapy. This suggests perhaps that symptomatic relief rather than longevity has always been the main benefit driving demand for revascularization. A percutaneous procedure is less traumatic, safer, and less costly than open surgery. If the same results could be achieved, PTCA would probably be preferred to CABG by patients, funding bodies, and cardiologists (who perform the procedure themselves).

Table 16.3 An international comparison of percutaneous transluminal coronary angioplasty rates in 1990

Country	PTCA procedures per million population
US	1072
Belgium	569
Holland	545
West Germany	543
Canada	453
France	400
Switzerland	354
Austria	229
United Kingdom	148
Italy	79
Spain	60

Source: Intervention Ltd. 1 Redman Court, Bell Street, Princes Risborough, Buckinghamshire, UK.

Given the attraction of PTCA, an effect on CABG rates might have been expected. Although certain patient groups make a smaller contribution to the bypass population, namely those with single-vessel disease, there has not been a straightforward transfer of patients from CABG to PTCA with a reduction in demand for CABG as a consequence. There could be a number of reasons for this. The availability of PTCA has contributed to the increase in the rate of coronary catheterization, which in turn has identified more patients who would benefit from CABG. In the US, the need to provide PTCA has also led to more hospitals offering CABG. The latter is considered to be an essential back-up facility for the former, approximately 2% of patients undergoing PTCA need urgent CABG. Many of the patients that now receive CABG have complex abnormalities of the coronary vessels currently beyond the scope of balloon angioplasty. In one study 62% of patients undergoing CABG were found to be unsuitable for PTCA (29). Most patients treated by PTCA are thought to be those that would otherwise have been managed medically rather than by CABG. Finally, the CABG rate is being sustained by the increasing demand for repeat procedures.

One of the randomized controlled trials of PTCA versus CABG that has produced results at the time of writing is the RITA study (30). There was no difference in survival between the two groups after 2.5 years of follow-up, or in the rate of non-fatal myocardial infarction. However, angina was more prevalent in the PTCA group. Trials comparing PTCA and CABG have recently been reviewed (31). One problem will be the difficulty of keeping up with the rapid development of PTCA technology and practice. Whatever the trials show, it will be impossible to know whether the same results apply to newer PTCA techniques, for example the use of stents.

Access to CABG surgery in the UK and US

Much of the debate about the provision of CABG has been about inequality of access to the procedure. Differences in rates of use have been found between racial groups (32), between the sexes (33), according to income (31) and between geographical regions of the same country.

Geographical variation

In studies that have examined CABG rates by locality, variation has generally been found which does not appear to be principally related to the need for surgery (34). For example in Canada, in 1986–87, CABG rates varied from 195 per million in Saskatoon to 469 in Montreal (35). This variation is often greater in the elderly than in other age groups. In the US, rates were found to be lowest in the north east and highest in the west, which is the inverse of variation in mortality from IHD (36). One difficulty with such studies is the identification of non-resident patients. Most routine databases do not allow true population-based rates to be calculated. For example it is known that a number of Canadian residents travel to the US for cardiac surgery.

Those undertaking the recent British study took a great deal of trouble to identify all CABG surgery in defined resident populations of three regions in Britain (37). Private and NHS surgery were both included. The CABG rate per million varied from 68 to 617 for District Health Authority populations within these three regions. Only a small proportion of this variation could be accounted for by random variation. It was apparent from a simple geographical analysis that the districts close to cardiothoracic units had much higher CABG rates. A weak inverse correlation was found between mortality from IHD and the CABG rate. There is some evidence from repeat studies that the variation is decreasing but the continuing inequality in access to CABG across the UK is still a serious concern.

An important question is the extent to which these geographical differences in use in the UK and elsewhere are accounted for by differences in criteria for surgery in different areas. This is analogous to the question posed about the difference between rates of use in the US and the UK. There is evidence of disagreement among expert panels on the appropriateness of CABG in specific clinical situations. It is possible that variation in surgical rates is caused mainly by differences in severity thresholds at which clinicians consider CABG to be indicated. Little direct evidence is available to test this hypothesis, although more studies are underway. In a study of the use of coronary angiography (38), rates in Medicare beneficiaries varied among counties in one US state from 13 to 158 per 100 000. Differences in the rate of inappropriate use of the procedure accounted for 28% of this variation. In centres such as Toronto and the Cleveland Clinic with relatively high CABG rates the proportion of patients that have severe IHD, and clear indications for CABG (such as three-vessel disease and left ventricular impairment) is also high. This may be partly because they are referral centres but it also suggests that areas with high rates of use are not served by clinicians with low thresholds for surgery. The most recent study of the appropriateness of CABG surgery, from New York (39), showed that very little variation was due to levels of inappropriate surgery. These levels were generally lower than in previous studies.

Thus, although the literature is incomplete, it is likely that variation in the use of CABG conforms to a general model put forward by the RAND Corporation investigators to explain variation in use of specialized health services (40). This model proposes that variation in the intervention rate is mainly explained by underuse of interventions in low use areas rather than differences in criteria for surgery and large numbers of 'inappropriate' operations in high use areas. The number of inappropriate interventions increases, but only a little, as the overall rate increases. The presence of a finite level of inappropriate cases in a low use area, as was the case in Trent, is to be expected and does not mean that all appropriate cases are being treated.

What are the implications of this model for the UK? If access in all districts was to approach that in districts close to cardiothoracic units, the overall CABG rate would rise to the level in those districts, i.e. around 600 per million per year. This increase in activity would be expected without any change in criteria for surgery or in the characteristics of the bypass population.

Assessment of the need for CABG surgery in populations

The demand for CABG surgery is greatly influenced by the level of access to cardiac surgical services. For this reason establishing the true requirement for CABG in any population is difficult. A number of approaches have been tried in the UK to determine an appropriate CABG rate in order to plan the provision of specialist cardiac services.

The first King's Fund consensus conference, held in 1984, considered the size of the pool of potential patients for CABG (41). Despite the panel's wish to be entirely objective they were limited by the lack of data on contemporary British cardiac surgical practice and on the underlying epidemiology of IHD in the UK. They were, however, aware that the surgical rate in the UK was very low compared with the US. A short term target of 300 operations per million population was recommended, providing for 'high-benefit' patients only. At the time the highest rates in the UK were about half that figure. This incremental approach was probably justified given the lack of good data on the true requirement. Even now some districts in Britain have not achieved the King's Fund target. However, a minimum acceptable target is no longer adequate. The role of surgical management in IHD is better understood and the process by which resources are allocated for high technology health care has become much more explicit. It is not enough to say that any rate above 300 per million is acceptable.

Instead of asking a panel of experts, another common approach to determining need is the normative or comparative method. Here it is assumed that need approximates to the actual level of use in a situation where access is optimal and utilisation conforms to current standards of appropriate use (42). The weakness of this method is that the underlying assumption that the norm corresponds to correct practice is rarely tested. A CAB rate of 470 per million was reported in North West Surrey in 1989 (24). It was suggested that this represents a minimum requirement for the UK as the population of Surrey has a low incidence of IHD compared with the rest of the country. Comparisons are often made between CABG rates in the UK and countries where access to surgery is not restricted by limited supply, for example the US. These generally suggest that the requirement for CABG is very much greater than 300 per million (see Table 16.1). Evidence that US surgeons operate on few inappropriate cases adds weight to these observations. However, the US is arguably a special case with respect to the use of high technology treatments because of the nature of the American health care industry. A more useful comparison is that between the UK and Canada, where most health care is funded by central government from a finite overall budget. In three Canadian provinces combined, the rate of CABG surgery in 1989 was 624 per million adults over 20 years of age, compared with 1 125 in California and 884 in New York (31). This Canadian rate, of approximately 450 CABGs per million total population (note different denominator), appears to be similar to that in areas of the UK with good access to specialist cardiac services. If a normative target rate is required, then that of 450 CABGs per million would seem an appropriate one to adopt for the UK population, superseding the current target of 300 CABGs per million.

The Canadian rate is inadequate to prevent the development of waiting lists for CABG surgery — evidence that it does not represent over provision relative to demand. Waiting lists for CABG surgery have also been reported from New Zealand (43), and the Netherlands (44). In the UK the median time from angiogram to CABG was 127 days in one study (6) but can be much longer.

Waiting times for CABG appear to be increasing in some parts of the UK (45) and have recently been included in the range of Patient's Charter standards with which all NHS hospitals should comply. The presence of waiting lists for a potentially life-saving operation is a bleak reminder that the resources available for cardiac surgery will not be sufficient in most countries to treat all those who might benefit from CABG.

Normative targets at whatever level (unless they are truly minimum targets) may lead to patient quotas for the procedure. There is then a danger that the likelihood of surgery being offered could depend as much on the phase of the financial year as on clinical severity (46). The pragmatic and equitable response to this situation should be to assess the relative priority of patients considered eligible for surgery in order to ensure that those treated are the ones likely to benefit most. An explicitly utilitarian approach to the rationing of CABG services might, however, create more ethical problems than it solves. How should the value of symptom relief in a 75 year old patient be compared with that in a 60 year old? Should priority be given to those likely to derive survival benefit even if they are asymptomatic?

Naylor et al. have demonstrated that it is feasible to rank patients according to relative urgency of the need for revascularization (47). They used a consensus method based on objective clinical factors — mainly the features of the patient's presenting pain and its response to treatment, and the angiographic findings. Although there was some disagreement between members of the panel, the level of agreement was more striking. The criteria generated by the Canadian consensus study have also been successfully applied to patients in New Zealand. Actual waiting times were compared with those considered acceptable by the panel for each clinical group. In the UK, there is little information on the clinical severity of patients undergoing CABG. It would be extremely useful to apply the Canadian consensus criteria to a group of British patients undergoing, and waiting for, CABG.

Frankel has suggested that the requirement for elective surgical procedures should be determined by careful surveys of defined populations using instruments which can be interpreted in terms of the current indications for surgery (48). Most epidemiological data available on the incidence and prevalence of chronic diseases, for example osteoarthritis of the hip, has not been collected in these terms. Unfortunately this approach cannot be adopted easily for CABG because the criteria for surgery are partly defined by an invasive test, namely angiography. An indication of the need for revascularization could, however, be obtained from a survey based on exercise electrocardiograms (49). Although not ideal, a survey of this kind is possibly the only way of obtaining information on need for CABG that is independent of the level of supply of services.

The information that is available on the epidemiology of IHD in the UK includes estimates of the number of new cases of angina presenting in general practice and of the number of myocardial infarctions treated in hospital. An algorithm was developed by Yorkshire Regional Health Authority which used information from published studies to estimate the number of CABGs that would be expected given the existing incidence of IHD in the UK (50). The rate suggested was 426 CABGs per million. This figure is a dubious estimate of need as the algorithm simply applies proportions based on current practice to the incidence data. There was no independent justification of the appropriateness of that practice. The main value of this method is in estimating the implications for other services, for example cardiology, of different levels of CABG activity.

Future trends in the need and demand for CABG

The study commissioned by the Clinical Standards Advisory Group has shown levels of variation in access to CABG in the UK which are inconsistent with the equitable principles of the NHS (7).

The apparent need for CABG in the UK could increase considerably as health authorities try and reduce this inequity. If this takes place without an increase in the resources available for cardiac surgery, the clinical urgency of patients allocated to receive CABG must rise — possibly to an unacceptable level. It is important, therefore, to monitor the clinical characteristics of those undergoing bypass operations.

It seems likely that the number of elderly people referred for angiography will increase. Any triage system based on objective clinical criteria will give priority to this group as they tend to have more severe disease although the extent to which CABG improves survival in the elderly is uncertain. The average age of the CABG population will increase and the proportion of females will probably also increase.

Finally, age-specific prevalence rates of the indications for revascularization are expected to rise. Accurate data on which to make predictions are sparse, but it seems that patients are more likely to be admitted to hospital after a myocardial infarction than in the past. The hospital case-fatality from myocardial infarction has been falling for some time, a trend which is likely to accelerate with the widespread use of thrombolysis. Thus, the number of surviving prevalent cases of IHD known to the health service and therefore likely to be investigated will probably rise. On the other hand, the incidence of IHD is thankfully decreasing in many countries as shown by the fact that death rates from IHD are falling. Alas, the reduction in deaths is numerically far too great to be accounted for by the rising rate of revascularization and appears to be mainly due to a decline in the number of sudden out-of-hospital deaths.

Acknowledgements

I would like to thank Mr Ravi Pillai for supplying data from the UK Cardiac Surgical Register. Dr Cyril Nair and Dr Ed Graves for providing similar information for Canada and the USA respectively, and Carol Ashton and David Taylor for their helpful comments on an earlier draft.

References

1. Favaloro RG. Saphenous vein autograft replacement of severe segmental coronary artery occlusion: operation technique. *Ann Thorac Surg* 1968;**5**:334–9.
2. McIntosh HD. Aortocoronary bypass grafting, an internist's perspective. *Circulation* 1982;65(Suppl II):77–81.
3. Goldman L, Cook EF. The decline in ischaemic heart disease mortality rates: an analysis of the comparative effects of medical interventions and changes in lifestyle. *Ann Int Med 1984;***101**:825–36.
4. Bates MS. A critical perspective on coronary artery disease and coronary bypass surgery. Soc Sci Med 1990;**30**:249–60.
5. English TA, Bailey AR, Dark JF *et al*. The UK cardiac surgical register, 1977–82. Br Med J 1984;**289**:1205–8.
6. Black N, Langham S, Petticrew M. *Coronary artery bypass grafting and coronary angioplasty: access to and availability of specialist services.* London:HMSO, 1993.
7. Black N, Langham S, Coshall C, Parker J. Impact of the 1991 NHS reforms on the availability and use of coronary revascularisation in the UK (1987–1995). Heart 1996; (Supplement 4), **76**:1–30.

8. Graves EJ. *National Hospital Discharge Survey: annual summary, 1991*. Hyattsville: National Center for Health Statistics, 1993.

9. Ugnat A-M, Naylor CD. Trends in coronary artery bypass grafting in Ontario from 1981 to 1989. *Can Med Assoc* 1993;**148**:569–75.

10. Lytle BW, Cosgrove D, Loop FD. Future implications of current trends in bypass surgery. *Cardiovasc Clin* 1991;**21**:265–78.

11. Braunwald E. Coronary artery surgery at the crossroads. *New Engl J Med* 1977;**297**:661–3.

12. Blustein J. High-technology cardiac procedures: the impact of service availability on service use in New York State. *JAMA* 1993;**270**:344–9.

13. Jones EL, Weintraub WS, Craver JM, Guyton RA, Cohen CL. Coronary bypass surgery: is the operation different today? *J Thorac Cardiovasc Surg* 1991;**101**:108–15.

14. Feinleib M, Havlik RJ, Gillum RF, Pokras R, McCarthy E, Moien M. Coronary heart disease and related procedures: national hospital discharge survey data. *Circulation* 1989;**79**(Suppl I):13–18.

15. Weintraub WS, Clements SD, Ware J *et al.* (1991) Coronary artery surgery in octogenarians. *Am J Cardiol* 1991;**68**:1530–4.

16. Tobin JN, Wassertheil-Smoller S, Wexler JP, Steingart RM, Budner N, Lense L, Wachspress J. Sex bias in considering coronary bypass surgery. *Ann Intern Med* 1987;**107**:19–25.

17. Langa KM, Sussman EJ (1993) The effect of cost-containment policies on rates of coronary revascularisation in California. *New Engl J Med* 1993;**329**:1784–9.

18. *Cardiac surgery 1990*. Report No. 28. Canberra:National Heart Foundation of Australia, 1992.

19. *European survey on cardiac interventions in 1992*. Salzburg: Institute for Cardiac Survey of the European Academy of Sciences and Arts, 1993.

20. World Health Organisation *European HFA Database*. Copenhagen: WHO, 1992.

21. Brook RH, Kosecoff JB, Park RE, Chassin MR, Winslow CM, Hampton JR. Diagnosis and treatment of coronary disease: comparison of doctors' attitudes in the USA and the UK. *Lancet* 1988; **I**:750–3.

22. Bernstein SJ, Kosecoff J, Gray D, Hampton JR, Brook RH. The appropriateness of the use of cardiovascular procedures: British versus US perspectives. Int J Tech Assess in Health Care 1993;**9**:3–10.

23. Gray D, Hampton JR, Bernstein SJ, Koescoff J, Brook RH. Audit of coronary angiography and bypass surgery. *Lancet* 1990;**33**:1317–20.

24. MacRae CA, Marber MS, Keywood C, Joy M. Need for invasive cardiological assessment and intervention: a ten year review. *Br Heart J* 1992;**67**:200–3.

25. Black N, Langham S, Petticrew M. Trends in the age and sex of patients undergoing coronary revascularisation in the United Kingdom 1987–93. *Br Heart J* 1994;**72**:317–20.

26. Elder AT, Shaw TRD, Turnbull CM, Starkey IR. Elderly and younger patients selected to undergo coronary angiography. *Br Med J* 1991;**303**:950–3.

27. Lessof MH, Evans JG, Joy MD *et al.* Cardiological intervention in elderly patients: report of a working group of the Royal College of Physicians. *J Roy Coll Physicians* 1991;**25**:197–205.

28. Hubner PJB. Cardiac interventional procedures in the United Kingdom during 1990. *Br Heart J* 1992;**68**:434–36.

29. Hollman J. The limited impact of percutaneous coronary artery angioplasty on bypass surgery. *Int J Cardiol* 1988;**20**:193–200.

30. RITA Trial Participations. Coronary angioplasty versus coronary artery bypass surgery: the Randomised Intervention Treatment of Angina (RITA) trial. *Lancet* 1993;**341**:573–80.

31. Anderson G, Grumbach K, Luft H, Roos LL, Mustard C, Brook R. Use of coronary artery bypass surgery in the United States and Canada: influence of age and income. *JAMA* 1993;**269**:1661–6.

32. Whittle J, Conigliaro J, Good CB, Lofgren RP. Racial differences in the use of invasive cardiovascular procedures in the Department of Veterans Affairs medical system.*New Engl J Med* 1993;**329**:621–7.

33. Ayanian JZ, Epstein AM. Differences in the use of procedures between women and men hospitalised for coronary heart disease. *New Engl J Med* 1991;**325**:221–5.

34. Chassin MR, Brook RH, Park RE *et al.* Variations in the use of medical and surgical services by the Medicare population. *New Engl J Med* 1986;**314**:285–90.

35. Naylor CD, Ugnat A-M, Weinkaupf D, Anderson GM, Wielgosz A. Coronary artery bypass grafting in Canada: what is its rate of use? Which rate is right? *Can Med Assoc J* 1992;**146**:851–9.

36. Gillum RF. Coronary artery bypass surgery and coronary angiography in the United States, 1979–1983. *Am Heart J* 1987;**113**:1255–60.

37. Black N, Langham S, Petticrew M. Coronary revascularisation: why do rates vary geographically in the UK? *J Epid Comm Health* 1995;**49**:408–12.

38. Leape LL, Hilbourne LH, Park RE. *et al.* The appropriateness of use of coronary artery bypass graft surgery in New York State. *JAMA* 1993;**269**:753–60.

39. Leape LL, Park RE, Solomon DH, Chassin MR, Kosecoff J, Brook RH. Does inappropriate use explain small-area variations in the use of health care services? *JAMA* 1990;**263**:669–72.

40. Park RE. 'Does inappropriate use explain small-area variation in the use of health care services?' Λ reply. *Health Services Research* 1993;**28**:401–10.

41. King's Fund Consensus Panel. Consensus development conference: coronary artery bypass grafting. *Br Med J* 1984;**289**:1527–9.

42. Relman AS. Determining how much medical care we need. *New Engl J Med* 1980;**303**:1292–3.

43. Fitzpatrick MA. Audit of prioritisation for coronary revascularisation procedures: implications for rationing. *N Z Med J* 1992;**105**:145–7.

44. Suttorp MJ, Kingma JH, Koomen EM, Tijgssen JGP, Defauw JAM, Ernst SMPG. Predictive characteristics for early mortality in patients awaiting coronary artery bypass. *Lancet* 1990;**336**:310–11.

45. Marber M, MacRae C, Joy M. Delay to invasive investigation and revascularisation for coronary heart disease in South West Thames region: a two tier system? *Br Med J* 1991;**302**:1189–91.

46. Olsburgh B. Medical education.*Br Med J* 1993;**306**:66.

47. Naylor CD, Baigrie RS, Goldman BS, Basinski A. Assessment of priority for coronary revascularization procedures. *Lancet* 1990;**335**:1070–3.

48. Frankel S. The epidemiology of indications. *J Epid Comm Health* 1991;**45**:257–9.

49. Mark DB, Shaw L, Harrell FE *et al.* Prognostic value of a treadmill exercise score in outpatients with suspected coronary artery disease. *New Engl J Med* 1991;**325**:849–53.

50. Yorkshire Regional Health Authority. *Implementing Health of the Nation: ischaemic heart disease*. London: Faculty of Public Health Medicine of the Royal Colleges of Physicians, 1991.

Further Reading

Califf RM, Harrell FE, Lee KL *et al*. The evolution of medical and surgical therapy for coronary artery disease: a 15-year perspective. *JAMA* 1989;**261**:2077–86.

Leape LL, Hilborne LH, Schwartz JS *et al*. The appropriateness of coronary artery bypass graft surgery in academic medical centers. Working Group of the Appropriateness Project of the Academic Medical Center Consortium. *Ann Intern Med* 1996;**125**(1):8–18.

Rothlisberger C, Meier B. Coronary interventions in Europe 1992. The Working Group on Coronary Circulation of the European Society of Cardiology. *Eur Heart J* 1995;**16**(7):922–9.

Talley JD, Mauldin PD. Publications concerning costs of various cardiovascular procedures and drugs. *Am J Cardiol* 1997;**79**(1):70–2.

Tu JV, Naylor CD, Kumar D *et al*. Coronary artery bypass graft surgery in Ontario and New York State: which rate is right? Steering Committee of the Cardiac Care Network of Ontario. *Ann Intern Med* 1997;**126**:(1):13–9.

Unger F. Open heart surgery in Europe 1993. *Eur J Cardiothorac Surg* 1996;**10**(2):120–8.

Index